Debat

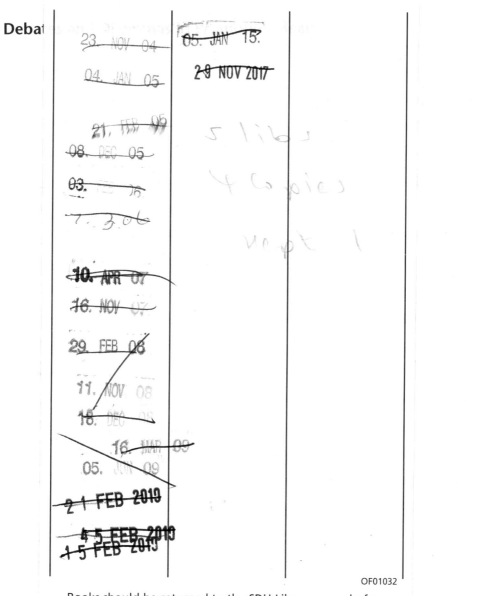

OF01032

Books should be returned to the SDH Library on or before
the date stamped above unless a renewal has been arranged

Salisbury District Hospital Library

Telephone: Salisbury (01722) 336262 extn. 4430 / 33
Out of hours answer machine in operation

This Reader forms part of The Open University course *Promoting Health: Skills, Perspectives and Practice* (K301), a 60-point Level 3 undergraduate course. K301 is an optional course for both the BA/BSc (Hons) in Health Studies and the BA/BSc (Hons) in Health and Social Care, as well as being a core course for the Diploma in Health and Social Welfare. Students who complete K301 successfully can apply for the Certificate in Health Promotion. The course was produced with support from the Health Education Authority for England and Health Promotion Wales, although the content of the course is the sole responsibility of The Open University.

The chapters in this book have been designed as a source for students during their study of this course. The collection of readings has been chosen to challenge pre-conceptions and to evoke a critical understanding of health issues. Opinions expressed in the Reader are not necessarily those of the Course Team or of The Open University.

If you are interested in studying the course or working towards a related degree or diploma please write to the Information Officer, School of Health and Social Welfare, The Open University, Walton Hall, Milton Keynes MK7 6AA, UK. Details can also be viewed on our web page at http://www.open.ac.uk.

Other texts required for the course, also published by Palgrave Macmillan in association with The Open University are:

- the first core text, *Promoting Health: Knowledge and Practice* (2nd edn), edited by Jeanne Katz, Alyson Peberdy and Jenny Douglas;

- the second core text, *The Challenge of Promoting Health: Exploration and Action* (2nd edn), edited by Linda Jones, Moyra Sidell and Jenny Douglas;

- the set book, *Health Promotion: Professional Perspectives* (2nd edn), edited by Angela Scriven and Judy Orme.

Debates and Dilemmas in Promoting Health
A Reader

Second Edition

Edited by

Moyra Sidell
Linda Jones
Jeanne Katz
Alyson Peberdy
and
Jenny Douglas

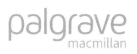

First edition 1997
Second edition 2003

Published by
PALGRAVE MACMILLAN
Houndmills, Basingstoke, Hampshire RG21 6XS and
175 Fifth Avenue, New York, N.Y. 10010
Companies and representatives throughout the world

PALGRAVE MACMILLAN is the global academic imprint of the Palgrave Macmillan
division of St. Martin's Press, LLC and of Palgrave Macmillan Ltd. Macmillan® is a
registered trademark in the United States, United Kingdom and other countries.
Palgrave is a registered trademark in the European Union and other countries.

ISBN 1–4039–0228–3

This book is printed on paper suitable for recycling and made from fully managed
and sustained forest sources.

A catalogue record for this book is available from the British Library.

10 9 8 7 6 5 4 3 2
12 11 10 09 08 07 06 05 04

Printed and bound in Great Britain by
Creative Print & Design (Wales), Ebbw Vale

Contents

Section Four: Looking forward – dilemmas in health promotion: Introduction

List of figures and tables

Figures

Tables

Acknowledgements

The editors and publishers wish to thank the following for permission to use copyright material:

Marlan Barnes, for material from 'User movements, community development and health promotion', from L. Adams, M. Amos and J. Munro, *Promoting Health: Politcs and Practice* (2002), by permission of Sage Publications Ltd.

Norman Beale and Susan Nethercott, for 'Job-loss and family morbidity: a study of a factory closure', *Journal of the Royal College of General Practitioners*, 35 (1985) pp. 510–14, by permission of the British Journal of General Practioners.

Dan Beauchamp, for 'Lifestyle, public health and paternalism' from S. Doxiadis (ed.) *Ethical Dilemmas in Health Promotion* (1987) pp. 69–83, by permission of John Wiley & Sons Ltd.

Michael L. Burr, for 'Explaining the French paradox', *Journal of the Royal Society of Health*, August (1995) pp. 217–19, by permission of the author.

Roger Burrows, Robin Bunton, Steven Muncer and Kate Gillen, for material from 'The efficacy of health promotion, health economics and late modernism', *Health Education Research*, 10:2 (1995) pp. 241–9, by permission of Oxford University Press.

Russell Caplan, for material from 'The importance of social theory for health promotion: from description to reflexivity', *Health Promotion International*, 8 (1993) pp. 147–57, by permission of Oxford University Press.

R. J. W. Cline and K. M. Haynes, for material from 'Consumer health information seeking on the Internet: the state of the art', *Health Education Research*, 16:6 (2001) pp. 671–92, by permission of Oxford University Press.

Trudi Collins, for material from 'Models of health: pervasive, persuasive and politically charged', *Health Promotion International*, 10:4 (1995) pp. 317–24, by permission of Oxford University Press.

Pete Connor, for material from 'Counselling people living with

HIV/AIDS' from Kim Etherington (ed.) *Counsellors in Health Settings* (2001) pp. 141–60, by permission of Jessica Kingsley Publishers.

Billie Corti, C. D'Arcy, J. Holman and Robert J. Donovan, for material from 'Using sponsorship to create healthy environments for sport, racing and art venues in Western Australia', *Health Promotion International*, 10:3 (1995) pp. 185–97, by permission of Oxford University Press.

Charlie Davison, Stephen Frankel and George Davey Smith, for material from 'The limits of lifestyle: re-assessing "fatalism" in the popular culture of illness prevention', *Social Science and Medicine*, 34:6 (1992) pp. 675–85, by permission of Elsevier Science.

Susan Denman, for material from *The Health Promoting School* by Susan Denman *et al.* (2002) Routledge, pp. 153–60, by permission of Taylor & Francis.

Allson Dines, for material from 'A case study of the ethical issues in health promotion – mammography screening: the nurse's position' in]. Wilson-Barnett and J. Macleod Clark, *Research in Health Promotion and Nursing* (1994) pp. 119–31, by permission of Palgrave Macmillan.

Angela Everitt and Pauline Hardiker, for material from *Evaluation for Good Practice* by Angela Everitt and Pauline Hardiker (1996) pp. 83–104, by permission of Palgrave Macmillan.

Wendy Farrant, 'Addressing the contradictions: health action in the United Kingdom', *International Journal of Health Services*, 21:3 (1991) pp. 424–39, by permission of Baywood Publishing Co., Inc.

Hilary Graham, for material from the Introduction, 'The challenge of health inequalities' from Hilary Graham (ed.) *Understanding Health Inequalities* (2000) pp. 3–20, by permisssion from The Open University Press; and for a figure from P. Gregg and J. Wadsworth, 'More work in fewer households' in J. Hills (ed.), *New Inequalities: The Changing Distribution of Income and Wealth in the United Kingdom*, included in the material, by permission of Cambridge University Press.

Penelope Hawe and Alan Shiell, for material from 'Social capital and health promotion: a review', *Social Science and Medicine*, 51:6 (2000) pp. 871–85, by permission of Elsevier Science.

Ronald Labonte, for material from 'Econology: Integrating health and sustainable development', *Health Promotion International*, 6:2 (1991) pp. 147–56, by permission of Oxford University Press.

R. Craig Lefebvre, for material from 'The social marketing imbroglio in health promotion', *Health Promotion International*, 7:1 (1992) pp. 61–4, by permission of Oxford University Press.

A. J. McMichael and R. Beaglehole, for 'The changing global context of public health', *The Lancet*, 356 (2000) pp. 495–99, by permission of Elsevier Science.

David V. McQueen and Laurie M. Anderson, for material from 'What counts as evidence: issues and debates' from *Evaluation in Health Promotion: Principals and Perspectives*, WHO Regional Publications, European Series 92, by permission of the World Health Organization.

John Middleton, for 'Crime is a public health problem', *Medicine, Confict and Survival*, 14 (1998) pp. 24–8, by permission of Frank Cass Publishers.

Keith Tones and Sylvia Tilford, for material from *Health Promotion*, 3rd edn, by Keith Tones and Sylvia Tilford (2001) pp. 49–51, 52–5, by permission of Nelson Thornes.

Peter Townsend, for material from his article, 'Think globally, act locally', *European Labour Forum*, June (1994) pp. 2–8, by permission of the author.

Charles Webster and Jeff French, for material from 'The cycle of conflict: the history of the public health and health promotions movement', from L. Adams, M. Amos and J. Munro, *Promoting Health: Politics and Practice* (2002), by permission of Sage Publications Ltd.

Every effort has been made to trace all the copyright-holders, but if any have been inadvertently overlooked the publishers will be pleased to make the necessary arrangement at the first opportunity.

Introduction

At Alma-Ata, in 1978 the World Health Organization (WHO) set the task of achieving 'health for all' by the year 2000. This landmark date has come and gone, and the hoped-for health for all has not been achieved. For some, this was in any case an impossible dream, naïvely optimistic and unrealistic. For others it was a vision thwarted by lack of political will, global economic recession, Third-World debt and the greed of the 'haves' over the 'have nots'. Perhaps the time scale was just too short. But we also need to question whether health for all will ever be an achievable goal, whether we yet have a shared understanding of priorities, or even a clear vision of 'what health is'. Part of the difficulty for health promotion has been that there are no straightforward answers to such questions.

Through the Ottawa Charter (WHO, 1986) and the Sundsvall Conference (1992) the health promotion movement has arguably set out more of a strategic checklist than a formal strategy for health promotion (Levin and Ziglio, 1996). In identifying five key priority areas – building healthy public policy, creating supportive environments, strengthening community action, developing personal skills and reorientating health services – it has offered scope for innovation and imagination but also for confusion and doubt. The discourse of health promotion has fuelled many debates and dilemmas; it has its advocates as well as its adversaries, there are believers and sceptics. Health promotion has sometimes been projected, rather like health itself, as an example of an unmitigated good. After all, which groups would not wish to have their health protected and promoted? Who would not want to live longer and live better? In this view, the rise of health promotion is unproblematic, a response to changing knowledge about epidemiology and risk. Whether engaged in modifying people's behaviour or protecting the public through regulatory change, health promotion emerges as a justifiable and necessary enterprise.

In contrast to this, health promotion has been seen by critics as being beset with problems. It has been criticized by those on the political right for its 'nanny state' attachment to policy interventions. Others have questioned its role in creating an apparatus of 'surveillance' which constructs and monitors the 'worried well' in its attempts to limit risk-taking. For some critics, health promotion approaches feed what is seen as an unhealthy contemporary consumerist obsession with health.

Much criticism has come from within health promotion itself, particularly about the narrow focus and superficiality of much health promotion work. One concern has been about its over-emphasis on modifying

1

individual behaviour and its construction of 'lifestyle' as a set of personal choices unrelated to the socio-cultural and economic influences on people's lives. Increasingly, the knowledge base on which people are being asked to change their behaviour is questioned as the advice becomes more complex and often conflicting. The overwhelming evidence of the influence of social and economic disadvantage on health and disease has led many health promoters to recognize that the choice to change behaviour is not an easy one for many people, and the phrase 'making healthy choices the easy choices' sums up the aim of health promotion. One identified way to do this is through influencing public policy at all levels to create supportive environments for health, an approach which resonates very much with the Ottawa Charter and Sundsvall agreement.

It is often said that health is everybody's business. But responsibility for the health of individuals, communities and populations is the subject of much debate. Tied up with notions of responsibility are notions of control. How far can people have responsibility for their health if the means to health are outside their control? Those who advocate empowerment as the most appropriate means to promote health see education and participation in the decisions which affect health as a means to that end. Sharing of knowledge and listening to people have long been the tradition within community development, but since the 1990s this has become increasingly advocated by government and policy makers.

Another focus of debate has been on the poverty of theory in health promotion, or rather the failure to make explicit the extent to which the health promotion agenda inevitably involves an acceptance of more thorough-going social, economic and political change. A related criticism has been of the vague and all-embracing nature of positive definitions of health, and of the difficulties encountered in using a 'social change' approach, once the notion of health as 'absence of disease' has been found to be lacking.

Health promoters increasingly are being asked to evaluate their activities in cost-effective terms. Yet the diverse nature of the activity and the uncertainty about its parameters make a simple cost–benefit analysis unrealistic. The dilemma for health promoters is to find indicators for their work which reflect the process as well as the outcome.

The thirty-eight articles that make up this collection testify to the fact that debate is alive and well in health promotion. Some of the articles are classics, while others represent new thinking at the cutting edge of theory. Section One addresses key issues about the foundations of health, and health promotion and the means through which it is practised. In Section Two questions are raised about the knowledge base of health promotion interventions. Evidence about the outcomes of such interventions and how they can be evaluated is subjected to scrutiny.

Section Three explores wider debates around the interplay between local action and public policy, and Section Four looks to the future and raises ethical, sociological and political dilemmas for health promotion in the twenty-first century.

This Reader was compiled to accompany an Open University Level 3 course 'Promoting health: skills, perspectives and practices', originally produced in collaboration with the Health Education Authority and leading to the Certificate in Health Promotion. While the Reader forms an essential element in the 'Promoting health' course, it also stands alone as a coherent and wide-ranging source book for those who would like to engage in some of the debates and dilemmas inherent in promoting health. Although purposely arranged in four coherent sections, the individual articles stand alone and the book could be consumed *à la carte*. The contributors come from a wide range of backgrounds and include academics, practitioners and policy makers. We would like to thank the authors for their co-operation in reviewing and agreeing the sometimes extensive edits, amendments and revisions. We are assured that the substance and style of the original papers has been retained. We hope that the articles in this book will engage the reader in the fundamental dilemmas about health and its promotion and stimulate yet more debate.

References

Levin, S. and Ziglio, E. (1996) 'Health promotion as an investment strategy: considerations on theory and practice', *Health Promotion International*, 11 (1), 33–9.
WHO (World Health Organization) (1986) *Ottawa Charter for Health Promotion*. Ottawa: WHO.

Key issues in health and health promotion: introduction

Promoting health will remain at best a diverse, complex and multi-faceted activity. At worst it can be irritatingly jargon-ridden, impossibly idealistic and seemingly confused. Section One of the Reader is designed to help explain, if not expunge, the jargon, temper the idealism of health promotion with hard ethical and political questioning, and shed some light on the confusion.

Underlying the confusion is a basic uncertainly about the parameters of health promotion work. What is health promotion, beyond the specialist health promotion service? What is its relationship to public health? What should they be doing, these health, welfare, education and environmental professionals, lay people, community groups and policy makers pressed into service in the name of 'intersectoral collaboration' and 'inter-agency working'?

One key response, introduced in Section One and expanded on in the rest of the book, is to argue that these generalist health promoters should be continuing to undertake their usual work – *but in a more health promoting way*. This requires process changes: improved communication skills, increased sensitivity to socio-cultural issues, heightened awareness of environmental constraints, greater clarity about ethical problems, a more robust assessment and evaluation cycle, and a more systematic understanding of concepts of health and its promotion. And add to this a clearer understanding of the contribution that others, lay or professional, might make that would complement and extend their own efforts. What it does not mean is a 'product' approach; that is, the addition of yet more tasks and roles, more clinics, visits, inspections, interactions, collaborations, undertaken to demonstrate that health promotion is 'really happening'. The articles that follow address some of these central issues.

Section One starts with a chapter that lays the foundation for many of the debates and dilemmas discussed in this volume. Charles Webster and Jeff French trace historically the relationship between public health and health promotion, and set the scene for analysing contemporary health promotion. One of the major challenges facing public health and health promotion in the twenty-first century is the continuing increase in inequalities in health. Hilary Graham, in Chapter 2, points out that health inequalities based on income, education, housing employment and area increased steadily in the last quarter of the twentieth century. She suggest that health inequalities arise from the cumulative and inter-acting effects of material conditions, and behavioural and psychosocial factors throughout the life-course. A life-course perspective as well as attention to spatial patterning are discussed as strategies for tackling health inequalities.

The life-course perspective is nowhere more evident than in old age. In Chapter 3, Moyra Sidell draws on Antonovsky's salutogenic paradigm and 'sense of coherence' theory to understand the cumulative effects of social inequalities on older people's health. She explores how meaning-fulness, comprehensibility and manageability in people's daily lives can assist in maintaining their health.

The concept of social capital attempts to absorb both a life-course and spatial perspective on health inequalities. In Chapter 4, Penelope Hawe and Alan Shiell discuss the contested nature of the concept and draw out the implications for health promotion. The next two chapters move on to unravel the conceptual basis for health promotion itself. Russell Caplan in Chapter 5, and Trudi Collins in Chapter 6, focus on health promotion models and challenge the prevailing view that a 'pick and mix' approach to models is realistic. Both emphasize the (often inexplic-itly) political and economic agendas that underlie contemporary models, arguing that models and theories inevitably express deep-seated beliefs about the social world. Health promotion models should be connected to wider social theories, with the complexity of socio-cultural and eco-nomic relationships at an individual and community level identified more clearly.

Andrew Tannahill makes a plea in Chapter 7 for the integration of thinking and action, and presents a broad vision for the planning and delivery of health promotion in the context of the modern day United Kingdom. He explores different orientations for health promotion pro-grammes, and argues for a high priority to be put on reducing inequali-ties in health that are related to socio-economic and social environmental factors.

In contrast to this broad agenda, health promotion has often appeared to be preoccupied with narrow individual behavioural change. In Chapter 8, Charlie Davison, Stephen Frankel and George Davey Smith are critical of the 'victim blaming' approach, arguing that it ignores the influence of heredity, social conditions and environment on health, and is seriously out of step with popular culture and lay beliefs about illness. This criticism finds a response in the new agenda in health education advocated by Keith Tones and Sylvia Tilford in Chapter 9. Invoking the work of Paulo Freire (Section Three contains an extract from his work), they argue that the fundamental focus of health education should now be on the empowerment of individuals and communities. A major aspect of health promoters' work must be to raise public consciousness of health issues, to enable people to gain autonomy and to provide them with information and support to work for radical change at a local and policy level. This is a far cry from behaviour modification, and opens up more general issues about health promotion practice.

The next two chapters focus on practice issues. Both are concerned with the impact of communication on dis-empowered individuals and communities. Pete Connor in Chapter 10 sensitively explores the use of counselling for people affected by HIV and AIDS. In Chapter 11, Yasmin Gunaratnam addresses the dilemmas involved in communicating across cultural boundaries, and explores the use of techniques such as 'ethnic matching' that have been employed in health and social care.

Communication at a very different level is the subject of Ralph Lefebvre's contribution in Chapter 12. He questions whether mass communication of health promotion messages through 'social marketing' is realistic or even ethical. Should health promoters be in the business of selling health in the same way that other producers market their goods? Is it ethically justifiable to convince people to change their habits through persuasive media messages? And on what evidence are the media messages based? These issues are picked up in Section Two of the Reader, which questions the evidence base of health promotion.

1 The cycle of conflict: the history of the public health and health promotion movements*

Charles Webster and Jeff French

Although the immediate sources of both health promotion and the 'New Public Health' are located in the 1970s, many of the ideas associated with these movements have much deeper roots. This short review sets the development of health promotion and the 'New Public Health' in a wider historical framework. Although we are concerned mainly with the UK, the key features are common to many other national contexts. Most histories of the development of public health, and more recently of health promotion, fail to acknowledge that, while methods and motivations may vary, co-ordinated community action to ensure a better life is as old as civilization and remains a feature of every community today. In histories of public health there has been a tendency to assume that concern for better health as a prerequisite for better life is a relatively new, medically-led and Eurocentric concept. This assumption is symptomatic of a historic interpretation that seeks to medicalize what has been, and remains, a complex and contested social phenomenon. What is required is a reassessment of the development of public health and health promotion that takes account of the social conflict inherent in these movements. In doing so, it should-not be taken as self-evident that we have necessarily built up a sophisticated and objective understanding of the contribution of public health and health promotion to better health. Finally, it is also necessary to bear in mind the fundamental purposes of health promotion and public health, and the extent to which they represent different conceptions of the aspiration to health.

The phrase 'public health' as currently used embodies many of the confusions, vested interests and singular interpretations that have resulted from a simplistic interpretation of its historical development. It could even be argued that the term public health is often used in a spirit of what might be described as conspiratorial confusion – a point made by Alan Milburn, as UK Secretary of State for Health:

> 'Public health' understood as the epidemiological analysis of the patterns and causes of population health and ill health gets con-

---

* From Adams, L., Amos, M. and Munro, J., (eds) 2002 *Promoting Health: politics and practice*, London: Sage.

fused with 'public health' understood as population-level health promotion, which in turn gets confused with 'public health' understood as public health professionals trained in medicine. So by series of definitional sleights of hand, the argument runs that the health of the population should be mainly improved by population level health promotion and prevention, which in turn is best delivered, or at least overseen and managed, by medical consultants in public health. The time has come to abandon this lazy thinking and occupational protectionism. (Milburn, 2000)

The minister's evident frustration testifies to the current confusion over definitions of purpose and territorial responsibility among health professionals. Implicit in the above quotation, and most other current discussions of public health, are elements of a definition that have, in fact, been in widespread use over the last seventy-five years. The goals of public health are usually stated to be 'preventing disease and promoting health', and the mechanism for realizing these objectives are to be organized interventions directed at particular groups or the community as a whole. Clearly, therefore, public health has always been associated in some way with health promotion. While this dual identity has been a source of strength, as noted below, it has also proved to be an effective source of friction. Even before the terms public health and health promotion came into use, dilemmas in defining the objectives of such interventions were apparent. In Britain, the first public health manifesto was issued on 25 January 1796, in response to the social upheavals associated with the Industrial Revolution. This remarkable 'Heads of Resolutions for the consideration of the Board of Health' in Manchester resisted the invitation to censure the labouring people for their moral delinquency; instead, it called for their protection through state intervention involving 'a system of laws for the wise, humane, and equal government' of working conditions (Maltby, 1918, pp. 121–2). Looking forward to the thinking of a much later date, the Manchester manifesto firmly located the root cause of ill health in the prevailing economic system. Although this episode demonstrates that general social activism and a strong liberation philosophy pre-date modern conceptions of public health, in the event such movements failed to bring about widespread improvements in health, owing to the absolute dominance of forces of economic production.

During the 1840s, the early public health movement predominantly focused on sanitary conditions, motivated by a desire to reduce Poor Law support and promote economic efficiency. However, at the same time, an alternative perspective which saw patterns of disease as a reflection of social conflict was being put forward by writers such as Friedrich Engels. In *The Condition of the Working Class in England*, in 1844, Engels (1973) cited the mode of economic production as the principal cause of ill health. His justification for public health intervention was one based on notions of social justice rather than efficiency of production.

Most histories of public health label this supposed start of the modern public health movement in the 1840s as the *sanitation phase*, a period characterized by adoption of a medical perspective and concentration on environmental issues such as housing, working conditions, the supply of clean water and the safe disposal of waste. Under the supervision of the newly-invented Medical Officers of Health (MOH), the sanitarians focused on improving the health of working people by bringing about changes in their conditions of everyday living. The motivating forces of this early public health movement were economic advantage and, to a lesser extent, the maintenance of social cohesion between the working poor and the middle and upper classes.

A more critical perspective is provided by Turshen (1989), who suggests that attempts by some historians to portray public health doctors as the health champions of working people are misplaced. Turshen argues that what working people themselves wanted was radical social and economic change, not environmental engineering or minor social legislation designed to mitigate the worst effects of capital production.

The safe disposal of waste and the supply of uninfected water yielded real and measurable reductions in infectious disease, but the inadequacy of the sanitarian approach to health was exposed by the Interdepartmental Committee on Physical Deterioration, which reported in 1904. This committee revealed the enormous extent of ill health associated with poverty and economic exploitation, but rather than resulting in significant changes to the social and economic determinants of health, the committee's findings became the springboard for what is often termed the second, *personal hygiene*, era in public health intervention. Winslow (1952) characterizes this as focusing on education and hygiene, which relocated the responsibility for health improvement with individuals, as opposed to collective community action or state intervention. Newsholme's report of 1913 typifies the then prevailing medical public health attitude that poverty was not in itself a cause of infant deaths (Newsholme, 1936, pp. 179–82). Instead, this report maintained that it was the removable evils of 'motherhood ignorance' about infant care and 'poor personal hygiene' that were to blame.

The second stage of public health, occupying the first half of the twentieth century, generated a vast array of clinics and other institutional services to deal with the needs of such vulnerable groups as mothers, infants, schoolchildren, and those suffering from particular diseases such as tuberculosis. Inevitably, these services required the employment of a large workforce, with the result that this period became the heyday of the MOH and public health departments of local government. These services brought about greater contact with individuals and families, and 'health education' figured prominently in this work. Increasingly in the

UK, the conceptualization of health promotion was dominated by health education in schools. While this state-sponsored health education was underpinned by what we would now call a 'victim blaming' philosophy, an alternative 'liberation and empowerment approach' to health education was also being developed by lobbying groups such as the Children's Minimum Council, the Committee Against Malnutrition and the National Unemployed Workers Movement (Lewis, 1991).

The achievements of public health in the first part of the twentieth century were heavily publicized, not least by figures such as Sir Arthur Newsholme and Sir George Newman, Chief Medical Officers of the time. Both conducted their apologetics in the language of missionary zeal and in a paternalistic spirit, which invited uncritical admiration rather than objective understanding (Newsholme, 1936; Newman, 1939). As in the sanitarian phase, the personal hygiene era brought genuine health gains, but also disadvantages. On the eve of the Second World War, we might characterize public health professionals as bureaucratic, complacent, eugenic and preoccupied with national economic objectives. Worse, in the light of evidence relating to health during the interwar depression, was not only that public health professionals had made little impact on the problems identified by the Interdepartmental Committee on Physical Deterioration, but also that its elite had manipulated the official statistics to disguise the limitations of its competence (Webster, 1982).

In sum, although the public health establishment during its second phase made every effort to show that its health education services embodied a genuine attempt to empower and liberate the population, this was only true to the most limited extent, and the limitations were recognized by social activists on both the right and left. In the late 1930s, new thinking about public health emerged from such sources as the maverick Peckham Health Centre, from the eugenicist Richard Titmuss, and in the form of 'Social Medicine' as advocated by John Ryle (Ryle, 1948). The idea of Social Medicine was to apply a biomedical paradigm to populations. At least in the UK, this was largely an academic construct limited to an intellectual elite and not extending its influence beyond a few university public health departments, with the result that it was ignored by the dominant medical public health establishment.

For a short time, planners looked to Social Medicine as the means to revitalize public health. In fact, Social Medicine failed to consolidate its influence, with the result that, in the UK, epidemiology was its only long-term legacy. This approach is, in turn, being increasingly challenged as embodying a simplistic, biomedical and professionally dominated idea of health (Peterson and Lupton, 1996). None the less, the abortive Social Medicine movement underlined the limitations of the previous era and, in this respect, prepared the ground for health promotion and was one of the factors causing the medical profession to invent the 'new public health'.

Social Medicine accepted that 'health' implied a 'positive' condition, representing much more than freedom from communicable diseases. Achievement of positive health implied a changed attitude to the causes of ill health, involving reference to the 'whole economic, nutritional, occupational, educational, and psychological opportunity or experience of the individual or community' (Ryle, 1948, pp. 11–12). The success of Social Medicine depended on a new form of collaboration, in which all medical personnel, 'ordinary health workers and the general public', engaged in genuine teamwork (Leff, 1953, p. 15). Where necessary, this form of medical intervention also required commitment to social and political action (Crewe, 1945). Although Social Medicine was a British product, it was influenced by thinking elsewhere, particularly in America, and especially by Henry Sigerist, who is generally credited with having been the first to attach special importance to 'health promotion' and to the principles later embodied in the Ottawa Charter (WHO, 1986). Sigerist believed that the primary task of medicine was to 'promote health', and declared that medicine should be seen as a social science. It was 'merely one link in a chain of social welfare institutions', central to which was 'socialised medicine', for which he was also a leading advocate (Sigerist, 1941; Sigerist, 1943, p. 241). Although Social Medicine made little impact in the UK, it was more influential in North America and WHO circles, which ultimately became the main sources for igniting the health promotion movement in the 1970s.

The introduction of the National Health Service (NHS) in 1948 revolutionized health care in the UK. However, the benefits were distributed unevenly, and the activities most relevant to health promotion were located in the most neglected corners of the new service. As one of its most radical changes, the NHS reduced the functions of public health departments, thereby turning the once powerful MOH into a minor functionary in charge of only a small rump of preventive services. While health care was transformed, public health professionals were launched into a phase of disorientation.

In a move that seemed symbolic of this collapse of influence, the government abandoned its health centre programme. This had been the only important new function promised to the MOH, and many of the hopes for the realization of Social Medicine's potential had depended on the creation of health centres (Lewis, 1986; Webster 1988, pp. 381–8).

At the time of the NHS reorganization of 1974, which completely eliminated local government involvement in the health service, an attempt was made to rescue public health activity from extinction by repackaging it as community medicine, but this too was a failure (Lewis, 1986). In particular, the 1974 changes deprived community medicine specialists of their control of environmental health departments, and shifted them back into hospital administration and also abandoned the annual reports that were a key component of the watchdog role of the

MOH. Continuing erosion of confidence led to a further rescue effort in 1988, based on the recommendations of the Acheson Report (1988), which reintroduced public health medicine as the name of the specialty.

Alongside the decline in medically dominated conceptions of public health during the 1960s and 1970s, the empowerment conception of health education continued to grow in influence. It was not until 1976–7 that the UK government issued its first prevention policy documents, but these timid efforts made no permanent mark (Webster, 1996, pp. 660–86). They simply restated the contention that ill health was largely the responsibility of individuals whom, through ignorance, were not looking after themselves. It was implied that ill health, rather than being related to poverty, was attributable to affluent lifestyles. Reflecting the barrenness of thinking about promotion, the commentary on health education of the Royal Commission on the NHS was also entirely lacking in insight (Royal Commission on the NHS, 1979, pp. 44–7). With respect to prevention and promotion, perhaps the most important changes were incidental features of the 1974 NHS reorganization, which gave environmental health officers new professional autonomy under local government, and established health education as an embryonic specialism in the NHS.

Under the NHS, public health medicine limped along with its traditional routines, but it failed to respond to new challenges and avoided confronting the continuing problems of ill health associated with poverty. The mounting economic crisis of the 1970s prompted new concern about poverty and public health, and stimulated yet another rebirth of Social Medicine. The new social awakening centred around the problem of 'inequality' (Townsend and Bosanquet, 1972). In the field of health. this concern reached its classic expression in the Black Report (1980) (Townsend and Davidson, 1982). The findings of the Black Report drew together a great deal of evidence that highlighted appalling, inequalities in health, maldistribudon of resources, and irrational disparities in the provision of seemingly every type of service, including, those relating to prevention and promotion (Hart, 1971; Culyer, 1976; Dowling, 1983).

In light of the above brief history, it is not surprising that the impetus for new thinking about public health and health promotion came from outside the UK. The context of this reappraisal was provided by a confluence of forces: first, the rising tide of radical critiques of the medical establishment and the health industry in the Western economies; second, a mood of self-criticism within health services concerning their shortcomings, especially with respect to the needs of the poor and the developing world; third, growing concern in Western governments over the escalating cost of health care; and finally, the dramatic impact of the oil price rises introduced by OPEC states at the end of 1973. This date marked the end of the golden age of the welfare state, introduced an era of retrenchment, and provoked a rethinking of every aspect of health care. One of the early products of this rethinking was the development of empowerment models of health education and the concept of 'health promotion'.

The three seminal documents that launched the heath promotion movement were the Lalonde Report New Perspectives on the Health of Canadians (1974), and the WHO's *Global Strategy for Health for All by the Year 2000* (1981) and the *Ottawa Charter for Health Promotion* (1986). Together, they set out a vision for health improvement that went beyond sanitation engineering, lifestyle health education and preventive and caring health services, and mark the advent of the *health promotion* phase of public health. Health promotion was concerned principally with empowering citizens so that they could take control of their health and in doing so attain the best possible chance of a full and enjoyable life. The principal methodologies included community development, empowerment, social marketing, advocacy, organizational development and the formulation of integrated health strategies. Bunton (1992) contended that health promotion represented a new form and conception of health intervention: it 'deliberately tried to address issues of power, political, economic and social structures and processes'. MacDonald (1997) suggested that, because health promotion is intrinsically revolutionary, governments have, since its conceptualization, been trying by elaborate means to accommodate it and have displayed great ingenuity in appearing to absorb its radical ideas without in reality disrupting the *status quo*. As governments seek to embed health promotion within the existing medical and health-care dominated agenda, attention is drawn away from the challenges that it presents for society – most radically to set health, rather than the creation of wealth, as the overarching goal of society. As we have seen, this is not a new idea, but rather a re-emergence of much earlier calls for health to take priority over wealth creation.

Kelly and Charlton (1995) have, however, pointed out that health promotion is characterized by a difficulty that arises from the failure by its advocates to address their unspoken assumptions about the relationship between social autonomy and social structure. They suggest that this is especially problematic when considering the effects of social inequality on oppressed groups: 'Here the emphasis is on social determinism among the oppressed while maintaining a place for the idea of free will among non-oppressed groups. Empirically, this may seem to be the way the world operates, and politically it may make sense to construct things in this way, but theoretically and epistemologically it does not work' (1995, p. 89).

Stevenson and Burke (1991) are even more critical of health promotion, arguing that it weakens struggles for social equity and political change to the extent that 'with its emphasis on organic harmony and consensus among diverse identities and its tendency to develop methodological 'resolutions' to political problems, health promotion mystifies rather than clarifies the nature of social barriers to meaningful change' (1991, p. 281).

Health promotion and the 'New Public Health' possess common characteristics. Both are closely associated with the WHO *Health for All* strategy, and both seem to consist of multiple and disparate stands. Draper believes that the new public health takes a 'comprehensive view of health hazards in the human environment, from the physical, chemical and biological to the socio-economic' (Draper, 1991, p. 10). Baum (1990) has argued that the 'new' public health carries the same flaws as many understandings of health promotion, in that it is underpinned by the assumption that change can be achieved through consensus building, while history teaches us that it is conflict and challenges to existing power structures that promote health.

If health promotion and the new public health have a major distinguishing feature, it would appear to be the conviction that health is a right – opposed to older ideas of health as a necessity for national efficiency, or as a moral duty of citizens. However, even this claim does not withstand critical examination. The 'health as a right' concept can be traced back for thousands of years and, like 'health as a means to efficient production', represents a recurrent theme. The health as a right concept has, however, continuously been subordinated to a more politically and capital sensitive paradigm that emphasizes individual and environment solutions to poor health over social and economic ones.

Yet it is possible to make an even more critical assessment of the new public health movement. It is arguable that the new public health – concept developed largely by medical practitioners working in the public health field – represents an assault by the medical profession, intent on recapturing the commanding heights which were lost to the globally developed and more inclusive notion of health promotion. Evidence of this reassertion of public health is evident in much of the UK government's recent health strategy. The term 'health promotion' is noticeable by its absence, despite the fact that, internationally, the phrase is used as an umbrella term that includes the subset of public health. As indicated in the quotation from Alan Milburn earlier in the chapter, it seems that the case for interdisciplinary and intersectoral partnerships to promote health is now accepted by the UK government. The Health Development Agency established in 2000 in England seems to be a concrete expression of this acceptance, although only time will tell whether the agency receives the governmental support it will need to be effective.

The public health and health promotion professions embody – and tolerate – conflicting ideas of why and how health should, and could, be improved. The meaning of public health and health promotion are themselves contested and open to a range of understandings. The origins of these conflicts lie in the contested nature of health itself, of the causes of ill health, of the methods for reducing ill health and promoting well-being, and fundamentally, in the motivation for such interventions. The historical record suggests that one expression of these conflicts has been through the cyclical invention, abandonment and reinvention of the 'social model' of health and disease which, when advocated, quickly falls out of favour due to the fact that inevitably it brings its supporters into direct conflict with the state and existing economic interests. Alongside this, the history of public health has also been one of a long battle for occupational domination by the medical profession. Given a widespread acceptance of the complexity of improving health, and the UK government's moves to develop multidisciplinary public health leadership, the traditional hegemony of the medical profession is clearly no longer sustainable.

The promotion of health depends on the engagement of a wide number of sectors and professions. Public health promotion has always been, and remains, a collective activity. Only if we are prepared to recognize the historic conflict, and the contested nature of health promotion and public health, will it be possible to develop a deeper understanding of how the battle could be more effectively fought on behalf of those currently deprived of their rights to health. In the light of history, it is clear that the fundamental test of health promotion is yet to come as it struggles to exercise any influence at all in a world increasingly shaped by global economic forces.

References

Acheson, D. (1988) *Independent Inquiry into Inequalities in Health*, London, HMSO.

Baum, F. (1990). The new public health: force for change or reaction?, *Health Promotion International*, 5(2).

Bunton, R. (1992). More than a woolly jumper: health promotion as social regulation, *Critical Public Health*, 3(2), 4–11.

Crewe, F. A. E. (1945). *Social Medicine. An academic discipline and an instrument of social policy*. Edinburgh: Graduates' Association.

Culyer, A. J. (1976). *Need and the National Health Service. Economics and social choice*. Oxford: Martin Robertson.

DHSS (Department of Health and Social Security) (1980). *Inequalities in Health. Report of a research group*. London: DHSS.

Dowling, S. (1983). *Health for a Change. The provision of preventive health care in pregnancy and early childhood*. London: Child Poverty Action Group.

Draper, P. (ed.) (1991). *Health through Public Policy. The greening of public health*. London: Green Print.

Engels, F. (1973). *The Conditions of the Working Class in England*. Moscow: Progress Publishers.

Hart, J. T. (1971). The Inverse Care Law, *Lancet*, i, 405–503.

Kelly, M. and Charlton, B. (1995). The modern and the post-modern in health promotion. In Bunton, R., Nettleton, S. and Burrows, R. (eds), *The Sociology of Health Promotion: Critical analysis of consumption, lifestyle and risk*. London. Routledge.

Lalonde, M. (1974). *A New Perspective on the Health of Canadians*. Ottawa, Ministry of Supply and Services.

Leff, S. (1953). *Social Medicine*. London: Routledge.

Lewis, J. (1986). *What Price Community Medicine? The philosophy, practice and politics of public health since 1919*. Brighton: Harvester/Wheatsheaf

Lewis, J. (1991). The origin and development of public health in the UK. In Holland, W. W., Detels, R. and Know, G. (eds), *Oxford Textbook of Public Health*. Oxford: Oxford Medical Publications.

MacDonald, T. (1996). Health promotion, ancient and modem and their relationships to biomedicine, *Bulletin of the International Council of Psychologists*, 207–24.

MacDonald, T. (1997). Holism and reductionism – their role in mediating health promotion and biomedicine, *Report on the 7th National Health Promotion Managers Conference*. Carlisle: North Cumbria Health Development Unit.

Maltby, S. E. (1918). *Manchester and the Movement for National Elementary Education*. Manchester: Manchester University Press.

Milburn, A. (2000). Health and economics, Speech at the London School of Economics, 8 May.

Newman, Sir G. (1939). *The Building of a Nation's Health*. London: Macmillan.

Newsholme, Sir A. (1936). *The Last Thirty Years of Public Health*. London: Allen & Unwin.

Peterson, A. and Lupton, D. (1996). *The New Public Health*. London: Sage Publications.

Royal Commission on the National Health Service (1979) *Report*. Cmnd. 7615. London: HMSO.

Ryle, J. A. (1948). *Changing Disciplines*. London: Oxford University Press.

Sigerist, H. (1941). *Medicine and Human Welfare*. New Haven, Conn.: Yale University Press.

Sigerist, H.(1943). *Civilisation and Disease*. Ithaca, NY: Cornell University Press.

Simon, J. (1890). *English Sanitary Institutions*. London: Cassell.

Stevenson, H. and Burke, M. (1991). Bureaucratic logic in new social movement clothing: the limits of health promotion research, *Health Promotion International*, 6, 281–9.

Townsend, P. and Bosanquet, N. (eds) (1972). *Labour and Inequality: Sixteen Fabian essays*. London: Fabian Society.

Townsend, P. and Davidson, N. (1982). *Inequalities in Health: The Black Report*. Harmondsworth: Penguin.

Turshen, M. (1989). *The Politics of Public Health*. London: Zed Books.

Webster, C. (1982). Healthy or hungry Thirties?, *History Workshop Journal*, 13, 110–29.

Webster, C. (1988). *The Health Services since the War. I, Problems of Health Care: The National Health Service before 1957*. London: HMSO.

Webster, C. (1996). *The Health Services since the War. II, The Government of Health Care. The British National Health Service 1958–1979*. London: The Stationery Office.

WHO (World Health Organization) (1981). *Global Strategy for Health for All by the Year 2000*. Health for all series, No. 3. Geneva: WHO.

WHO (World Health Organization) (1986). *Charter for Health Promotion: An international conference on health promotion – the move towards a New Public Health*. Ottawa: WHO.

Winslow, C. E. A. (1952). *Man and Epidemics*. Princeton, NJ: Princeton University Press.

2 The challenge of health inequalities*

Hilary Graham

Introduction

This chapter turns the spotlight on the link between social inequality and individual health. It does so by focusing on socio-economic inequality: on the fact that how well and how long one lives is powerfully shaped by one's place in the hierarchies built around occupation, education and income . . .

Health inequalities: patterns and trends

Evidence of an association between socio-economic position and health dates back to ancient China, Greece and Egypt and is apparent today in societies for which data are available (Krieger, 1997; Whitehead 1997). Table 2.1 captures this association in mid-nineteenth-century England. It highlights, too, how the scale of these socio-economic differences varied across the country. In Liverpool, for example, the average age of death for labourers was 15, less than half that recorded for gentry in the city (35 years) and for labourers in rural Rutland (38 years).

Mid-nineteenth-century England was a rapidly industrializing society in which infectious diseases of childhood and early adulthood kept life expectancy low. Since then, death rates have fallen by half and it is the chronic diseases of later life, like coronary heart disease (CHD) and cancer, which dominate the mortality statistics. Despite these changes, the distribution of ill-health continues to follow the contours of disadvantage.

The map of regional mortality still marks out the poorer industrial and rural areas of northern UK from the richer rural and suburban areas of the south (see Figure 2 1). The spatial patterning of health is repeated at area level. For example, the prevalence of limiting long-standing illness varies from under 10 per cent in areas of the country characterized by growth and prosperity to over 20 per cent in the coalfields and industrial ports (Wiggins *et al.*, 1998).

* From Graham, H. (2000) *Understanding Health Inequalities*, Buckingham, Open University Press, pp. 3–20.

Table 2.1   Average age of death by social class and area of residence, 1838–41

District	Gentry and professional	Farmers and tradesmen	Labourers an artisans
Rutland	52	41	38
Bath	55	37	25
Leeds	44	27	19
Bethnal Green	45	26	16
Manchester	38	20	17
Liverpool	35	22	15

Source: Whitehead (1997) adapted from *Lancet* 1843, Office for National Statistics © Crown Copright 1997

Inequalities between places are matched by inequalities between individuals. Each step down the class ladder brings an increased risk of premature death (see Figure 2.2). The gradient is less steep for women but, as for men, higher socio-economic status (SES) protects against premature death. Major causes of death also display strong socio-economic gradients. CHD, is the leading single cause of death in the UK. Among men, death rates from CHD are about 40 per cent higher among manual workers than among non-manual workers; the death rate for wives of manual workers is about twice the rate for wives of non-manual workers (Marmot, 1998). Like mortality, morbidity from CHD also displays a socio-economic gradient, with angina and heart attacks (myocardial infarction – MI) more common among manual than non-manual groups. Less is known about recovery from myocardial infarction, and whether socio-economic disadvantage slows the recovery process.

Statistics on disease and death provide a negative picture of the health of the population. Subjective measures, where individuals are invited to assess their physical and psychosocial health, again reveal a socio-economic gradient. While self-rated health has been regarded as a less accurate measure of health, it predicts mortality and is associated with other clinically- based measures of disease (Power *et al.*, 1998).

The inequalities captured in Figures 2.1 and 2.2 are widening. Life expectancy has continued to rise for men and women in all socio-economic economic groups, but the differential has become more pronounced. Between 1972 and 1996, life expectancy for men in social class I increased by 5.7 years: among men in social class 5, the gain was 1.7 years (Hattersley, 1999). Mortality rates tell a similar story. While death rates have fallen, the decline has been greater in higher socio-economic groups. Figure 2.3 captures the trend among men of working age using standardized mortality ratios (SMRs) which take into account differences in the size and age composition of different classes. If there were no class inequalities, men in each social class would have an SMR of 100. An SMR below the line indicates a lower than average death rate; one above the line reflects a greater than average death rate. In recent decades, class differences in mortality have widened. In the 1970s, death

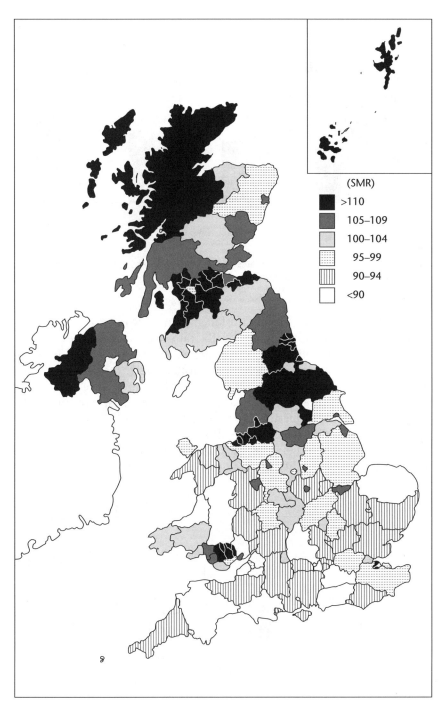

Figure 2.1   Standardized mortality ratios (SMRs) in the UK, by country and unitary authorities, 1997

Source: *Regional Trends* 34, Office for National Statistics © Crown Copyright 1999

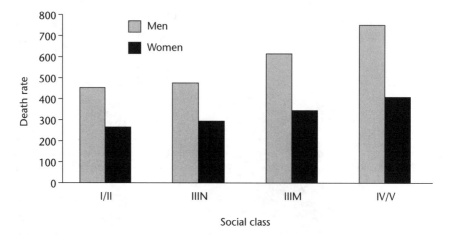

Figure 2.2   Age standardized death rates per 100,000 people by social class, men and women aged 35–64, England and Wales, 1980–92
Note: Women are classified by partner's occupation details or, if absent, by their own.
Source: Harding *et al.* (1997), Office for National Statistics © Crown Copyright 1997

rates were twice as high among unskilled manual workers as among professionals; by the 1990s, the death rate was three times higher. Underlying this widening class divide are widening differentials in major causes of premature death, including coronary heart disease, stroke and lung cancer. Among children, falling mortality rates have again been associated with widening inequalities in major causes of mortality, including accidents (Roberts and Power, 1996).

Spatial inequalities in health are also increasing, as the poorer areas of Britain are left behind in the general improvement in health. Poorer areas which had mortality rates 20 per cent above the national average

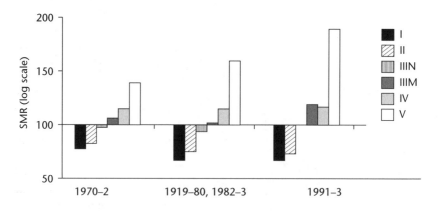

Figure 2.3   SMRs by social class (based on occupation), males, England and Wales 1970–2, 1979–80, 1982–3 and 1991–3, all causes
Source: Drever *et al.* (1996), Office for National Statistics © Crown Copyright 1996

in the 1950s like Oldham, Salford and Greenock, had mortality rates 30 per cent above the national rate by the 1990s (Shaw *et al.* 1998). The result is a concentration of premature deaths in areas of high (and often increasing) deprivation . . .

Socio-economic inequalities: patterns and trends

Analyses of health inequalities – between individuals and between areas – are set against the backdrop of broader economic and social change. Again, trends in the UK capture patterns evident in other older industrial societies.

The economic base has shifted away from the traditional manufacturing industries which provided full-time manual jobs for men, to the service industries which have opened up part-time work for women. The result has been a sharp rise in unemployment among men in unskilled manual groups (to 20 per cent in the late 1990s compared with 1 per cent in professional households) and a continuing rise in women's employment. Seventy per cent of women are now in paid work, but their hourly wages are 25 per cent lower than men's (ONS, 1998; Harkness and Waldfogel, 1999). Gaining entry to this changing labour market increasingly turns on educational qualifications. Those with qualifications are more likely to be employed in a well-paid job, while lack of qualifications is linked to unemployment and low-paid work. Although overall levels of educational attainment are improving, the gap between the highest and lowest attaining pupils widened through the 1990s (Sparkes, 1999).

While education is increasingly determining access to employment, employment is increasingly determining access to housing. Since the 1970s, there has been a rapid rise in owner-occupation, and a sharp decline in the availability of social housing (homes to rent from local authorities and housing associations). The result is that housing tenure, and the neighbourhoods in which tenants and owner-occupiers live, are increasingly patterned by SES. In the owner-occupied sector, eight in ten heads of household are in paid employment; but in the social housing sector, six in ten are economically inactive (ONS, 1998). Polarization in the housing market has been associated with an increase in the number of households excluded from it, in a sharp rise in homelessness, and in households in temporary accommodation.

Changes in the labour and housing markets are fuelling a spatial polarization of poverty and wealth. The industrial conurbations, like Greater Manchester, Merseyside and Tyne and Wear, have seen their populations fall as the manual jobs on which working-class men relied have been lost, with those left behind concentrated in local authority housing (Power, 1998)

Changes in access to employment and to housing have coincided with changes in family structure. In the 1950s and 1960s, social class made little difference to the domestic pathways which women and men negotiated as they moved through their adult lives. Across the class spectrum, the vast majority of men and women married in their early twenties, had their first baby within three years of marriage and remained married until separated by death (Kiernan, 1989). Today, this uniform progression through marriage and parenthood has given way to domestic trajectories which are strongly patterned both by social class and by gender. Young people who grow up in non-manual families and out of poverty are deferring – perhaps indefinitely – both marriage and parenthood, while it is those exposed to disadvantage in childhood who are most likely to marry and have children before their mid-twenties (Ferri and Smith, 1997; Harding et al., 1999). These divergent socio-economic pathways take a gendered form, with early parenthood and lone parenthood marking out the trajectories of working-class women. Figure 2.4, based on the 1958 birth cohort study, describes the domestic circumstances of young adults by their social class at the age of 23 (in 1981). Among men in the highest social class, less than one in ten are fathers by the age of 23; among women in the lowest social class, more than six in ten are mothers. Single parenthood shows even more pronounced gender and class differences. Few men in any social class are lone fathers by the age of 33; the proportions are significantly higher among women and are finely graded by social class. Among women in social classes IV and V, nearly four in ten are lone mothers by the age of 33.

Changes in people's working and domestic lives are fuelling a redistribution of employment between households. Through the 1980s and 1990s there was a rapid shift away from households containing a mix of employed and non-employed adults, and a corresponding increase in two-earner and no-earner households (Gregg and Wadsworth, 1996).

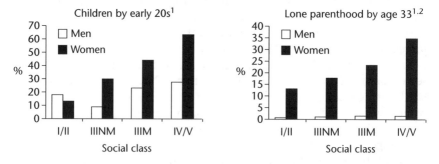

Figure 2.4   Domestic pathways by social class at age 23
Notes:
1   p < 0.001.
2   Ever been a lone parent (greater than 1 month).
Source: Unpublished analysis of data from the National Child Development Study by Sharon Matthews, Institute of Child Health

The growth in single adult and single parent households explains some of the growth in no-earner households. Figure 2.5 is therefore restricted to two-adult (male/female) households, which make up about 60 per cent of all households in Britain. As it indicates, male earner households are being replaced by two-earner and no-earner households.

The changing distribution of work is changing the distribution of income. The clumping of households on incomes in the middle of the income range is giving way, as the incomes of working households rise and non-working households struggle to make ends meet. The result is an increase in poverty and income inequality. Figure 2.6 plots the proportion of the UK population below the European Union (EU) poverty line, a line represented by a household income below half the average for all households, adjusted for size and composition. In the mid-1970s, less than one in ten (7 per cent) were in poverty; by the mid-1990s one in four (25 per cent) were. The increase in poverty has impacted disproportionately on households with children. One in three children (35 per cent) lives in poverty, a rate which dwarfs those elsewhere in the EU. In France, for example, less than one in six children live in poverty (HM Treasury, 1999).

Income inequality has been identified as an important determinant of health in richer societies. A series of studies have found that population health is related less to how wealthy a society is, and more to how equally or unequally this wealth is distributed. Life expectancy is higher in more equal societies: the USA, for example, has a gross domestic product (GDP) per capita over twice as high as that of Greece, yet life expectancy is higher in Greece than in the USA (Wilkinson, 1999).

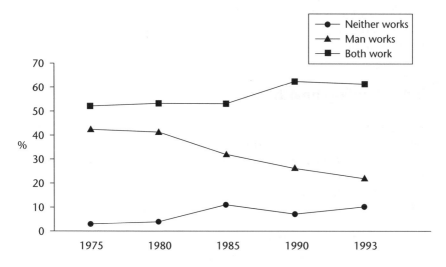

Figure 2.5 Employment in two-adult households, Britain, 1975–93
Source: Gregg and Wadsworth (1996)

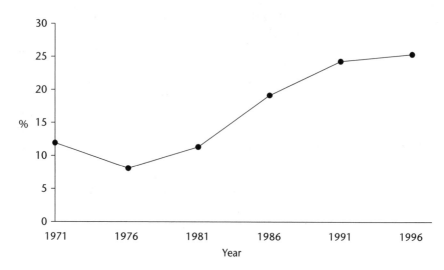

Figure 2.6 Proportion of the population below 50 per cent of average income (after housing costs), UK, 1971–96/7

Source: Goodman and Webb (1994); Department of Social Security (1998). (Crown copyright material is reproduced with the permission of the Controller of The Stationery Office)

An increase in poverty and income inequality is not the inevitable consequence of social and economic change. A key factor is the extent to which the living standards of households are dependent on the labour market position of their adult members (as they are in the UK). In countries with redistributive fiscal and social policies – for example, with progressive taxation and social security benefits pegged to average incomes – poverty and income inequality have not increased inexorably with the rise in unemployment . . .

Understanding health inequalities

How can the enduring association between SES and health be understood? In seeking answers to this question, researchers have been aware that the association may be a statistical artefact: an illusion resulting from flaws in the measurement of SES and in the statistical techniques through which its health effects are calculated. It is now accepted that such statistical inaccuracies are insufficient to account for the consistency and scale of the gradient (Davey Smith *et al.*, 1994). Researchers have been mindful, too, that an individual's health is a determinant as well as an outcome of socio-economic circumstances. Those in better health are more likely to move up the occupational ladder, amplifying the health advantages associated with higher socio-economic status.

Conversely, the downward mobility of those in poorer health is likely to increase the rates of morbidity and mortality in lower socio-economic groups. While health selection is contributing to the socio-economic gradient, its contribution is modest (Power *et al.*, 1996).

With neither statistical errors nor health-related mobility providing the answer, attention has turned to the pathways through which SES might exert an influence on health. A single pathway would, of course, simplify the explanatory task and provide a 'clear steer' to policy makers seeking to reduce health inequalities. However, the evidence points to multiple chains of risk, running from the broader social structure through living and working conditions to health-related habits like cigarette smoking and exercise. Different factors are likely to combine in different ways for different health outcomes. For example, health-related habits are known to play a larger part in the socio-economic differentials in lung cancer and CHD than in accidents, where environmental hazards, and exposure to road traffic in particular, are major causes.

The chains of risk have been uncovered primarily through surveys of individuals. However, a small seam of research is beginning to locate individuals in the places in which they live and to suggest that both individual factors and area influences have their part to play in the aetiology of health inequalities.

Factors at the individual level

The search for causes has focused on factors whose distribution varies in line with socio-economic position, and which have proven or plausible health effects. These factors are typically grouped under three broad headings: material, behavioural and psychosocial, although it is recognized that many health influences fall between and across these categories.

Material factors include the physical environment of the home, neighbourhood and workplace, together with living standards secured through earnings, benefits and other income. Behavioural factors are the health-related routines and habits which display a strong socio-economic gradient, like cigarette smoking (see Figure 2.7), leisure-time exercise and diet. While these lifestyle factors have been a major focus of national strategies to improve health, they make a relatively small contribution to health inequalities. Recent estimates suggest that between 10 per cent and 11 per cent of the socio-economic gradient may be explained by socio-economic differentials in health-related behaviour (Lantz *et al.*, 1998).

Alongside these material and behavioural determinants, research is uncovering the psychosocial costs of living in an unequal society. For example, perceiving oneself to be worse off relative to others may carry a

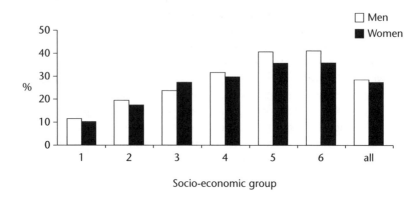

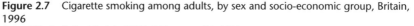

Socio-economic group

Figure 2.7   Cigarette smoking among adults, by sex and socio-economic group, Britain, 1996
Source: Office for National Statistics (1998), © Crown copyright 1996

health penalty in terms of increased stress and risk-taking behaviour. Attention has also focused on the health effects of the work environment, and particularly on the control that individuals exercise over the pace and content of work (Marmot *et al.*, 1997).

Material, behavioural and psychosocial factors cluster together, and those in lower socio-economic groups are likely to be exposed to risks in all three domains. Health-damaging factors also accumulate: children born into poorer circumstances clock up more by way of material, behavioural and psychosocial risks as they grow up and grow older. For example, girls and boys born into social classes IV and V are more likely than those in higher social classes to grow up in overcrowded homes, to develop health-damaging habits like smoking, and to be exposed to stressful life events and work environments (Power *et al.*, 1998).

Such analyses lend weight to what has become known as the 'life-course perspective'. This perspective suggests that health inequalities are the outcome of cumulative differential exposure to adverse material conditions, and to behavioural and psychosocial risks. Longitudinal studies are uncovering how the socio-economic structure becomes inscribed in the biographies and bodies of individuals. The emphasis in these quantitative studies is on how individuals are shaped by class-related 'exposures' and 'insults'. Qualitative studies focus less on the exposures and more on the experiences of those who endure them. They explore how people act against, as well as within, their class circumstances. Rather than plotting life-courses, these studies record people's life narratives: the biographical accounts through which we thread together understandings of the influence of the past and the impact of the present. This biographical approach is also uncovering how class relationships and class identities are expressed through health habits . . .

Area influences

Statistical advances, like multi-level modelling, are enabling researchers to locate individuals in the areas in which they live and to measure the contribution which people and places make to health inequalities. These new analyses confirm that poorer people in poorer health raise the rates of morbidity and mortality in poorer areas, while richer people in better health keep rates below average in more prosperous areas. However, while individual factors are the primary cause of spatial inequalities in health, areas also have an effect. In other words, poorer people may have poor health in part because they have to live in places which are health damaging (Macintyre, 1997).

How can places damage health? Both material and psycho-social pathways have been suggested. For example, the areas populated by poorer people score higher on material hazards, like environmental pollution, traffic volume and rates of road traffic accidents (Acheson, 1998). These areas are also less well-resourced in terms of shops, recreational facilities, public transport and primary healthcare services than those serving better-off neighbourhoods (Macintyre, 1997).

With respect to psychosocial pathways, research has focused particularly on the ways in which communities operate to resource and suport the well-being of residents. Community support is typically measured by aggregating data from individuals – on their involvement in voluntary organizations and with neighbours, for example, or their feelings of trust in those who lives around them – but it is seen to operate independently of the individuals whose lives are influenced by it (Lochner *et al.*, 1999). The concept of social capital has gained particular currency in research concerned with these social dimensions of areas. The concept was popularized by Putnam (1993), in his study of people's engagement in community life in different regions of Italy. His finding that income inequality is associated with lower levels of social capital has prompted research on the contribution it may make to health in richer societies (Wilkinson, 1996) . . .

Research into policy

Reducing health inequalities is moving up the policy agenda of national governments and international agencies. Older industrial countries like the UK are seeking 'to improve the health of the worst off and to narrow the health gap' (Secretary of State for Health, 1999), and are looking to research to guide the development of new public health strategies. An appreciation of both life-course and area influences is evident in the flagship policies of the 'New Labour' government.

A lifecourse perspective frames a raft of interventions designed to lift those heading for a lifetime of disadvantage on to more advantaged trajectories. The New Deal programme seeks to provide a ladder out of dependency on social security benefits and into paid work for disadvantaged young people and adults. On a smaller scale, Sure Start, an area-based intervention targeted at children aged 0 to 3 in disadvantaged areas, is designed to improve their health and development in the run-up to school, and provide a springboard into better health and higher SES in adulthood. Other area-based interventions to tackle health inequalities and social exclusion include the New Deal for Communities and a range of 'zoned' interventions like Health Action Zones. These area interventions typically operate within the framework of universal services – like education, health, policing and housing – to enforce basic standards of provision and to provide additional resources designed to improve the social and physical fabric of disadvantaged areas.

The effectiveness of these policies is likely to turn on the extent to which their positive impact is blunted by trends which are increasing poverty and income inequality like the continuing collapse of demand for low-skilled workers and the continuing fall in the living standards of claimant households. Further, the targeted nature of many of the interventions limits their reach and impact; while there are areas with high and increasing levels of disadvantage, most poor people do not live in disadvantaged areas . . .

Acknowledgements

This chapter draws on research funded by the Economic and Social Research Council (ESRC) under the Health Variations Programme (L128341002) and on analyses presented in Graham (2000). I am grateful for permission to reproduce data from the Office of National Statistics (Table 2.1, Figures 2.1, 2.2, 2.3, 2.7); Cambridge University Press (Figure 2.5, taken from J. Hills (ed.) New Inequalities, 1996); the Institute for Fiscal Studies and Her Majesty's Stationery Office (Figure 2.6); unpublished analyses by Sharon Matthews from the National Child Development Study (Figure 2.4); and from regional mortality data by Mary Shaw (Figure 2.1).

References

Acheson, D. (1998). *Independent Inquiry into Inequalities in Health*. London: The Stationery Office.

Davey Smith, G., Blane, D. and Bartley, M. (1994). Explanations for socio-economic differentials in mortality, *European Journal of Public Health*, 4, 131–44.

Department of Social Security (DSS) (1998). *Households Below Average Income, 1979 to 1996/97*. Leeds: DSS.

Drever, F., Whitehead, M. and Roden, M. (1996).Current patterns and trends in male mortality by social class (based on occupation), *Population Trends*, 86, 15–20.

Ferri, E. and Smith, K. (1997). Where you are and who you live with. In Bynner J., Ferrie, E. and Shepherd, P. (eds), *Twenty Something in the 1990s*. Aldershot: Ashgate.

Goodman, A. and Webb, S. (1994). *For Richer, For Poorer: The changing diststribution of income in the United Kingdom*. London Institute of Fiscal Studies.

Graham, H. (2000). Socio-economic change and inequalities in men and women's health in the UK. In Hunt, K. and Annandale, E. (eds), *Gender Inequalities in Health*. Buckingham: Open University Press.

Gregg, P. and Wadsworth, J. (1996). More work in fewer households. In Hills, J. (ed) *New Inequalities: The changing distribution of income and wealth in the United Kingdom*. Cambridge: Cambrdige University Press.

Harding, S., Bethune, A., Maxwell, R. and Brown, J. (1997) Mortality trends using the longitudinal study. In Drever, F. and Whitehead, M., (eds), *Health Inequalities* (Series DS No. 15). London: The Stationery Office.

Harding, S., Brown, J., Rosaro, M. and Hattersley, L. (1999). Socio-economic differentials in health: illustrations from Office for National Statistics Longitudinal Study, *Health Statistics Quarterly*, 1, 5–11.

Harkness, S. an Waldfogel, J. (1999) *The Family Gap in Pay: Evidence from seven industrialised countries* (Casepaper 30). London: London School of Economics.

Hattersley, L. (1999) Trends in life expectancy by social class – an update, *Health Statistics Quarterly*, 2, 16–24

HM Treasury (1999). *The Modernisation of Britain's Tax and Benefit System: No. 4, Tackling Poverty and Social Exclusion*. London: HM Treasury.

Kiernan, K. (1989). The family: formation and fission. In Joshi, H. (ed.), *The Changing Population of Britain*. Oxford: Blackwell.

Krieger, N. (1997). Measuring social class in US public health research, *Annual Review of Public Health*, 18, 341–78.

Lantz, P. M., House, J. S., Lepkowski, J. M. *et al.* (1998). Socio-economic factors, health behaviours and mortality, *Journal of the American Medical Association*, 279(21), 1703–8.

Lochner, K., Kawachi, I. and Kennedy, B. P. (1999). Social capital: a guide to its measurement, *Health and Place*, 5, 259–70.

Macintyre, S. (1997). What are spatial-effects and how can we measure them? In Dale, A. (ed.), *Exploiting National Survey and Census Data: the role of locality and spatial effects* (CCSR occasional paper 12). Manchester: University of Manchester.

Marmot, M. (1998). The magnitude of social inequalities in coronary heart disease: possible explanations. In Sharp, I. (ed.), *Social Inequalities in Coronary Heart Disease*. London: The Stationery Office.

Marmot, M. G., Bosma, H., Hemingway. H., Brunner, E. and Stansfeld, S. (1997). Contribution of job control and other risk factors to social variations in coronary heart disease incidence, *Lancet*, 350, 235–9.

Matheson, J. and Holding, A. (1999). *Regional Trends 34*. London: The Stationery Office.

ONS (Office for National Statistics) (1998). *Living in Britain: results from the 1996 General Household Survey*. London: The Stationery Office.

ONS (Office for National Statistics) (1999). *Regional Trends 34*. London: The Stationery Office.

Power, A. (1998). The relationship between inequality and area deprivation. In Centre for Analysis of Social Exclusion, *Persistent Poverty and Lifetime Inequality: The evidence*. London: HM Treasury.

Power, C., Matthews, S. and Manor, O. (1996). Inequalities in self-rated health in the 1958 birth cohort: life time social circumstances or social mobility?, *British Medical Journal*, 313, 449–53.

Power, C., Matthews, S. and Manor, O. (1998). Inequalities in self-rated health: explanations from different stages of life, *Lancet*, 351, 1009–14.

Putnam, R. D. (1993). *Making Democracy Work: Civic traditions in modern Italy*. Princeton, NJ: Princeton University Press.

Roberts, I. and Power, C. (1996). Does the decline in child injury vary by social class? A comparison of class specific mortality in 1981 and 1991, *British Medical Journal*, 313, 784–6.

Secretary of State for Health (1999). *Saving Lives: Our Healthier Nation*, Cm. 4386. London: The Stationery Office.

Shaw, M., Dorling, D. and Brimblecombe, N. (1998) Changing the map: health in Britain 1951–91, in M. Bartley, D. Blane and G. Davey Smith (eds) *The Sociology of Health Inequalities*. Oxford: Blackwell.

Sparkes, J. (1999) *Schools, Education and Social Exclusion* (Case paper 29). London: London School of Economics.

Whitehead, M. (1997) Life and death across the millennium, in F. Drever and M. Whitehead (eds) *Health Inequalities* (Series DS No. 15). London: The Stationery Office.

Wiggins, R. D., Bartley, M., Gleave, S. *et al.* (1998) Limiting long-term illness: a question of where you live or who you are? A multi-level analysis of the 1971–1991 ONS longitudinal study, *Risk, Decision and Policy*, 3(3): 181–98.

Wilkinson, R. G. (1996) *Unhealthy Societies: The Afflictions of Inequality*. London: Routledge.

Wilkinson, R. G. (1999) Putting the pieces together: prosperity, redistribution, health, and welfare, in M. Marmot and R. G. Wilkinson (eds) *Social Determinants of Health*. Oxford: Oxford University Press.

3   Older people's health: applying Antonovsky's salutogenic paradigm*

Moyra Sidell

Introduction

If we take morbidity data as the yardstick, older people's health on the whole is not very good. Evidence from the General Household Survey has, since the start of the 1990s shown that about 60 per cent of all people over the age of 65 suffer from some form of chronic illness or disability (Walker *et al.*, 2001). Yet, when asked in similar surveys how they rate their health, less than 25 per cent of people rate it as poor. One possible explanation is that they are using different accounts of health. When asked to define 'health', well over half talked in terms of psychological well-being or feeling good, another 12 per cent said that it was about having energy (Blaxter, 1990). Only about 12 per cent saw health as the absence of disease, with about a quarter defining health as the ability to function.

Accounts of health

Morbidity statistics which describe 60 per cent of the older population as diseased operate within a biomedical account of health. This is still the most influential of the health accounts of Western societies. It sees health as the absence of diagnosed disease. This view of health is both sanctioned and supported by the healthcare system. Biomedical explanations relate to the physical body, and health is explained in terms of biology. It is a mechanistic view which concentrates on the structure of the body, its anatomy, and the way it works, its physiology. This functional view of health sees the human being as a complex organism which can best be understood by breaking it into isolated parts, each with a 'normal' way of working. Disease can then be narrowed down to the malfunction of a particular part of the body. Medical treatment focuses on the diseased part and the tendency is to concentrate on dis-

---

* Commissioned for this volume. This chapter draws on material published by the author elsewhere (see Sidell, 1995).

33

crete parts or organs and pay less attention to the whole or the interaction of the parts.

This mechanistic and disease-orientated view of health inevitably paints a bleak and negative view of the prospects for health in old age. Later life is portrayed as a time of declining strength and increased frailty as organs and tissues wear out or succumb to disease and degeneration. It views individuals narrowly in terms of their bodies, which are in decline as the natural consequence of growing older. Hope for better health in old age will come from maintaining the body in better shape, eradicating the diseases to which the ageing body is prone, and replacing defective organs. Increasingly, medicine is accepting wider social and psychological influences on health and reflecting elements of other models of health, but most doctors and research scientists still believe that the way our bodies work can be understood within a biological framework and that a cause and therefore a treatment can be found for all disorders, whether physical or mental.

But biomedicine, with its emphasis on the functioning of individual bodies, has little to say about emotional and psychological health. Some strands of biomedicine have tended to see mental illness as some form of malfunctioning of the brain. Yet the separation of mind and body in explanations of health is a fairly recent phenomenon. In earlier historical periods in Western society and in some contemporary Eastern cultures mental and physical health are linked inseparably.

The humanistic psychology tradition developed the notion of a healthy personality with an ideal of health as a thinking, feeling and reflecting being, able to change and grow – a rounded, balanced personality (Stevens, 1990). A. Maslow and Carl Rogers have explored more positive aspects of psychological health, with an ideal of health moving from fulfilling basic human needs to reaching a state of 'self-actualisation' or 'becoming what one is capable of becoming' (Maslow, 1954). In this model, self-esteem and the ability to express one' emotions are important elements of healthy growth in people.

A holistic account of health is more concerned with the whole person as a unique individual. The older person is not seen as a collection of bodily ills but as a thinking, feeling, creative being who has strengths and weaknesses of body, mind and spirit. It is possible to be healthy in mind and spirit even though the body may be frail. Holism is often linked with equilibrium or a state in which body, mind and spirit are in balance. These are concepts drawn from ancient Eastern traditions and have become very popular in the West, particularly in the alternative health movement. But, as with biomedicine, the focus of attention is on the individual. Critics of a holistic account of health argue that this ignores the impact on the individual of the wider physical and social environment.

There is now widespread support for a more overarching social model of health which extends the medical model and draws attention to the adverse effects on health in the physical and social environment, such as poor housing, poverty, pollution, unemployment and poor working conditions (Heller *et al.*, 2001). This represents a challenge to orthodox medical views and puts health concerns on wider agendas, emphasizing the link between the economic, political and social environment and health.

The social model of health puts less emphasis on decline and decay of the organism and more on the interactions with the physical and social environment. So disease and decline are not inevitable in old age and not attributable to age *per se*, but to the conditions in which people age and in which they have lived their lives. Disease is never just 'due to your age' but to hostile forces in the environment, such as poverty and poor housing.

All the accounts of health explored so far see the normal state of affairs to be one of homoeostasis. Any disruption of this homoeostasis is considered to be abnormal, and if homoeostasis is not restored then the organism is said to be in a state of pathology or disease. Aaron Antonovsky (1984) has called this 'the pathogenic paradigm' and he claims that all our models of health, even the biopsychosocial models, are dominated by this paradigm.

Moving to a salutogenic paradigm

Antonovsky (1984) points out some of the consequences of the domination of the pathogenic paradigm. The first is that 'we have come to think dichotomously about people, classifying them as either healthy or diseased' (p. 115). Those categorized as 'healthy' are normal, while those categorized as non-healthy or diseased are deviant. If 60 per cent of older people have some form of chronic illness or disability then the majority of older people are not healthy. There is no place in this dichotomy for those who have a chronic illness yet are able to function perfectly well or for those who have a handicap yet are well satisfied with life. Second – and this echoes the holistic account – we have come to think of specific diseases such as cancer or heart disease instead of being in a state of disease. We have become obsessed with morphology instead of relating to generalised dis-ease and its prevention. This leads to Antonovsky's third concern, which is that we look for specific causes for these specific diseases so that the causes can be eradicated instead of accepting that 'pathogens are endemic in human existence' (p. 115). He believes that we need to explore the capacity of human beings to cope with pathogens. Fourth, the pathogenic paradigm deludes us into thinking that if we can eliminate 'disease' we will have health. This 'mirage of health' (Dubos, 1961) has been the driving force behind the 'technological fix' and 'magic bullet' attitude to eradicating disease. This attitude leads to the fifth consequence that Antonovsky identified, which is that the pathogenic paradigm concentrates on 'the case' and identifies high risk groups instead of studying the 'symptoms of wellness' (1984, p. 116). Adopting this approach would entail studying the smokers who do not get lung cancer, or the 'fat eaters' who do not have heart trouble.

Antonovsky believes that we should think 'salutogenically'. He claims that instead of assuming that the normal state of the human organism is one of homoeostasis, balance and equilibrium, it makes more sense to acknowledge that the 'normal state of affairs for the human organism is one of entropy, of disorder, and of disruption of homoeostasis' (1984, p. 116). He suggests that none of us can be categorized as being either healthy or diseased, but that we all can be located somewhere along a continuum which he calls 'health-ease-dis-ease'. He explains:

> We are all somewhere between the imaginary poles of total wellness and total illness. Even the fully robust, energetic, symptom-free, richly functioning person has the mark of mortality: he or she wears glasses, has moments of depression, comes down with flu, and may well have as yet nondetectable malignant cells. Even the terminal patient's brain and emotions may be fully functional. (p. 116)

This way of thinking would have profound effects on the way we view health in old age. It would discourage a percentage approach to assessing the health of older people. Instead of assuming that because 60 per cent have a chronic illness or disability they are therefore in poor health, while the other 40 per cent are in good health, we would need to look behind those figures to ask how those 60 per cent are actually affected by their chronic illness or disability, and to explore their wellness. We would have to ask questions such as why do some people cope while others do not, and why some consider themselves to be healthy in spite of their chronic illness while others do not. We would also need to ask about the dis-ease of the 40 per cent without chronic illness or disability. Do they have non-classifiable aches and pains, discomforts and feelings of unwellness?

Antonovsky is anxious that this reorientation towards health does not minimize the achievements of medical science, nor would he wish to impede the progress of technological change. Rather, his purpose is to redress an imbalance inherent in the way we view health; not to abandon the struggle against disease but to widen the armoury and explore other ways of achieving health. We need the availability of hip replacement surgery but we also need to understand why one person copes well with the operation and regains full mobility while another does not. We need to identify all the factors that might help us move along the continuum, and not just focus on the disease. We ask not so much how we can eradicate certain stressors but how we can learn to live with them, concentrating on the ability to adapt. This very much resonates with the empowerment approach of Keith Tones (2001), who states:

> (A)lthough we must acknowledge the specific illnesses and diseases to which older people are prey, it is both more ethical and more efficient to develop a positive approach and seek to enhance well-being of older people. The most useful way of encapsulating such an approach is in terms of empowerment. (p. xvi)

Antonovsky's salutogenic paradigm helps in our understanding of health in later life in that it turns on its head the notion that older people are a high risk group in terms of disease. As Antonovsky says, all of us 'by virtue of being human are in a high risk group' (p. 177). If we locate people dynamically along a continuum of health we are less likely to stereotype 'the elderly' as being diseased. By adopting a salutogenic paradigm we can reconceptualize questions about health in later life to concentrate on why and how people cope well with chronic illness and disability. The questions change from what stops people becoming sick to what helps them to become healthy in spite of disease.

In an attempt to define the mechanisms that help people to cope with adverse health conditions, Antonovsky developed a construct that he calls a *Sense of Coherence*, and abbreviates to SOC. He describes it as follows:

> The sense of coherence is a global orientation that expresses the extent to which one has a pervasive, enduring though dynamic feeling of confidence that one's internal and external environments are predictable and that there is a high probability that things will work out as well as can reasonably be expected. (Antonovsky, 1979, p. 123)

In a later refinement he identified three main components – comprehensibility, manageability and meaningfulness. Comprehensibility is the ability to see one's own world as understandable, to 'have confidence that sense and order can be made of situations' (p. 118). One views the future as being reasonably predictable rather than chaotic, disordered or unpredictable. Meaningfulness is the 'emotional counterpart of comprehensibility . . . life makes sense emotionally' (p. 119). Life is worth living for those who see their lives as comprehensible and meaningful. Manageability reflects the extent to which people feel that they have adequate resources, mental, physical, emotional, social and material to meet whatever demands are put upon them. He believes that wherever a person is located on the health-ease-dis-ease continuum at any particular time, those with a stronger SOC are more likely to move towards the health end of the continuum.

A person's SOC is built up from a range of experiences and sources through the life course and should be well developed by adulthood. Antonovsky sees the SOC developing from the degree to which our life experiences provide 'consistency', an 'underload/overload balance' and provide for participation in decision making. We experience consistency when a given behaviour results in the same consequences whenever we exhibit it, and when people respond to us in consistent ways. This allows us to predict the outcome of behaviour and therefore our lives seem reasonably predictable. Underload/overload balance is achieved when the demands made upon us are appropriate to our capacities. Underused capacity due to lack of challenges can be as harmful as not having sufficient capacity to meet the challenges with which we are faced. The extent to which we participate in decision making is important to the emergence of a strong SOC and is the basis of the meaningfulness component. When every things is decided for us and we have no say in the matter, when the rules are set by others without consultation, then the experience is alien to us. The issue is not so much having control over the events of our lives but in having some part in the decision making process.

Antonovsky's theory provides a useful framework for analysing the health status of older people, both collectively and individually. The health-ease-dis-ease continuum allows us to locate older people along the continuum rather than categorizing them in terms of either health or disease. It allows us to explore how people move along the continuum towards the health end in spite of chronic illness disability.

It is possible that Antonovsky's theory of SOC could be interpreted in a very individualistic way and thus be 'victim blaming': if only those older people with chronic illness had developed a strong SOC they would cope better with their lot. This was clearly not Antonovsky's intention, and in a paper presented at the WHO seminar on 'Theory in Health Promotion: Research and Practice' held in September 1992, he makes a case for seeing the SOC as a theoretical basis for health promotion. He asks, 'Can it be contended that strengthening the SOC of people would be a major contributor to their move toward health?' (1996, p. 16). He goes on to make it clear that this strengthening of the SOC is not aimed at individuals but at a given population, and frames the question for health promotion programmes:

> What can be done in this 'community' – factory, geographic community, age or ethnic or gender group, chronic or even acute hospital population, those who suffer from a particular disability, etc. – to strengthen the sense of comprehensibility, manageability and meaningfulness of the persons who constitute it?

It is important to remember that older people are a very diverse group, each with a unique biography and different life experiences and access to social and economic resources. But old age is a time when the threat to a sense of coherence can be great. Manageability, comprehensibility and meaningfulness can be hard to maintain in the face of much loss and change. This is particularly true of those old people who spend their last years in institutions, where it is likely to be even more difficult to maintain any sense of coherence.

Antonovsky's theory presents ways of both understanding health in old age and of helping older people to move towards the health end of the continuum whatever their circumstances. In order to do this they require ageing-friendly environments which must be both prosthetic and stimulating at the same time. Unfortunately, many older people experience extremely ageing-unfriendly or ageist environments which are a threat to any sense of coherence.

References

Antonovsky, A. (1979). *Health, Stress and Coping: new perspectives on mental and physical well-being*. San Francisco: Jossey-Bass.

Antonovsky, A. (1984). The sense of coherence as a determinant of health. In Matarazzo, J. P. (ed.), *Behavioural Health*. New York: Wiley.

Antonovsky, A. (1996). The salutogenic model as a theory to guide health promotion, *Health Promotion International*, 11(1), 11–18.

Blaxter, M. (1990). *Health and Lifestyles*. London, Routledge.

Dubos, R. (1961). *Mirage of Health*. New York: Andor Books.

Heller, T., Lloyd, C. and Sidell, M. (2001). *Working for Health*, Level 2 distance learning course K203. Milton Keynes: The Open University.

Maslow, A. (1954). *Motivation and Personality*. New York: Harper & Row.

Sidell, M. (1995). *Health in Old Age: myth, mystery and management*. Buckingham: Open University Press.

Stevens, R. (1990). Humanistic psychology. In Roth, I. (ed.), *Introduction to Psychology*. Milton Keynes: The Open University and Lawrence Erlbaum Associates.

Tones, K. (2001). Foreword. In Chiva, A. and Stears, D., *Promoting the Health of Older People: the next step in health generation*. Buckinham: Open University Press.

Walker, A., Maber, J., Coulthard, M., Goddard, E. and Thomas, M. (2001). *Living in Britain: Results from the 2000 General Household Survey*. London, The Stationery Office.

4 Social capital and health promotion*

Penelope Hawe and Alan Shiell

Introduction

. . . In her recent book on community organising, Meredith Minkler (1997) quoted the work of political scientist Richard Couto, who suggested that 'because Americans have so little sense of community, we pay a great deal of attention to it'. Couto went on to refer to the term *grassroots* 'as if it were a herbal medicine for current public problems'. The sentiment echoes something said by Australian sociologists, Lois Bryson and Martin Mowbray, who referred to 'community' as a 'spray-on solution' to the complex social problems that emerged in the late 1970s and early 1980s (Bryson and Mowbray, 1981). Substitute the words 'social capital' for 'grassroots' or 'community' in these quotations and a present-day feeling arises.

We quote these authors not because we wish to represent the post-modern cynicism of our times, but rather to inject a sense of perspective into the current enthusiasm for the notion of social capital, particularly as it relates to those who would wish to use it to promote health. We agree with others who have observed that social capital is on the brink of being used so widely and diversely that its power as a concept may be weakened (Wall *et al.*, 1998). The concept of social capital needs to be positioned relative to other concepts, such as sense of community and capacity-building, thus linking it to a broader, cross-disciplinary history. Interrogation of the concept should better clarify what it is that social capital will bring us, over and above current thinking about the ways to explain and advance population health.

In this chapter, we begin with a brief overview of the history and definitions of the term social capital . . . before going on to adopt the perspective of the change-agent – that is the interventionist or health promoter – in order to draw attention to what it is about social capital that may be open to influence or amenable to intervention. This literature includes reflections on the broader ethical and political considerations involved when health promoters try to help build better societies.

---

* From *Social Science and Medicine*, vol. 51, issue 6, 15 September 2000, pp. 871–85.

What is social capital and where did it come from?

Social capital is a relatively recent addition to the social sciences, though there is little that is new in the idea. The central elements of what is now called social capital, namely that membership of a social group confers obligations and benefits on individuals, can be traced back to both classical sociology and economics (Portes, 1998; Wall *et al.*, 1998).

The renewed interest in social capital is typically traced to one of three sources: Pierre Bourdieu, James Coleman and Robert Putnam. Each of these authors provides a similar definition of the term 'social capital', but there are significant differences in meaning and the implications that follow. Coleman attributes first use of the term to the economist Loury (1977). Portes and Landolt (1996) suggest Bourdieu was using the term before this. Bourdieu (1986) defined social capital as 'the aggregate of the actual or potential resources which are linked to possession of a durable network of more or less institutionalized relationships of mutual acquaintance and recognition – or in other words to membership of a group'. Coleman defined it functionally as 'not a single entity, but a variety of different entities having two characteristics in common: They all consist of some aspect of social structures, and they facilitate certain actions of individuals who are within the structure. Like other forms of capital, social capital is productive, making possible the achievement of certain ends that would not be attainable in its absence' (Coleman, 1988). According to Putnam, social capital refers to 'features of social organization, such as trust, norms, and networks, that can improve the efficiency of society by facilitating coordinated actions' (Putnam, 1995). These differences have been amplified in a growing research literature that has sought to operationalize the concept of social capital in fields as diverse as economic theory, social control, family behaviour, community life, and democracy and governance (Woolcock, 1998; Portes and Landolt, 1996).

In order to synthesize the growing literature, Portes (1998) suggests that social capital has come to mean 'the ability to secure benefits through membership in networks and other social structures'. This definition distinguishes two components, namely a relational element residing in the social organizations of which the individual is a member, and a *material* one that relates to the resources to which that individual has claim by virtue of his/her membership of the group. The central relationship is one of trust and reciprocity, which in turn generates a system of expectations and obligations. Trust between members of a network 'oils the wheels' of social and economic exchange, reducing transaction costs, allowing group members to draw on favours, circulate privileged information, and gain better access to opportunities.

Portes also stresses the need to distinguish the *sources* of social capital from its *consequences*. Among the beneficial consequences of social capital, he lists social control, the provision of parental or kinship support, and the benefits derived from network membership. Social capital is not without its downside, though, and it may also be used to constrain opportunities to non-network members; to place excessive demands on network members; to restrict individual freedom and to reinforce delinquent behaviour where this is the defining characteristic of group membership.

Woolcock (1998) also stresses the difference between what social capital *is* and what it does, but he goes further than Portes in classifying the nature of network relations and the levels at which social capital applies. Two different but complementary forms of relational social capital are identified – embeddedness and autonomy, each of which might apply at the micro-level, with which Coleman and Bourdieu were primarily concerned, or at the macro-level more consistent with Putnam's use of social capital.

The two varieties of network relationship take on different forms at each of these levels setting up a two-by-two classification table (see Figure 4.1). At the micro-level, embeddedness refers to dense, intra-community ties or the extent to which individual members are *integrated* into their networks. Autonomy refers to an individual's looser, extra-community ties, or the freedom they have to interact with others outside the immediate group (*linkage*). At the macro level, embeddedness refers to state–society connections, or the extent to which there is *synergy* between the state's actions and the interests of its populace. Autonomy here refers to the capacity of institutions and organizations to act independently, free from the influence of vested interests, a property that Woolcock labels *integrity*.

Clearly, therefore, social capital is not 'one thing'. It has relational, material and political aspects, and it may have positive or negative effects. It can refer to both dense and loose networks and it takes on a different form depending on whether one is concerned with the individual and his or her immediate group membership, or the interaction between social institutions . . .

	Micro-level	Macro-level
Embeddedness	Intra-community ties INTEGRATION	State – society connections SYNERGY
Autonomy	Extra-community ties LINKAGE	Institutional capacity and credibility INTEGRITY

Adapted from Woolcock (1998)

Figure 4.1   Levels and types of social capital

Social capital and health promotion

In Australia in 1999, the 11th National Health Promotion Conference took social capital as its theme and attracted a record number of local and international participants. Many presenters cast their current research and/or practice into social capital terminology, perhaps to increase the chance that their abstracts would be accepted for the conference. In some cases, this was clearly an adoption of the rhetoric. In others, it was apparent that the conference provided an opportunity for people whose work had hitherto been relatively hidden to be seen and appreciated in a new light. The sophistication of research and practice in social health promotion has been largely unrecognized in an era where the most prominent programmes have been in cardiovascular disease prevention.

Our purpose in this section is to give a brief overview of some insights and accomplishments of a broad spectrum of workers who have been striving to understand and harness properties of communities, environments and relationships to improve health or well-being. These insights have been hard won, and have led to critical reformulation of theory and a reassessment of the goals and values that drive interventions. At a time when the enthusiasm for social capital is running high and many new players are entering the field, we feel that it is essential to signpost literature that documents what we already know. This includes contributions which outline the limits of what can be done by 'health promoters' funded from health budgets, reminding us that the broader social capital agenda is, of necessity, intersectoral. What is special about this literature is that the contributors come with an intervention-level perspective – that is, from researchers and practitioners who focus on amenable factors to change and who have had the opportunity to contemplate the practice and ethics of (community-worker driven) involvement in macro-level change processes. These are people who have already taken up Marmot's challenge to direct interventions at the social environment (Marmot, 1998). McLeroy et al., (1993) refer to this as the insights that come uniquely from those working with the 'theory of the solution' instead of the 'theory of the problem'.

Analysis of power

Perhaps the strongest message that has come from those who have been dealing thoughtfully with the complexities of community or social environmental intervention is about power. Not only is power and powerlessness implicated as a variable in the production of health inequalities but practitioners who would seek to promote health have been conscious of the way they work, lest they reinforce status hierarchies and the oppression of some groups over others (Minkler and Cox, 1980;

Israel, 1985; Minkler, 1989; Minkler *et al.*, 1994; Robertson and Minkler, 1994). Even common methods of needs assessment in a community can act simply to reinforce the status quo (Marti-Costa and Serrano-Garcia, 1983; Hawe, 1996). Structural analyses of this type are present in the general health literature (Ryan, 1972; Nettleton and Bunton, 1995; Krieger, 1994; Seedhouse, 1997; Tesh, 1997), but they take on a special quality among those workers presenting case studies from locales that many of us would place in the 'too hard basket' (Schulz *et al.*, 1997; Minkler, 1992). In these settings, Putnam's romantic, essentially middle-class view of social capital quickly evaporates and Bourdieu's analysis sits more comfortably. Supportive relational ties are not a sufficient antidote to material deprivation and learned helplessness.

Workers in these settings have argued that interventions cannot be developed without the people running them being open to challenge about their worldview/values, their interpretation of power and empowerment, the ethics that will govern their decision making and power sharing, and the means by which success will be defined (Mondros and Wilson, 1994; Minkler, 1997; Serrano-Garcia, 1994; Hawe, 1994; Hawe, 1998). In other words, public health practitioners who wish to promote social capital and tackle social environments have to take a stand and recognize that they are political actors.

Building relational ties

The creation of settings (for example, schools, classrooms, agencies, communities and neighbourhoods) that foster a sense of community has been a primary goal of community psychology since the early 1970s (Sarason, 1974). Accordingly, measurement of this construct is well established (Davidson and Cotter, 1986) and sense of community has the status of an outcome variable in community interventions (Hawe and Farish, 1995). Community development has a long tradition of strengthening natural helping networks and there are many examples in the social work and broader literatures (Gottlieb, 1981; Whittaker and Garbarino, 1983). Use of natural or lay helping strategies in health promotion is best associated with the extensive works by Eng *et al.*, (1993; 1997) and Israel (1985). This includes an acute awareness of not upsetting the local helping ecology in networks. That is, recognizing the need to maintain reciprocity across the network and of not replacing indigenous helping styles with professional helping styles (Gottlieb, 1987). It is crucial that the sophistication that has evolved in this field is recognized as new players with a 'social capital agenda' might do more harm than good. The capacity of ill-conceived network interventions to create an unhealthy exclusivity and homogeneity among members has been noted (Sidel and Sidel, 1976; Stevens, 1976). In Woolcock's terminology (Figure 4.1), integration can be too easily promoted at the expense of linkage, both horizontal (across diverse networks) and vertical (across multiple levels of power).

Empowerment and capacity building

Health promoters typically may start by building relational ties, but then move beyond this to promote problem-solving capacities within the community (capacity-building) (Eng and Parker, 1994; Israel, 1985). Thus, capacity-building could be seen as activities that address a continuum from micro- to macro-level dimensions of social capital. Wallerstein (1992) describes empowerment as a social action process that promotes participation of people, organizations, and communities towards the goals of increased community control, political efficacy, improved quality of life and social justice. Community development strategies of this kind have been guided by the work of the Brazilian educator Paulo Freire (1970). Central to this strategy is the process of *conscientization*, whereby people develop the skills of critical social analysis and recognise the roles they may take in changing their social conditions. Knowing when to link within the group and when to seek resources beyond it is an aspect of critical analysis. Compelling case studies of conscientization used with alcohol and substance abuse interventions among high risk youth are given by Wallerstein and Sanchez-Merki (1994). Significantly, for those interested in the processes involved in how 'the social' becomes 'the physical'. Wallerstein's model of intervention includes self-identity changes, in which one's relative place in the social environment is addressed specifically.

There are many other examples of capacity-building in health promotion (see Eade, 1997, for example). This literature documents how the process of working in partnership with communities (sharing power, building skills) on a particular issue can provide multiple flow-on benefits for other issues. For example, Eng *et al.* (1990) have shown how participatory approaches to building water supplies in Third World countries can simultaneously increase vaccination rates. This literature also recognizes that the concept of community competence, or problem-solving capacity, is intertwined with local culture and values. This highlights the need for measurement of outcomes in capacity-building to be tailored sensitively to local context (Eng and Parker, 1994; Jackson *et al.*, 1997; Hawe *et al.*, 1999) that is, that measures of community capacity (and hence social capital) are unlikely to be directly transferable from one context to another.

Creating 'healthy' public policies, 'healthy' cities and places

Enshrined in the Ottawa Charter for Health Promotion in 1986 is an emphasis on creating environments and public policies that promote health. Thus intersectoral approaches to health promotion through the worldwide Healthy Cities project and other related initiatives (Ashton, 1992) have been one of the main avenues that have been used to tackle health inequalities at the level of how basic services and infrastructure are provided in places. Again, this is a broad literature that we cannot give sufficient attention to here. Intersectoral action has become a sophisticated practice area with its own theories, practice guides and measurement tools (Gray, 1985; Butterfoss et al., 1993; Funnell et al., 1995; Gray, 1996; Goldstein, 1997; Scriven, 1998).

The influence of place on health, independent of the characteristics of individuals dwelling within it (Sooman and Macintyre, 1995; Macintyre et al., 1993; Kaplan, 1996) has led to a call for more place-related initiatives to address health inequalities coupled with a reconceptualization of 'place' in health research (Popay et al., 1998; Kearns, 1998). Accordingly, it has been suggested that the concept of setting in health promotion is evolving into new forms (Hawe, 1998a). More crudely, it has been the venue within which we 'capture target groups' and subject them to health interventions. A step up from this was the recognition that we can manipulate properties of settings to make 'healthy choices easy choices'. A third step in the evolution is the recognition that people's experience of themselves as persons with meaning, dignity, power to act on their own behalf and care respectfully for others happens in a social context and properties of that context can either encourage human interaction, connection, growth and respect or, conversely, foster alienation and despair (Hawe, 1998a). Theoretical models to explain and influence the properties of context and the relationships that arise within them have arisen in ecological community psychology (for example, O'Donnell et al., 1993). For example, interventions can be designed to elevate the importance of the symbol of a setting and, through this, the meaning of the setting for people within it by use of narrative methods (Hawe, 1998). In this way 'participatory place making' (Dovey et al., 1985), connection and cohesion is fostered using place-centred approaches to health promotion. Further development of these ideas is also occurring in sociology and geography (Popay et al., 1998; Curtis and Rees Jones, 1998; Kearns, 1998).

Concluding remarks

The question is, will social capital provide a new or better pathway to tackle health inequalities over and above what is currently being advanced? We have suggested that the concept of social capital may add little and may perhaps even act to dilute social health initiatives already in place (under the various names of community health promotion, community development, empowerment and capacity-building). Many of these lean towards the political and material aspects of social capital, whereas a great deal of social capital rhetoric pertains only to its relational aspects. An important conclusion in this literature is that psychological empowerment, although it may have direct effects on health, is not the same as real empowerment (Zimmerman and Rappaport, 1988) so it is critical to take a wide view.

An agenda for tackling inequalities in health in the UK has been outlined by Whitehead (1995), involving strengthening individuals, strengthening communities, improving access to essential facilities and services, and encouraging macroeconomic and cultural change. It would be important to make sure that commitments to this are enhanced and not distracted by social capital debates. Portes' distinction between the sources of social capital (networks and relationships) and the consequences of it (power and material benefits) (Portes, 1998) is important, but should not distract us from recognizing that material benefits also derive from how governments conduct themselves. Solutions to health problems lie in many places . . .

The other lesson that stands out when comparing the social capital literature with the broader literature in social health and health promotion is that about power. The general feel of the writing from contributors who have worked in community settings is that Bourdieu's view of social capital fits better than does Putnam's. It deals better with community complexity. Practitioners are alert to the realities of structural power and discourses that define what is a problem and who is at risk. As mentioned previously, the less radical definitions of social capital are the ones that are being promoted by major agencies and translated into sets of indicators . . .

Finally, we are working in a time when many literatures are coming together. The field of health promotion has much to gain from 'next generation' thinking within epidemiology and ecological-level studies that link social capital and health. This will alert health promoters to more sophisticated ways of conceptualizing and designing population-level and place-level interventions, and will challenge the way we conceptualize, measure and intervene in aspects of 'settings'. This may help to reverse the tendency of interventions aimed at redressing health inequality to focus too much on individual-level, remedial activities (Whitehead, 1995; Gunning-Schepers and Gepkins, 1996). The entry of place theorists, urban designers, sociologists, geographers and ecologists into public health interventions may serve to counterbalance the dominant influence of behavioural sciences. Established theories and models of intervention in these fields have been largely untapped (Sarason, 1972; Curtis and Rees Jones, 1998). Without these new influences, the emerging opportunities that the social capital debate provides for health promotion could be lost.

References

Ashton, J. (1992). *Healthy Cities*. Milton Keynes: Open University Press.

Bourdieu, P. (1986). The forms of capital. In Richardson, J. (ed.), *Handbook of Theory and Research for the Sociology of Education*, New York: Macmillan.

Bryson, L. and Mowbray, M. (1981). 'Community' – the spray-on solution, *Australian Journal of Social Issues*, 16, 255–67.

Butterfoss, F. D., Goodman, R. M. and Wandersman, A. (1993). Community coalitions for prevention and health promotion, *Health Education Research*, 8, 315–30.

Coleman, J. (1988) Social capital in the creation of human capital, *American Journal of Sociology*, 94 (Supplement), S95–S120.

Curtis, S. and Rees Jones, I. (1998). Is there a place for geography in the analysis of health inequality? In Bartley, M., Blane, D. and Davey Smith, G. (eds), *The Sociology of Health Inequalities*. Oxford: Blackwell Educational.

Davidson, W. B. and Cotter, P. R. (1986). Measurement of sense of community within the sphere of the city. *Journal of Applied Social Psychology*, 16, 608–19.

Dovey, K., Downton, P. and Missingham, G. (eds) (1985). *An ecology of place and place-making: structures, processes, knots of meaning*. Melbourne: Royal Melbourne Institute of Technology.

Eade, D. (1997). *Capacity-Building. An Approach to People-Centred Development*. Oxford: Oxfam.

Eng, E. (1993). The Save Our Sisters project A social network strategy for reaching rural black women, *Cancer*, 72, 1071–77.

Eng, E. and Parker, E. (1994). Measuring community competence in the Mississippi Delta: The interface between program evaluation and empowerment, *Health Education Quarterly*, 199–220.

Eng, E., Briscoe, J. and Cunningham, A. (1990). Participation effect from water projects on EPI, *Social Science and Medicine*, 30, 1349–58.

Eng, E., Parker, E. and Harlan, C. (1997). Lay health advisor intervention strategies: a continuum from natural helping to paraprofessional helping, *Health Education and Behaviour* 24, 413–17.

Freire, P. (1970). *Pedagogy of the Oppressed*. New York: Seabury Press.

Funnell, R., Oldfield, K. and Speller, V. (1995). *Towards Healthier Alliances. a tool for planning, evaluating and developing healthy alliances*, London: Health Education Authority.

Goldstein, S. M. (1997). Community coalitions: a self assessment tool, *American Journal of Health Promotion*, 11, 430–5.

Gottlieb, B. H. (1981). *Social Networks and Social Support*. Beverly Hills, Calif.: Sage.

Gottlieb, B. H. (1987) Using social support to promote and protect health. *Journal of Primary Prevention*, 8, 49–70.

Gray, B. (1985). Conditions facilitating interorganisational collaboration, *Human Relations*, 38, 911–36.

Gunning-Schepers, L. J., and Gepkins, A. (1996). Review of interventions to reduce social inequalities in health: research and policy implications. *Health Education Journal*, 55: 226–38.

Hawe, P. (1994). Capturing the meaning of 'community' in community intervention evaluation: some contributions from community psychology, Health Promotion International, 9, 199–210.

Hawe, P. (1996) Needs assessment must become more change-focussed. *Australian and New Zealand Journal of Public Health*, 20, 473–78

Hawe, P. (1998a). Making sense of context-level influences on health, *Health Education Research*, 13, I–IV.

Hawe, P. and Farish, S. (1995). Evaluation of the Victorian Healthy Localities Project, Chapter 7, Impact of the Benalla Healthy Localities project on community outlook, cohesion and participation. Melbourne: Municipal Association of Victoria, 295–311.

Hawe, P., King, L., Noort, M., Lloyd, B. and Jordens, C. (1999). *Indicators to Help with Capacity-Building in Health Promotion*. Sydney: Australian Centre for Health Promotion.

Israel, B. A. (1985). Social networks and social support: implications for natural helper and community level interventions, *Health Education Quarterly*, 12, 65–80.

Jackson, S. F., Cleverly, S., Poland, B., Roberston, A., Burman, D., Goodstast, M. and Salsberg, L. (1997). Half Full or Half Empty? Concepts and research design for a study of indicators of community capacity. Ontario, Canada: North York Community Health Research Unit, City of North York, Public Health Department.

Kaplan, G. A. (1996). People and places: contrasting perspectives on the association between social class and health, *International Journal of Health Services*, 26, 507–19.

Kearns, R. A. (1998). *Putting Health into Place. Landscape, identity and well being*. New York: Syracuse University Press.

Krieger, N. (1994). Epidemiology and the web of causation: has anyone seen the spider?, *Social Science & Medicine*, 39, 887–903.

Loury, G. C. (1997). 'A dynamic theory of racial income differences'. In Wallace, P. A. and La Monde, A. M. (eds) *Women, minorities and employment discrimination*. Lexington: M. A. Health

Macintyre, S., Maciver, S. and Sooman, A. (1993). Area, class and health: should we be focussing on places or people?, *Journal of Social Policy*, 22, 213–34.

Marmot, M. G. (1998). Improvement of the social environment to improve health. *Lancet*, 351, 57–60.

Marti-Costa, S. and Serrano-Garcia, I. (1983). Needs assessment and community development: an ideological perspective. *Prevention in Human Services*, 2, 75–8.

McLeroy, K. R., Steckler, A. B., Simons-Morton, B., Goodman, R. M., Gottlieb, N. and Burdine, J. N. (1993). Social science theory in health education: time for a new model?, *Health Education Research*, 8, 305–12.

Minkler, M. (1989). Health education, health promotion and the open society: an historical perspective, *Health Education Quarterly*, 16, 17–30.

Minkler, M. (1992). Community organizing among the elderly poor in the United States: a case study, *International Journal of Health Services*, 22, 303–16.

Minkler, M. (1997). *Community Organization and Community Building for Health*. New Brunswick, NJ: Rutgers University Press.

Minkler, M. and Cox, K. (1980) Creating critical consciousness in health: applications of Freire's philosophy and methods to the health care setting, *International Journal of Health Services*, 10, 311–22.

Minkler, M., Wallace, S. P. and McDonald, M. (1994). The political economy of health: a useful theoretical tool for health education practice, *International Quarterly of Community Health Education*, 15, 111–25.

Mondros, J. B. and Wilson, S. M. (1994). *Organizing for Power and Empowerment*. New York: Columbia University Press.

Nettleton, S. and Bunton, R. (1995). Sociological critiques of health promotion. In Bunton, R., Nettleton,. S. and Burrows, R. (eds), *The Sociology of Health Promotion*. London: Routledge

O'Donnell, C. R., Tharp, R. G. and Wilson, K. (1993). Activity settings as the unit of analysis: a theoretical basis for community intervention and development, *American Journal of Community Psychology*, 21, 501–20.

Popay, J., Williams, G., Thomas, C. and Gatrell, A. (1998). Theorising inequalities in health: the place of lay knowledge. In Bartley, M., Blane, D. and Davey Smith, G. (eds), *The Sociology of Health Inequalities*, Oxford: Blackwell.

Portes, A. (1998). Social capital: its origins and applications in modem sociology. *Annual Review of Sociology*, 24, 1–24.

Portes, A. and Landolt, P. (1996). The downside of social capital, *The American Prospect*, 26, 18–22.

Putnam, R. D. (1995). Bowling alone: America's declining social capital, *Journal of Democracy*, 6, 65–78.

Robertson, A. and Minkler, M. (1994). New health promotion movement: a critical examination. *Health Education Quarterly*, 21, 295–312.

Ryan, W. (1972). *Blaming the Victim*. New York: Vintage Books.

Sarason, S. B. (1974). *A Psychological Sense of Community. Prospects for a Community Psychology*. San Francisco: Jossey Bass.

Schulz, A. J., Israel, B. A., Becker, A. B. and Hollis, R. M. (1997). 'It's a 24-hour thing . . . a living-for-each-other concept': identity, networks, and community in an urban village health worker project, *Health Education & Behavior*, 24, 465–80.

Scriven, A. (1998) (ed.). *Alliances in Health Promotion. Theory and Practice*. London: Macmillan.

Seedhouse, D. (1997). *Health Promotion. Philosophy, Prejudice and Practice*. Chichester. John Wiley.

Serrano-Garcia, I. (1994). The ethics of the powerful and the power of ethics. *American Journal of Community Psychology*, 22, 1–20.

Sidel, V. W. and Sidel, R. (1976). Beyond coping, *Social Policy*, 7, 67–9.

Sooman, A. and Macintyre, S. (1995). Health and perceptions of the local environment in socially contrasting neighbourhoods in Glasgow, *Health and Place*, 1, 15–26.

Stevens, B. (1976). A fourth model for community work. *Community Development Journal*, 13, 86–94.

Tesh, S. N. (1997). *Hidden Arguments: Political Ideology and Disease Prevention Policy*. New Brunswick, NJ: Rutgers University Press.

Wall, E., Ferrazzi, G. and Schryer, F. (1998). Getting the goods on social capital, *Rural Sociology*, 63, 300–22.

Wallerstein, N. (1992). Powerlessness, empowerment and health: implications for health promotion programs, *American Journal of Health Promotion*, 6, 197–205.

Wallerstein, N. and Sanchez-Merki, V. (1994). Freirian praxis in health education: research results from an adolescent prevention program, *Health Education Research*, 9, 105–18.

Whitehead, M. (1995). Tackling inequalities: a review of policy initiatives. In Benzeval, M., Judge, K. and Whitehead, M. (eds), *Tackling Inequalities in Health. An Agenda for Action*. London: King's Fund.

Whittaker, J. K. and Garbanino, J. (1983). *Social Support Networks. Informal helping in the human services*. New York: Aldine.

Woolcock, M. (1998). Social capital and economic development: toward a theoretical synthesis and policy framework. *Theory and Society*, 27, 151–208.

Zimmerman, M. A. and Rappaport, J. (1988). Citizen participation, perceived control and psychological empowerment, *American Journal of Community Psychology*, 16, 725–50.

5 The importance of social theory for health promotion: from description to reflexivity*

Russell Caplan

Situating the problem

In trying to understand what health education/promotion is, and what those involved in it do, we have constructed various models. These models aim to capture in words some of the sense of what happens in practice. As such, they tend to describe in imaginative terms peculiar to the person doing the describing. The limitations of this form of understanding health education/promotion rest on the fact that people frequently use different terms/adjectives to describe similar health education/promotion situations or processes. Consequently, the more important similarities among health education/promotion models appear as differences, and fundamental differences are rarely considered. The net result of all this confusion is a failure to spell out more precisely what it is one means by health education/promotion, and more importantly what one is doing when one claims to be practising health education/promotion.

This confusion can be best understood as an inability to move beyond describing what one is doing to the more fundamental theoretical level, which explains more fully the nature and choice of particular models. In health promotion, as in many other fields of social intervention, descriptive models all too often take on the appearance of a theory. This blocks the possibility of deeper forms of understanding and evaluation. Access to knowledge about health education/promotion approaches, I believe, rests on a structure of abstract theoretical constructs and categories which serve to make up a theoretical map on which a wide range of health education/promotion approaches can be rationally located and explained as a series of paradigms or exemplars (Gallie, 1956; Kuhn, 1970; Chalmers, 1985). However, these exemplars or paradigms can only be uncovered through a rigorous analysis of those abstract theoretical and philosophical assumptions/categories which lie hidden in the terms health education/promotion is presented. This is what I shall call *reflexive analysis*, in the sense that these abstract categories or assump-

* From *Health Promotion International*. 8(2) (1993), pp. 147–57. Oxford University Press. © Oxford University Press 1993.

tions are read back from the initial descriptive terms in which health education/ promotion is presented (Holland, 1977). These abstract theoretical and philosophical assumptions constitute a basic structure which determines all our descriptions, concepts and theories about health education/promotion. This is the area of *social theory* proper.

The theoretical and philosophical assumptions

Theoretical and philosophical assumptions contained in the various health education/promotion models consist of two fundamental questions or dimensions.

The first question or dimension concerns the evidence or data on which we plan our interventions. Within health education/promotion the question revolves around the nature of scientific knowledge with competing theories of causality regarding individual and community health status laying claim to the mantle of scientific rationality. Does the medical view of health and illness as the presence or absence of an *objective* pathological entity provide the basis for a rational grasp of the causal links necessary to plan an effective programme of health promotion/education? Or, do we need to draw on less tangible categories of *subjective* human experience such as the cultural and personal meanings and definitions which would appear to connect with people's individual and collective health status?

Clearly, the question of causality within this latter position is much more complex and less linear and mechanical than its medical counterpart which has tried to bridge the gap by focusing on individual behaviour as an objective causal entity. But behaviour does not equate with this latter view of experience since it remains within the objectivist fold of medical explanations as a mechanical cause of health damaging effects, whereas the opposing position from the point of view of meaningful human experience would suggest individual human behaviour as a consequence or effect of a complex socio-economic, cultural and ecological system the rationality of which must be understood in different terms from that of the natural sciences. Thus, it can be argued that effective health education/promotion in reducing the incidence of coronary heart disease in the population needs to focus on categories of social and cultural experience which give meaning to the eating, drinking and smoking habits of people. Preventable heart disease cannot be addressed effectively as a consequence of unhealthy behaviour. Rather, unhealthy behaviour must be made intelligible in the light of people's experience of living in a social system defined by many layers of meaning ranging from family experience to the impact of social class.

The knowledge base around which we plan our programmes for action is thus a crucial dimension in determining what we do in the name of health promotion/education, how we do it and most importantly how

The SUBJECTIVIST approach	———————————	The OBJECTIVIST approach
social construction of experience	———— defining health ————	objective psycho-social type behaviour

Figure 5.1 Philosophical positions: the subjective–objective dimension about the nature of scientific knowledge

we compete for scarce resources. The problem of knowledge on which we base our programmes for action remains the fundamental philosophical question of immense practical import in the struggle over competing systems of rationality.

This struggle over competing systems of rationality in the design and adoption of health promotion policies and strategies can be represented on a horizontal plain as opposing views or polarities about the nature of scientific knowledge, and how we acquire knowledge about human affairs (see Figure 5.1).

The second dimension or question implicit in the various models of health education/promotion can be represented on a vertical plane which has to do with assumptions concerning the nature of society. These assumptions range from theories of Radical Change at the top to theories of Social Regulation at the bottom (see Figure 5.2).

Radical change
Views related to theories of *radical change* argue that our society is essentially unstable with a basic tendency towards change. It is governed by basic conflicts such as that between capital and labour, and the domination of ideas, rules and objectives of some groups over others. For example, the domination of men over women expressed in a patriarchal ordering of society, and, a Eurocentric value system which is both culturally and racially insensitive to ethnic and cultural differences, expressed in the many forms of discrimination and racism in our society. The consequences of this is the exploitation, deprivation and alienation of certain groups within our society.

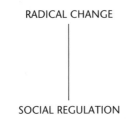

Figure 5.2 Assumptions spectrum

Theories of *radical change* are therefore concerned with finding explanations which demonstrate the need for fundamental change in the way our society is organised; that is, by social conflicts, tension and domination. Radical change, then, is concerned with emancipation from structures which constrain and limit human potential. It consequently focuses on questions which look at human deprivation in both social and psychological terms. Its major concern is with what is *possible*, more than with what *is* . . .

Social regulation

Ideas associated with theories of *social regulation* argue that we live in a predominantly stable society which is integrated and holds together well. This it is argued is reflected in a general consensus on rules and objectives. Social institutions such as the family, education, health and welfare all exist for the satisfaction of both individual and social needs.

Ideas about *social regulation* are therefore concerned with providing explanations of society in terms which emphasise its underlying unity and integration. This view seeks to understand why society holds together instead of falling apart. It is consequently concerned with the need for regulation in human affairs . . .

The two dimensions of Subjectivist and Objectivist approaches to knowledge and Radical Change or Social Regulation assumptions about the functioning of society, which all models of health education/promotion entail, can be combined as shown in Figure 5.3. Each quadrant represents a major approach or paradigm to the understanding of health and the practice of health education/promotion. It also provides the necessary concepts with which to assess more deeply and fundamentally what the differences are between the various health education/promotion models, and what they have in common with one another.

While Figure 5.3, and the more comprehensive map shown in Figure 5.4 is not a simple 'mechanical device' for piecemeal identification, categorizing and cataloguing of the various aspects of a model, it does nevertheless help us to assess whether there is anything of substance about a particular model, and its general direction. Again, while the approaches are not mutually exclusive with regard to certain assumptions, there are nevertheless certain limits beyond which to hold one position or approach must necessarily preclude the adoption of some other approaches . . .

By understanding the nature and purpose of health education/ promotion models in this way, it becomes possible to examine the degree of overlap and fundamental differences far more adequately and meaningfully.

The two abstract theoretical and philosophical dimensions (*Subjectivist–Objectivist* and *Radical Change–Social Regulation*) translate at a more concrete level into three pre-eminently practical questions which

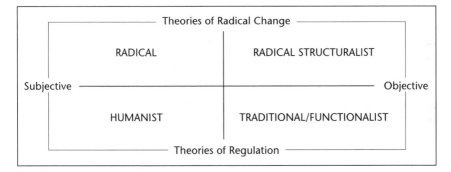

Figure 5.3 Major paradigms

Source: Burrell and Morgan (1985).

are implicit beacons, a type of cognitive compass guiding policy makers and practitioners alike in their quest to understand just what the determinants of health are, and what exactly constitutes a health promotion intervention.

Thus in each of the four approaches or paradigms which appear in Figure 5.4 the following questions provide the necessary evaluative mechanism by which various ideas, policies and plans can be properly analysed and mapped: (i) What is the core view of society? (ii) What are the principal sources of health problems? (iii) What are the health education/promotion aims? (Whittington and Holland, 1985).

Presented in this way, it becomes possible to construct a comprehensive map as set out in Figure 5.4, which summarizes the position of each of four approaches or paradigms. This systematized approach to theory in health promotion/education provides strong refutation of the conventional wisdom current within health promotion/education circles which argues that we are extremely unlikely to reach a point when a definitive map of health education will be possible (French and Adams, 1986).

Reflexivity in action–using social theory

The 'Ottawa Charter for Health Promotion' 1986, building on *Targets For Health For All 2000* (WHO, 1985), is the clearest statement of principles of a new public health movement which permeates much of the thinking and practice in the field. This statement of principles brings together a broad spectrum of descriptive terminology and categories which appear to be novel, radical and above all capable of providing the sort of understanding about health necessary for building effective action to promote it.

The view, however, as expressed in the Ottawa Charter, that you can

56

RADICAL HEALTH EDUCATION

Core view
Society is oppressive and alienating, It is characterized by hierarchical and authoritarian institutions of the state, business corporations, the professions, science, work and the family, which cognitively dominate people, (political and ideological domination). The very language we speak creates and sustains our participation in this form of oppression.

Sources of problems
Institutions we inhabit, which socialize and train us, and in which we work. The order which these institutions define devalues, discredits or invalidates alternatives. It affects human consciousness, relationships and potential, producing alienation and frustration of full personal and communal fulfilment.

Health education aims
Self-discovery through mutual aid and non-hierarchical cooperative projects which challenge the necessity of institutional processes. Radical self-help and deprofes-sionalism of health care which changes social control systems instead of so-called deviants. Reveal and challenge the 'political' in health.

RADICAL STRUCTURALIST HEALTH EDUCATION

Core view
Fundamental conflicts and contradictions arising from the economic system which give unequal wealth, power and opportunity to different classes. This determines broadly, the form of social institution and the state, of which the health and welfare services are but one example. Society is characterized by class conflict and struggle to redress the economic basis of class inequality.

Sources of problems
The demands of production and the reproduction of the conditions for capital accumulation (of which profits are part). Production – occupational diseases and injuries; unemployable and unemployed; occupational stress. Consumption – lifestyle patterns and consumer habits determined by what is produced, e.g. advertising which induces consumer preferences. Distribution – artificially maintained scarcity for basic needs, e.g. inadequate housing, heating, food and clothing.

Health education aims
Provide a theoretical analysis of the relationship between health, illness and the economic class structure. Link health education to those initiatives which challenge capitalism.

Subjective

Objective

Core view
Social life is meaningful and proceeds on the basis of the subjective interpretations of participants. Social struc-tures, institutions, roles and concepts of normality are socially created, sustained and changed by people through their interactions with one another. Implicit ori-entation to integrated, harmonious and enduring social units since it does not focus on political or economic consequences, or causes.

Sources of problems
Meanings and definitions that people give to their actions or identities are disrupted by events, or reinter-preted or so labelled by others that disorganized or deviant roles, identities and health careers are created. Loss and disruption of taken-for-granted reality produces disorientation and distress.

Health education aims
Improve understanding of self and others; improve com-munication by exploring the meanings of problems and events to all relevant parties, reconstruct identities by reframing accounts, representing unheard or unex-pressed versions, challenging key labellers, correcting stereotypes.

Core view
An enduring and integrated system based on a harmony of interests and common value system. Models and methods of natural science applied to the understanding of human affairs (medical science and epidemiology). The social whole is sustained by social institutions which function in the interests of individual and society, and which is adaptable to change.

Sources of problems
Pathological, maladaptive or incorrect (irresponsible) behaviour, habits or lifestyle; or pathological or faulty functioning of organizational and environmental processes.

Health education aims
Behaviour and attitude modification; or, administrative, legislative and environmental change (social engi-neering). Social change is not precluded so long as it is based on acceptance of the rules and legitimate institu-tions of liberal democracy.

HUMANIST HEALTH EDUCATION

FUNCTIONALIST HEALTH EDUCATION

Figure 5.4 Theoretical approaches in health education

Source: Caplan (1990), adapted from Whittington and Holland (1985)

build a new public health movement out of the rhetoric of disparate and contradictory ideological positions, constitutes an unwitting instrument for the imposition of an uncritical consensus incapable of mounting the necessary political and ideological challenges to the status quo so crucial for a health engendering society. In the final analysis the Ottawa Charter in the interests of consensus means all things to all people and precisely because of that is unlikely to provide the means for a clear strategy of action in raising the public health . . .

Much of what appears in the Ottawa Charter is an amalgamation of various models of health education/promotion which demand a proper analysis of their theoretical and philosophical underpinning. At least four models or methods which predate the Charter can be readily identified: the educational model, self-empowerment, the political economy model and the community development model (Tones, 1981, 1984, 1985; Beattie, 1984; Keeley-Robinson, 1984). While it is true that the terms in which they are presented are not always identical with that of the language used in the Charter, they nevertheless reflect with greater analytical precision the key notions embraced by the Charter. These notions relate to the development of personal skills as a means of self-empowerment through education and advocacy; the building of healthy public policy through political and economic means; and the empowerment of communities through community development (Ottawa Charter, 1987).

More often than not both the *educational* and *self-empowerment* notions or models, are presented as a radical antidote to the mechanical *objectivism* of the medical view based on simple disease prevention or individual behaviour change (Keeley-Robinson, 1984; Tones, 1985). However, if the preventive view of promoting health is 'by encouraging individuals to move away from unhealthy life styles and to adopt healthy behaviours' (Keeley-Robinson, 1984) then the educational and self-empowerment methods, while appearing to be more sensitive to the ideas of not imposing the professional's view of the right kind of health-related behaviour on individuals, nevertheless do not quite escape this line of reasoning.

Firstly, in the case of the educational model, who provides individuals with information, and secondly, who decides what informed decisions about health related behaviours are? This *objectivist* tendency within the self-empowerment framing of the model, while hidden by terms such as 'self-esteem' and 'informed healthy choices' (Keeley-Robinson, 1984; Ottawa Charter, 1987) is nevertheless all too present in the notion conveyed that there are *objectively identifiable skills*. Thus, it is argued that 'the purpose of health promotion is to enable people to achieve the personal skills and understanding of the environment that will allow them to exercise more control over their own health and make healthful choices' (Ottawa Conference Report, 1987).

What is clearly evident here on closer inspection is 'the existence of a priori concepts of the professional that are directive and strongly implicated in the succeeding action'. There is a preconceived model of 'how things should be which is implicit in the attitude of professionals' (Grace, 1991) and which is indicative of an *objective* purpose outside the individual . . .

In addition, the preventive model, like the other two models, focuses on 'encouraging individuals to move away from 'unhealthy life-styles' (Keeley-Robinson, 1984). In fact, I would strongly suggest that these three models are really aspects of a more complex *medical model* with *education* concerned with the ethics and obligations of the health educator, which is respect for and protection of individuals' health interests; prevention providing the scientific basis or *objective knowledge* about what has to be changed, health-related behaviour of individuals; and *self-empowerment* being the actual activity taught, conducted, or prescribed . . .

The *core view of society* which these approaches seem to hold is one of social integration and harmony where individuals need to change if their health status is going to be improved. The *principal source of health problems* lies somewhere between pathological, maladaptive or incorrect behaviour and disrupted life events forcing a dysfunctional set of roles and meanings to the behaviour of individuals. The *aim* conveyed here is a sense of individuals needing to be regulated or regulating themselves to a pre-defined goal of healthy behaviour. There is very little in these approaches which impresses upon the reader the sense of *collective action* borne of the essential class tensions and conflicts which is the real stuff of *radical change*. The overall position of these approaches lies somewhere between the Traditional or Functionalist and Humanist as set out in Figure 5.4 . . .

The Ottawa Charter also argues the case for combining 'diverse but complementary approaches including legislation, fiscal measures, taxation and organizational change' (Ottawa Charter, 1987). 'Public health legislation, better housing, an improved food supply and greater purchasing power are acknowledged as the most significant contributions to improvements in health status' (Keeley-Robinson, 1984). The view conveyed by this approach is that a package of legislative and administrative reforms is what is needed to improve people's health. Health education/promotion as *social engineering* is the strategy proposed to bring about the desired social changes.

The difference between this model and the educational and self-empowerment approaches is that the emphasis here is on administrative and legislative machinery to bring about the changes which will impact on the health related behaviour of individuals. The *objectivism* of individual behaviour has been substituted for the *objectivism* of public policy which is once again outside the locus of individual control.

And, even though 'powerful interests which profit from the products not conducive to health' (Keeley-Robinson,1984) are identified as part of the problem, they are nevertheless considered within an overall framework of a stable and enduring social consensus. They simply need to be reformed through the same legislative, administrative and fiscal measures which have been used in the past and even presently to secure these very same profits . . .

This fits quite easily into a *Functionalist* or *Traditional* approach. Political and economic indicators in this approach are a recapitulation of the traditional logic of incrementalism which simply adds 'new' indicators to an already bulging edifice of 'accumulated findings, like pebbles which if stacked up in sufficient quantity are bound to reach the sky eventually' (Ingleby, 1981). What is required is 'a "critical theory" that reconstitutes what needs to be indicated' (Stevenson and Burke, 1991) namely, radical *political economy*.

Perhaps the best attempt at constructing a truly radical practice in health education/promotion lay in the invocation of community action through *community development*. 'Community development draws on existing human and material resources in the community to enhance self-help and social support, and to develop flexible systems for strengthening public participation and direction of health matters. At the heart of this process is the empowerment of communities, their ownership and control of their own endeavours and destinies' (Ottawa Charter, 1987). 'The first step for the health educator/promoter' therefore 'would be to elicit the felt needs of the community. The formation of community groups would then be facilitated as a means of responding to identified needs' (Keeley-Robinson, 1984).

The *Radical* approach themes of domination in both its cognitive and institutional sense is implicit here (see Figure 5.4). In other words the community identifies what it considers to be its health problems (cognitive appropriation) and forms its own community groups (organisational ownership and control). However, while identifying health problems 'as one aspect of poverty and multi-deprivation' (Keeley-Robinson. 1984) it does not go further than this.

The *community development* model presented here is more readily identified with the *Humanist* approach, belonging with the other three models to a theory of *social regulation*. It is in the final analysis about competing more effectively within the defined social consensus. It is a piecemeal attempt at solving social and political issues of poverty and multi-deprivation through local community activity.

This is well demonstrated by the use of the term *community*. Community implies unity, togetherness, as opposed to social divisions which the *radical change* approaches are concerned with. Consequently, if a model is concerned with *radical change* then it cannot reflect the overall interests of everyone, as if they all had the same interest implied by the term *community*. This is because power, wealth and opportunity are unequally spread among the population, in the view of *radical change* adherents. If health is a consequence of this, then it is only the interests of a certain class or group of people that the *radical* or *radical structuralist* approaches are concerned with . . .

Conclusion

It would appear that all the models have a very similar view of society even though they seem to differ with regard to what they consider to be the *principal sources of health problems* and the *health education/promotion aims*. However, by showing how similar they are in their view of society we can come to an understanding of their differences at the level of sources of health problems and health education/promotion aims, as differences in degree and emphasis rather than fundamental differences of approach.

The analysis of the models is necessarily schematic. It does not represent a definitive analysis, but provides a common method and language through which to conduct a more thorough and informed debate. This points to, and draws on, a theoretical framework more definitive and enduring than has hitherto been realized within health education/promotion. This is not simply a matter of semantical refinement. For what is at stake is the very practice of health education/promotion and the positions it adopts based on a particular view of the world we live in.

Unless we understand more fully the theoretical and philosophical assumptions which underlie our methodological preferences, the link between health education/promotion and political processes remains unclear.

References

Beattie, A. (1984). Health education and the science teacher: invitation to a debate, *Education and Health* (January), 9–15.

Burrell, G. and Morgan, G. (1985). *Social Paradigms and Organisational Analysis*. Aldershot: Gower, 18.

Chalmers, A. F. (1985). *What Is This Thing Called Science?* Milton Keynes: Open University Press.

French, J., and Adams, L. (1986). From analysis to synthesis: theories of health education, *Health Education Journal*, 45, 71–4.

Gallie, W. B. (1956). Essentially contested concepts, *Reports of meeting of the Aristotelian Society* (21 Bedford Square, London, 12 March).

Grace, V. M. (1991). The marketing of empowerment and the construction of the health consumer: a critique of health promotion, *International Journal of Health Services*, 21, 329–43.

Holland, R. (1977). *Self and Social Context*. London: Macmillan, 267.

Ingleby, D. (ed.) (1981). *Critical Psychiatry: The politics of mental health*. Harmondsworth: Penguin.

Keeley-Robinson, M. (1984). Adult education issues for health promotion, *Occasional Paper, 1*. Hull University, 12–14.

Kuhn, T. S. (1970). *The Structure of Scientific Revolutions*. Chicago: University of Chicago Press.

Ottowa Charter for Health Promotion (1987). *Health Promotion*, 1, iii–v.

Ottowa Conference Report (1987). First International Conference on Health Promotion, *Health Promotion*, 1, 443–62.

Stevenson, H. M. and Burke, M. (1991). Bureaucratic logic in new social movement clothing: the limits of health promotion research, *Health Promotion International*, 6, 281–9.

Tones, B. K. (1981). Health education: prevention or subversion?, *Journal of the Royal Society of Health*, 3, 114–117.

Tones, B. K. (1984). Health education: present prospects and future potential, *TACADE Monitor*, 66, 6–9.

Tones, B. K. (1985). Health promotion – a new panacea? *Journal of the Institute of Health Education*, 3, 17–422.

WHO (1985). *Targets For Health For All 2000*, Copenhagen: World Health Organization.

Whittington, C. and Holland R. (1985). A framework for theory in social work, *Issues in Social Work Education*, Summer, 1–54.

6 Models of health: pervasive, persuasive and politically charged*

Trudi Collins

Introduction

The use of models clearly has the potential to be problematic. Each user has their own (or their agency's) political agenda and will interpret the model in their own, and possibly in their class, interest. Model developers can do little to protect against this except to include detailed explanations/interpretations of the model. Even then, the model developer's intentions can be ignored, misunderstood or misinterpreted. It is useful, therefore, to consider some established models of the determinants of health and to explore both the ways it appears that their developer intended their use and some other possible interpretations. The implications of the political ideology underpinning these models and its explicitness will also be addressed. The intent of this exercise is to consider ways in which models can be 'safeguarded' from misuse (if, indeed, that is possible) and, in addition, to assist in the development of an alternative way to conceptualise the determinants of health.

An established model of health

Hancock (1993) has been involved in the development of three ecological models of health, human development and the community. The third and most comprehensive of these, the model of health and the community ecosystem (Hancock, 1993), attempts to show the interactions between community, environment and the economy as they relate to health (see Figure 6.1). It emphasizes concepts such as conviviality in communities (social support, public participation, equity), generation of adequate wealth by the economy in a manner that is both socially and environmentally sustainable, and a liveable and viable built and natural environment (Hancock, 1993). This model has a clear emphasis on economics, being required to meet standards of environmental sustain-

* From *Health Promotion International*, 10 (4) (1995), 317–24. Oxford: Oxford University Press. © Oxford University Press 1995.

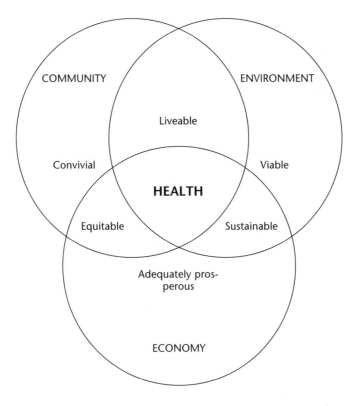

Figure 6.1 Interactions between community, environment, economy and health

Source: Hancock (1993)

ability and thus implicitly rejects the concept of economic growth at any cost, which has been gaining popularity in the wake of the ongoing recession experienced in the industrialized world. However, the model is less clear about the political implications of constraints on economic activity. For example, the notion of an *adequately* prosperous economy which is equitably distributed, as described by Hancock, is anathema to competitive, profit-motivated capitalist production. As noted in Tesh (1990), there are implicit political assumptions in the *status quo* (individualism, *laissez-faire* government, control by technocrats rather than lay people) and in challenges to the *status quo*. None of these issues or considerations of the impact and potential resolution of the political conflict suggested by this concept of environmental sustainability, are made explicit in Hancock's (1993) description of his model of health and the community ecosystem. Thus, while Hancock's model is an innovative and attractive attempt to link macro factors such as economic growth, environment and community conviviality to health, its silence on the public-policy implications of adopting such a model may restrict its utility as a tool for change.

A similar but less pronounced de-politicizing of the equity concept occurs in Hancock's (1993) description of his model. Thus while there is mention made of the need to distribute wealth more fairly, the political implications of this statement are not made explicit and neither are the appropriate policy items that would follow from such an understanding. While to some extent these implications may be self-evident, they become a question of interpretation rather than intent, as each user applies their own political understanding and agenda in deciding what appropriate programmes or policy would look like. Again, by not making explicit a political ideology for the model to be interpreted within, Hancock essentially locates his model within the *status quo* and falls short of making the political connections between a society organized on an understanding of the determinants of health as he has shown them and the one we currently inhabit.

This is not to say that Hancock does not possess that understanding, merely that he has not made it explicit. Indeed, his models represent an excellent attempt to introduce the concept of sustainability of economic and environmental practices to the health debate. Yet they fall short of their potential as a result of Hancock's failure to 'root' them in an explicit political ideology or explanatory account for why we do not have a 'healthy' society. As a result of this, it is not clear if structural socio-economic change is even on Hancock's agenda, or whether his models are calling for a conceptual re-ordering rather than a political re-structuring. This leaves their interpretation to the undeclared biases of the user . . .

It is from the context of the analysis of [this] established model of health (and others not described in this paper) that an alternative approach to conceptualising health has been developed.

An alternative way to conceptualize health

A model within a model

This model of health is composed of two 'levels' of activity at which health interventions could occur: the individual and the community (see Figure 6.2). This division was created primarily with the intention of 'forcing' model users to be aware of both the target and type of health determinants on which they are focusing their intervention *and* the other determinants (and level) that they are not addressing, i.e. to make explicit the limitations of their chosen intervention. This structure is intended to discourage programme developers from focusing on the least contested determinants of health (e.g. social support) to the exclusion of other less tractable but equally important areas (e.g. political and economic factors related to equity).

The intent of the 'model within a model' construction shown in

INDIVIDUAL MODEL

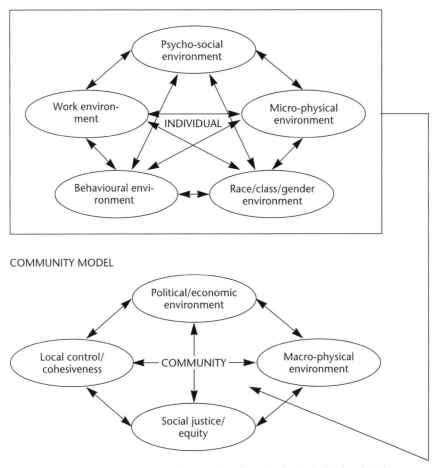

Figure 6.2 A nested model of health (note that the individual is located within the Community model)

Figure 6.2 is, then, to ensure that users are *explicitly* aware of the focus of their programme and the political implications of what that focus both includes and excludes. This is in direct contrast to the established models of health discussed above, which allow the user to focus on any determinant of heath and which do not address the individual–community interaction. Conceptually, the 'individual' portion of the model is located *within* the 'community' at the centre of the community model. The 'model within a model' concept asserts the importance of the structural factors such as the economic and political environment without suggesting a deterministic hierarchical structure. In addition, this 'nested' concept emphasizes the effects of social justice and equity within the community on both community and individual health. A consideration of the individual determinants of health is expected to lead to an evaluation of the community determinants of health and then a re-consideration of the individual level. [O]ne level of the model cannot be considered without also contemplating the other, for they are logically linked and inter-dependent.

The model's nested format also addresses the issue of reconciling a 'personal' model of health with a political model of health. The 'individual' part of the model relates well to the lived experiences of test cases used in model development, while the 'community' part of the model provides an avenue by which the over-riding macro or societal determinants of health can be emphasized. The intent of the model's construction is, therefore, to make it both personally and politically relevant, without being internally contradictory.

What is community?

In using the category 'community', however, one must be careful to be explicit as to its meaning. In the model described above, community is simply used to represent an aggregation of individuals with some shared experience. Therefore it could refer to a geographic community (towns, neighbourhoods), cultural community (ethnic groups, women's groups) or societal community (for example, Canadians). This concept has been deliberately left broad in order to encompass all levels of group behaviour and thus to make the model's application as wide as possible.

It is also noted that the nested construction is culturally specific to Western 'developed' societies, in that it accentuates a division between the individual and the community. In other societies less suffused with individualism, this division would probably not be appropriate. This approach to conceptualizing health arises from the context of an industrialized, advanced economy country and may not be appropriate for application in a developing country setting.

Model components

Individual model

The individual model is comprised of five broad categories or 'environments' of health determinants. These include the psycho-social environment (e.g. social support), the micro-physical environment (e.g. quality of indoor air, individual housing, etc.), the race/class/gender environment (e.g. the social construction of an individual's race, class or gender, education level, socio-economic level, effect of culture, etc.), behavioural environment (e.g. alcohol use, smoking behaviour, fitness, sexual practices, etc.) and the work environment (including workplace physical and chemical hazards, level of control over work scheduling and workplace demands). Each of these environments is thought to have influence on each other and also to both influence and be influenced by the individual in question. The health of the individual located at the centre of the model, will, then, be affected by some combination of these factors plus that person's biological makeup.

Thus, fitness behaviour is known to be affected by the class (Calnan and Williams, 1991) and gender (Saltonstall, 1993) environment as well as the safety of one's location (micro-physical environment). The micro-physical environment is, in turn, expected to be affected by one's socio-economic status (class environment), both of which have an effect on one's psycho-social environment. The simple schematic representation in Figure 6.2 can be seen, therefore, to mask a complex and changing set of interactions between factors. It is further expected that the 'environments' will differ in importance for different individuals and for the same individual over time. Therefore the model is expected to be temporally dynamic and to be able to accommodate the experience of a wide variety of people.

Community model
The individual model is then 'nested' within the community at the centre of the community determinants of health model. This community model consists of four broad categories of influential factors. These include the political and economic climate within which the 'community' is located (e.g. this may be as broad as global political trends and as specific as local by-laws, local unemployment levels or power-sharing within a support group), the macro-physical environment (e.g. outdoor air quality, transportation options, availability of good quality subsidized housing, global climate change, contamination of food sources, sustainable local environment, etc.), the degree to which there is a social justice and equity in the community (e.g. fair income distribution, a robust social security net, publicly insured health care, etc.) and the extent of community control and cohesiveness (e.g. the existence of vibrant community groups addressing community-identified needs, community involvement in local planning, an ethic of mutual-aid rather than competition).

Again, the linkages between each of these key categories of social determinants of health are designed to suggest the inter-relatedness of the categories. It is further conceptualized that there will be reciprocal interactions between the determinants of a healthy community and the community at the centre of the model. In addition, the determinants of a healthy community are expected to have an impact on the determinants of individual health and, thus indirectly on individuals themselves. Again, this is perceived as a reciprocal relationship, with individual change leading to community change as well. Hence the model has been designed to allow a role for human agency (Arnoux and Grace, 1991; City of Toronto, 1991) while still maintaining an explicit political stance regarding macro-economic, political and equity issues.

Again, the established model of health reviewed earlier does not provide a way to conceptualize this interaction between 'levels' of health.

A discussion of the implications of the model for both health promotion practice and policy development is provided here, but first it is necessary to locate the model in a theoretical context. This essentially outlines the model developer's 'agenda', an issue not always made explicit in published models.

Brief theoretical underpinnings

Using Caplan's (1993) framework of health education as a guide (see Chapter 5 in this volume), the overall model can be located towards the radical change end of the spectrum. What is important about this theoretical location is its recognition of the surfacing of the political, both in the model's inclusion of the political/economic climate as a determinant of community health and, hence, individual health, and also in the model structure which makes explicit to the user the areas both selected and avoided in designing health-promotion programmes or public policy, thus reducing the user's ability to omit a consideration of the political and economic determinants of health.

This inclusion of political/economic factors provides a direct link between the dominant political ideology and community and individual health. This is strengthened by the inclusion of the social justice/equity compartment, which is designed to encourage the user to consider the mitigative effects of the welfare state and social democracy on health in capitalist societies (Navarro, 1992). The inclusion of the community control/cohesiveness compartment is also designed to focus attention on issues of local rather than corporate control. Together, it is hoped that these elements will orient the user to challenge the political and economic *status quo*.

Implications for health promotion practice

From the perspective of health-promotion practice, the model has a number of implications, some of which follow directly from its theoretical base discussed above. Thus health-promotion programmes challenging the political and economic *status quo* at either level of the model would be expected to be developed by model users. For example, planned socio-political change as described in McKinlay (1993), programmes designed to increase equity in the society by providing economic activity for marginalized groups usually excluded from mainstream employment, and environmental health-promotion projects advocating for changes to environmental legislation or company operating procedures, would all constitute appropriate health-promotion programmes based on this model.

It is hoped that programme developers with a strict behaviour focus (e.g. smoking cessation) would be prompted by the model structure to consider other aspects of the issue. For example, a programme developer might consider the psycho-social (class-specific) benefits of smoking as well as the political and economic aspects of tobacco production and cigarette advertising and thereby propose a multi-faceted approach to the issue rather than the more common focus on individual behaviour. As with the other models reviewed, however, the focus of any programming developed with the aid of the model remains at the discretion of the user.

Implications for healthy public policy

The four influential categories of health determinants at the community level (political/economic, macro-physical environment, social justice/ equity, local control/cohesiveness) are expected to provide the main focus for policy makers using the 'model within a model' concept. Thus, like Hancock's (1993) model of health and the community ecosystem, equity, adequate economic prosperity and environmental sustainability might be key policy goals. Local control that truly involved power-sharing and local skills development would also be an appropriate policy development using the model.

In keeping with the political orientation of the model, it is intended that state regulation would be given precedence over free-market policies, although this would likely occur within the constraints of balancing the contradictory roles of the state (Fitzpatrick, 1987). Healthy public policy developed using the 'model within a model' concept is expected to extend to market regulation, environmental protection and equity measures.

Use of models: problems or panacea?

. . . The strength of the 'model within a model' conceptualisation of health arises not from its components, which can be found in many ecological health models of health, but in the way these determinants of health are organized into interactive, nested 'levels' of activity. The nested model attempts to provide a fluid representation of both individually and societally relevant determinants of health and tries to keep the user aware of the multiple 'levels' of health determinants and their implications for health-promotion practice and policy development.

It is worthwhile, however, to consider the more general utility of attempting to develop models of health. Indeed, models are, by their nature, reductionist generalizations that obscure detail and invite interpretation. They can be viewed as a product of positivist thinking that seeks a single or defined 'truth' to the problem' of the determinants of health.

They provide a simple representation of a situation that is both temporally and spatially varying (i.e. from person to person and with time).

Further, since health and its determinants are vexedly complex issues, in the face of increasing (or increasingly touted) financial insecurity of the state and rising health costs, a 'simple' understanding of health that allows resources to be moved from the expensive medical care system to other model-validated (and presumably less expensive, although undoubtedly less tried) determinants, is by its nature attractive. All models, including the 'model within a model', can be seen in this broader political and economic context of the crisis of the welfare state and they need to be interpreted with care as a result of this context . . . How better to justify change than by using theory as exemplified by a satisfyingly simple model? Models of health therefore have the potential to become dangerous political tools.

This analysis notwithstanding, models have many uses, some of them relatively benign. These include education, planning and conceptualization of health. Beyond these formalized uses, unarticulated 'models of health' underpin our understanding of health as health workers, policy makers and health-care receivers, and inform our approach to health-related matters in an unconscious but powerful manner. Indeed, one can attempt to develop, safeguard and use models in a manner that remains true to their developers' intent, and explicitly surfaces the ideology intrinsic to every model.

Recommendations

A number of possible approaches to 'safeguarding' models of health have been provided below. These are intended as a starting point for 'critical' health-model building and include:

- The need to make explicit both the political underpinnings and the policy or health-promotion practice implications of the model;
- The need for accompanying text detailing the theoretical basis of the model, its anticipated use, and contraindicated uses;
- A consideration of the potential for models to be applied in such a manner as to emphasize some determinants of health over others;
- The provision of examples of the contrary or ambiguous application of the model with respect to its goals. For example, does a model with an emphasis on community-based care provide some consideration of both the positive aspects of this approach (humanized health care, preservation of client's independence, etc.) and the potential negative consequences (potential for privatization and 'feminization' of care leading to an unhealthy burden on women as caregivers)?;
- A clear representation of the goals (beyond mere representation of the determinants of health) of the model;

- And, in the absence of such a clear representation on the part of the model developers, a critical analysis by the model user of the policy implications suggested by the model structure.

It is not enough, therefore, to merely provide a schematic representation of one's current understanding of the social determinants of health without qualifiers about what informs those beliefs, and a clear indication of the agenda the model intends to advance.

References

Arnoux, L. and Grace, V. (1991). From physical to critical epidemiology. New Zealand Public Health Association presentation, mimeo.

Calnan, M. and Williams, S. (1991). Style of life and the salience of health: an exploratory study of health related practices in households from differing socio-economic circumstances. *Sociology of Health and Illness*, 13, 506–29.

Caplan, R. (1993). The importance of social theory for health promotion: from description to reflexivity, *Health Promotion International*, 8, 147–57.

City of Toronto (1991). *Advocacy for Basic Health Prerequisites*. Toronto: Department of Public Health.

Fitzpatrick, R. (1987). Political science and health policy. In Scambler, G. (ed.), *Sociological Theory and Medical Sociology*. New York: Methuen.

Hancock, T. (1993) Health, human development and the community ecosystem: three ecological models, *Health Promotion International*, 8, 41–7.

McKinlay, J. P. (1993). The promotion of health through planned sociopolitical change, *Social Science and Medicine*, 36, 109–17.

Mustard, J. F. and Frank, J. (1991). *The Determinants of Health*, CIAR Publication, 5. Toronto: Canadian Institute of Advanced Research.

Navarro, V. (1992). Has socialism failed? An analysis of health indicators under socialism. *International Journal of Health*, 2, 583–601.

Premier's Council on Health Strategy (1991). *Nurturing Health: A framework on the determinants of health*. Toronto: The Ontario Premier's Council.

Saltonstall, R. (1993). Healthy bodies, social bodies: men's and women's concepts and practices of health in everyday life, *Social Science and Medicine*, 36, 7–14.

Tesh, S. (1990). *Hidden Arguments*. New Brunswick, NJ: Rutgers University Press, 154–77.

7 Planning and delivering health promotion: integration challenges*

Andrew Tannahill

The purpose of this chapter is to consider how best to plan and deliver health promotion in the context of the modern-day UK. There are many competing demands for attention. The major preventable diseases and health-related behaviours jockey for position as priorities for action. At the same time, thought has to be given to what should be done in a range of community settings, with different population groups (including people at different stages in the life-course), and using the numerous available methodologies (Hanlon *et al.*, 1995).

The chapter starts by identifying and appraising possible orientations for health promotion. It goes on to consider implications for health promotion *programmes*. The final section examines the place of health promotion as a *function* within the wider health improvement effort, with its strong emphasis on locality-centred plans and initiatives. The central theme throughout is *integration* of thinking and action.

Disease-orientated approach to health promotion

While it is important to make a distinction between health promotion and the narrower concept of prevention (Downie *et al.*, 1996a) a major aim of health promotion is to prevent ill-health. Historically – and still often today – the defining of health promotion priorities in terms of the prevention of specific major disorders has led directly to disease-centred health promotion programmes, with action in each directed at a group of risk factors associated with the disease in question (Figure 7.1).

Advantages of a focus on specific diseases are as follows:

- It helps to put, and keep, major preventable health problems on political, professional, organizational and public agendas;
- It enables health promotion policy makers, planners and 'doers' to ensure a coherent and relatively comprehensive package of preventive measures for each major category of ill-health;

---

* Commissioned for this volume.

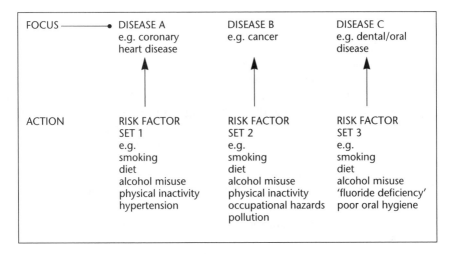

Figure 7.1   Disease-orientated approach to health promotion.

- A programme that is 'labelled' with, and 'flies the flag' for, a particular disease can help to motivate individuals, groups and communities and the population as a whole to play their part in the common cause of tackling the disease in question; and
- It demonstrates to all concerned that something is being done against particular problems.

On the other hand, a number of problems arise if health promotion efforts and programmes are driven purely by the disease-orientated approach (Tannahill, 1990; Tannahill, 1994; Downie *et al.*, 1996a; Downie *et al.*, 1996b).

- *Incomplete view of health.* The disease-orientated approach neglects the positive dimension of health (Downie *et al.*, 1996c). It is illogical to 'plough the single furrow' of prevention when well-being and fitness feature prominently in people's views of their own health and in what motivates them (Tannahill, 1992). The underlying vision of health is also incomplete in the sense that it is a 'top-down', professionally-dominated one in which self-assessment of health and health priorities by individuals and communities is not allowed for. To borrow from the vocabulary of clinical practice, the approach can amount to professionals' making a community diagnosis and issuing a population prescription, without any public consultation – and expecting mass compliance.
- *Incomplete view of the determinants of health.* It is too easy for the emphasis to be unfairly and squarely placed on individuals' health-related behaviour, viewed in absolute or relative isolation from the life

circumstances (Tannahill, 1998) that shape it. This issue is considered in more detail later in the chapter.

- *Duplication and over-saturation.* As illustrated in Figure 7.1, diseases share risk factors. Thus, for example, if there were to be individual programmes respectively centred on each of the UK's 'big 3' killers – cancer, coronary heart disease (CHD) and stroke – all three programmes would need to address smoking, diet, physical inactivity and alcohol misuse. If we have a number of disease-centred programmes, with the best will in the world it is unlikely that the content and timing of the efforts of the highly-focused teams delivering each programme can be co-ordinated sufficiently to maximize mutual added value, or even to avoid wasteful duplication across the disease topics. Accompanying this are risks of confusion among all concerned, and perceptions of over-saturation leading to a 'switch-off' response by professionals, organizations and members of the public alike.

- *Risk of inconsistency.* Also arising from the overlaps in risk factors between diseases is a danger of inconsistency of health education 'messages' that can damage overall professional–community communication, cause widespread confusion, and give some members of the public, and indeed some professionals, just the excuse they may be looking for to justify not changing their behaviour or practices.

- *Access difficulties and 'gatekeeper' concerns.* If we have a number of disease-centred programmes, all have to try to harness the mass media and gain access to communities and a range of settings – such as schools, the workplace and healthcare services. To do this they have to win the support of 'gatekeepers', i.e. the people who can provide or deny access to communities and settings. Such gatekeepers are faced with a whole succession of individuals and teams urging them to give time, attention and effort to tackling their own specific diseases of interest. For example, school headteachers may feel besieged by bids for time and space in already-crowded curricula. They may reasonably feel aggrieved at not having been involved at the earlier stages of programme development. They may be concerned that the disease-orientated approach is an unsatisfactory way of covering the spectrum of health-related topics – disjointed, piecemeal, inefficient and potentially counterproductive. They may recognise the incompleteness of the inherent model of health: the absence of the positive dimension and the fact that a whole view of health cannot be synthesized from a set or succession of separate topic-orientated inputs.

- *Neglect of general development.* Another source of concern for gatekeepers, if a purely disease-centred approach to programmes is adopted, is the propensity to neglect the need to develop infrastructures, methods and skills (e.g. among schoolteachers and pupils) that are of relevance across topics. This is associated with duplication and inefficiency: for example, there may be separate offers to provide training for schoolteachers on tobacco, alcohol and drug misuse, with each individual package devoting much of its time to the same sorts of educational skills.

- *Competition.* A common consequence of the programmes having to reach the same communities and settings is that, whereas they should be functioning as allies in the drive for better health, they effectively compete with each other for attention and action (Tannahill, 1998).

Risk factor-orientated approach to health promotion

A logical development from disease-orientated health promotion is risk-factor-orientated. In this case, action is directed towards tackling particular risk factors, primarily in order to prevent diseases with which they are linked (see Figure 7.2). The approach helps to put the risk factors 'on the map' and has the following advantages over the disease-orientated model (Tannahill, 1990; Downie *et al.*, 1996b):

- It reflects the recognition that a single risk factor will often have an impact on more than one disease category. For example, an anti-smoking programme can highlight associations with cancer, CHD and chronic obstructive airways disease. This reduces (but does not eliminate) duplication, inconsistency and the resulting problems arising; and
- It provides scope for highlighting positive health (well-being +/– fitness) benefits of certain 'lifestyle' behaviours such as regular physical activity. That said, in practice, positive health aims tend to be largely or totally eclipsed by the preventive, hence the representation in Figure 7.2.

Otherwise, the approach is associated with the same problems as those already described for disease-orientated health promotion. Not least, it

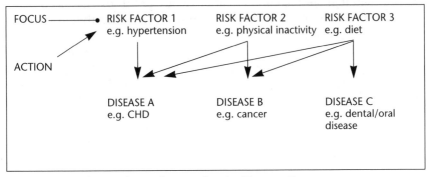

Figure 7.2   Risk-factor-orientated approach to health promotion

shares with that approach a real risk of viewing lifestyle behaviours in isolation from the life circumstances; and with both approaches, when life circumstances *are* acknowledged, they tend to be treated as though they have an impact on health more or less exclusively through influencing heath-related behaviour. It is important to recognize that life circumstances have major influences on lifestyle behaviours such as smoking, eating and physical activity, and through health promotion try to break the links between adverse circumstances and damaging behaviour. However, it is also important to be aware that an excess of serious diseases and premature deaths is still found in socio-economically disadvantaged groups, relative to more advantaged groups even when differences in behaviour between the two populations are allowed for. There is increasing recognition of plausible biological pathways whereby an accumulation of mutually compounding psycho-social stressors can increase susceptibility to behavioural risk factors and contribute more directly to physical disease processes (Wilkinson and Marmot, 1998).

Combined (disease- and risk factor-orientated) approach to health promotion

In practice, it is common to have a combination of disease- and risk-factor-centred health promotion programmes (Tannahill, 1990; Tannahill 1994; Downie *et al.*, 1996a; Downie *et al.*, 1996b). Thus, for example, in a single geographical location there may be separate topic-centred programmes for smoking, CHD and cancer. This gives rise once again to problems of duplication and potential inconsistency.

Health-orientated approach to health promotion

The shortcomings described in relation to the disease-orientated, risk factor-orientated and combined approaches point to the need for a model of health promotion that more fully captures health and its determinants, and is more integrated (see Figure 7.3).

Here, the focus is a dual one: the promotion of positive health and the prevention of ill-health. Thus the positive (as well as preventive) benefits of a healthy lifestyle are stressed, and the myth that 'it has to be hell to be healthy' is actively dispelled. For example, a healthy diet is presented (accurately) as rich, varied, enjoyable and satisfying, rather than as something that inevitably involves a sense of self-sacrifice to be tolerated for some speculative deferred benefit. The interlinked physical, mental and social components of positive health and ill-health (Downie *et al.*, 1996c) are recognized.

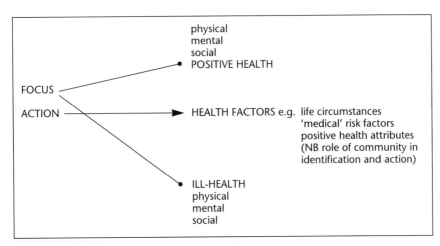

Figure 7.3   Health-orientated approach to health promotion

Action is directed at 'health factors' that include, but go well beyond, 'medical' risk factors. A 'salutogenesis' perspective takes its place along-side the more conventional 'pathogenesis' one (Antonovsky 1987; Kelly, 1989; Tannahill, 1992). In other words, efforts are made to identify and reinforce influences that produce and preserve health as well as attending to those that lead to disease. Action on specific 'medical' risk factor topics is built on the foundations of a concerted attack on adverse life circumstances (Tannahill, 1998; Scottish Office, 1999) that recog-nizes the tangled and shared roots of ill-health problems and health-damaging behaviour. Alongside this go efforts to promote life circumstances and behaviours that actively cultivate good health (Tannahill, 1998).

The positive perspective is reflected in the fostering of 'positive health attributes' (Downie *et al.*, 1996a) – healthy levels of self-esteem, self-belief and self-confidence among individuals, families, groups and com-munities, and a set of skills that helps people to take action to safeguard and promote their own health and that of others. Promotion of these empowering attributes should be combined with the nurturing of citi-zenship (Tannahill, 2000) and caring for others; qualities that enhance and protect the health of communities and societies.

The vision of health factors and the determination of priorities for action are not kept in the hands of professionals and others with tradi-tional position-derived power. Members of the public and groups and communities as a whole are involved in identifying health issues and in deciding upon, and implementing, health promotion action. The com-munity development approach to health promotion (Labonte, 1998) is seen as important.

Arena-centred programmes

We can see from the earlier part of this chapter that disease- and risk factor-centred health promotion programmes involve numerous individuals or teams seeking to gain access to the mass media and a range of settings, and running the risk of wasteful duplication of effort, mixed messages and competition between programmes. In the illustrative exploration of the possible perspective of the school headteacher as a gatekeeper, other problems and concerns were highlighted. The various described pitfalls of topic-centred programmes can be avoided by centring programmes on 'arenas' for health promotion (Tannahill, 1994; Downie *et al.*, 1996a). The word 'arenas' was introduced in health promotion in the 1990s to cover the notion of integrating efforts on health and behavioural topics through the mass media; in formal settings and sectors such as schools, the workplace and health services; and in other formal and informal community settings, with community development having an important part to play. A strategically co-ordinated mass media programme provides a backdrop for, and is complemented by, a set of strategic setting-based programmes.

Arena-centred programmes should be health-orientated. They allow for a broad view of health and of health factors. The importance of life circumstances can be highlighted and acted upon, and action on particular health and behavioural topics can take into account social, economic and cultural influences. Also, by providing everyday influences where people live, learn, work, spend leisure time or seek help, the programmes themselves contribute directly to life circumstances (Tannahill, 1998).

Multi-disciplinary and intersectoral collaboration is facilitated. Gatekeepers, e.g. to schools, primary care, workplaces and informal community settings, can be involved in developing the programmes from the earliest of stages, instead of having a hotch-potch of overlapping and possibly conflicting and competing initiatives dropping on them 'from above'. The right things can be done by the right people, in the right place, and at the right times. And the capacity of the settings to promote health in the round can be developed in a coherent and efficient way.

Crucially, the strategic arena-centred approach lends itself to building systematically and achieving sustainability. In it most fully developed form, it goes beyond notions of 'dropping in' health promotion to arenas topic-by-topic or project-by-project, or 'bolting on' a 'block' of health promotion to the everyday life of arenas. Rather, health promotion is 'built into' the arenas. Seen in this light, health promotion is development for health, and as such it can be conceptually – and practically – integrated with organizational development (e.g. in workplaces and the NHS) and community development. That said, it is important to be sensitive to 'where people are at' in a given setting in any particular location, so that gatekeepers and others are not put off or overwhelmed by unrealistic expectations to adopt the 'full-blown' setting model. A relatively modest initiative, e.g. on a topic seen as being of especially high priority in the place concerned, can be of value both in their own right and as an entry point and confidence-builder for subsequent broadening out and development.

An important challenge, if arena-centred health promotion programmes are adopted, is to co-ordinate and integrate topic-centred efforts *across* the arenas. It is helpful in this regard to have strategies, informed by available evidence and enlightened by robust theoretical frameworks, that take an overview of the policies, services and health education interventions needed in relation to particular health and risk factor topics. This is not to suggest that, in delivery terms, there should be both topic-centred and arena-centred programmes. Rather, the issue at stake is to ensure that arena-centred programmes are adequately informed by topic-centred strategies, and that the programmes taken as a whole cover the action points in these strategies comprehensively enough, but that the 'top-down' topic-centred dynamic is balanced by 'bottom-up' influences representing the perspectives of community members. The arenas can serve as vehicles for topic-specific pilot or demonstration projects, and for previously unplanned topic-focused work when urgent new priorities, needs or opportunities arise (e.g. the emergence of HIV/AIDS or chlamydia, new patterns of drug misuse or drug-related illness, or the availability of new screening services, vaccines or smoking cessation aids).

In addition to topic-centred strategies, it is helpful to have 'overview' strategies relating to particular stages in the 'life-course', e.g. early childhood, adolescence/early adult life, and later life, 'meshing' with arena-centred programmes.

The bigger picture

The first and foremost implication of the health-orientated approach is that the span of what can reasonably be included under the term 'health promotion' is huge, encompassing efforts to promote quality of life and social cohesion (Wilkinson and Marmot, 1998) or 'social capital' (Gillies, 1998) in communities, and the enhancement and protection of health through overlapping policies and strategies on social justice (Scottish Executive, 1999a) and social inclusion (Wilkinson and Marmot, 1998, Scottish Executive, 2000a), economic and social development and regeneration, poverty, employment and unemployment, general (not just health) education, housing and the built environment, crime and so on. This is entirely consistent with the action areas of the World Health Organization's Ottawa Charter (World Health Organization, 1986) (build healthy public policy, create supportive environments, strengthen community action, develop personal skills, reorient health services), which are often enthusiastically cited as defining health promotion while in practice a narrower view is manifest. The policies, strategies and actions that have the most fundamental bearing on people's and society's health prospects will not – and indeed need not – necessarily come under the banner of health or health promotion (Tannahill, 1998). Vital tasks for those whose work *is* 'labelled' health promotion are to foster awareness among those who are responsible for such policies and strategies of the potential for their decisions to affect health favourably or adversely; to encourage and enable them to subject their decisions to health impact assessment (Scottish Executive, 1999b); and to help them feel motivated to make policy and strategy choices that will safeguard and promote the public's health.

Consistent with the reasoning behind the health-orientated approach to health promotion, community planning (or community strategies) has been identified as a crucial vehicle for health improvement (Scottish Executive, 2000b). Developed by councils in partnership with the health, enterprise, police/criminal justice, private and voluntary sectors, and with local communities, community plans provide a framework for integrating social, economic and health development at local levels.

In today's vocabulary, the term 'health improvement' rather than health promotion tends to be used in connection with the health enhancement dimension of community planning and a plethora of locality-centred initiatives that have come into being in recent times in Scotland and elsewhere in the UK. This, together with the emergence of the term 'health development' and the modern use of 'public health', has led to some semantic confusion, to a reinforcement of narrower interpretations of health promotion than that applied in this chapter, and indeed in some places to the demise or near-demise of the term 'health promotion'. Arguably, however, the new language can be helpful if it is used to draw a distinction between health improvement action and health promotion as a specialist *function* within the wider public health function. Stepping beyond the scope of this chapter, distinguishing between health improvement and health promotion also helps to separate the health promotion function from the clinical effectiveness dimension of health improvement and public health.

The remainder of this chapter is concerned with how the specialist health promotion function can be deployed to stimulate, encourage, inform, enable and support the wider health improvement effort, with particular reference to health improvement action in localities.

Locality-centred health improvement initiatives and the health promotion function

The health-orientated approach to health promotion adds weight to the logic of having health improvement efforts centred on the needs of specific localities. The latter makes particular sense when viewed in the light of the substantial health inequalities that exist between localities, as the highest priority can be given to action in those places that have the greatest health needs. A locality focus can lend itself to a holistic way of working, with partnership between agencies and community members directed at a common goal, with a strong 'bottom-up' dynamic, and with prospects for the integration of action *within* given localities. Given the explosion of locality-centred initiatives funded from various budgets within the UK – social inclusion partnerships, health action zones, healthy living centres and the rest – integration is by no means automatic or guaranteed. It requires cohesive approaches to planning and delivery, across all sectors, organizations and communities within each locality. Community planning has an important part to play in this. So too does the specialist health promotion function, as evidenced by the fact that there has been a growth in health promotion specialists with geographical remits.

Locality-centred efforts need a supporting infrastructure of appropriate policies and strategies (e.g. in the overlapping areas of economic and social development, education and learning, and health) on a larger scale – at international, national, regional and area levels. Integration across national and local government departments is essential, as is co-ordination between the various levels.

I suggest that locality-centred initiatives also need to be able to benefit from health promotion function inputs planned and devised on a larger scale if they are not to become too much of a 'cottage industry' of small producers distracted by the wasteful and unreliable business of reinventing wheels. An important point here is that, if health improvement action is to be comprehensive in any locality, it needs to reach the various settings within it. National and regional/area arena-centred programmes can be key enablers of this. They can provide coherent frameworks for developing health promoting settings rather than leaving all localities to develop their own; and they can provide a mass media backdrop as well as health education materials (preferably provided such that they can be adapted to, and/or 'branded' for, local purposes) for use in different community settings.

Programmes can usefully be centred on the arenas listed below. The arena-centred programmes deployed in a given locality can reflect the key settings within it:

- Mass media – providing a national/regional/area strategic backdrop, and promoting the use of local media;
- Preschool and school education – including application of the health-promoting school concept;
- Further and higher education – applying the health-promoting college/university concept;
- Workplace – involving the health-promoting workplace concept, and award schemes such as Scotland's Health at Work;
- Health care – implementing the health-promoting health service and hospitals concepts;
- Social care:
- Prisons; and
- Other community settings – providing specialist health promotion function support for efforts in the areas of strengthening communities, building social capital, developing community capacity, community-based projects and community development.

The health promotion function can also feed in the strategies referred to earlier that integrate action on health and risk factor topics and at different stages in the life-course. Earlier discussion in this chapter has drawn attention to the advantages of delivering such strategies by 'meshing' them into arena-centred programmes. Feeding these strategies into localities through arena-centred programmes is perfectly feasible if the set of arenas involved is as comprehensive as the list above.

Figure 7.4 represents the suggested relationship between locality health improvement strategy/action and larger-scale health promotion function inputs set within the wider policy and strategy environment. The larger-scale health promotion inputs provide for pooling and concentration of specialist expertise, and an appropriate degree of integration *across* localities.

Health promotion specialists with geographical (e.g. local authority area) remits have complementary roles to play to the larger-scale health promotion function inputs referred to above, working as members of, and supporting, multi-disciplinary and multi-agency local health improvement teams. As well as providing a direct health promotion function input at local levels, these specialists can act as bridges between localities and the above health promotion function inputs, and can help to ensure that the latter are deployed in ways that are sufficiently sensitive to localities' needs and circumstances. The health promotion function can thus be seen as comprising arena-centred, topic-centred, life-course-centred and geographically-centred inputs, and together these inputs can promote sustainability of health improvement efforts in localities, in the face of a 'projects culture'.

Last, but certainly not least, the programmes and initiatives, and wider policies and strategies, should place a high priority on reducing inequali-

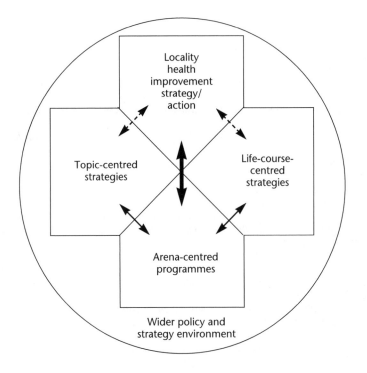

Figure 7.4 Integrating the health promotion function with wider health-improvement efforts

ties in health related to socio-economic/social environmental factors, ethnicity, disability, sex and age, and should identify and meet the special needs of particular population groups.

References

Antonovsky, A. (1987). *Unravelling the Mystery of Health*. San Francisco: Jossey Bass.

Downie, R. S., Tannahill C. and Tannahill, A. (1996a). *Health Promotion: Models and values*, 2nd edn. Oxford: Oxford University Press (ch. 4).

Downie, R. S., Tannahill C. and Tannahill, A. (1996b). *Health Promotion: Models and values*, 2nd edn. Oxford: Oxford University Press (ch. 3).

Downie, R. S., Tannahill C. and Tannahill, A. (1996c). *Health Promotion: Models and values*, 2nd edn. Oxford: Oxford University Press (ch. 2).

Gillies, P. (1998). Effectiveness of alliances and partnerships for health promotion, *Health Promotion International*, 13, 99–120.

Hanlon, P., Tannahill, C. and Tannahill, A. (1995). 'The planning compass': a tool for creative health promotion, *Public Health*, 109, 417–20.

Kelly, M. (1989). Some problems in health promotion research, *Health Promotion*, 4, 317–30.

Labonte, R. (1998). *A Community Development Approach to Health Promotion: A back-*

ground paper on practice tensions, strategic models and accountability requirements for health authority work on the broad determinants of health. Edinburgh: Health Education Board for Scotland and Research Unit in Health and Behavioural Change.

Scottish Executive (1999a). *A Scotland Where Everyone Matters – Our Visions for Social Justice.* Edinburgh: The Stationery Office.

Scottish Executive (1999b). *Review of the Public Health Function in Scotland.* Edinburgh: The Stationery Office.

Scottish Executive (2000a). *Social Inclusion – Opening the Door to a Better Scotland.* Edinburgh: The Stationery Office.

Scottish Executive (2000b). *Our National Health – a Plan for Action, a Plan for Change.* Edinburgh: The Stationery Office.

Scottish Office, The (1999). *Towards a Healthier Scotland – a White Paper on Health.* Edinburgh: The Stationery Office.

Tannahill, A. (1990). Health education and health promotion: planning for the 1990s, *Health Education Journal*, 49, 194–8.

Tannahill, A. (1992). Epidemiology and health promotion. In Bunton, R. and Macdonald, G. (eds), *Health Promotion: Disciplines and diversity.* London: Routledge, ch. 5.

Tannahill, A. (1994). *Health Education and Health Promotion: From priorities to programmes,* World Health Organization Regional Office for Europe Health Promotion Country Series, No. 1. Edinburgh:Health Education Board for Scotland and World Health Organization.

Tannahill A. (1998). The Scottish green paper: beyond a healthy mind in a healthy body, *Journal of Public Health Medicine*, 20, 249–52.

Tannahill, A. (2000). Integrating mental health promotion and general health promotion strategies, *International Journal of Mental Health Promotion*, 2, 19–26.

Wilkinson, R. and Marmot, M. (eds) (1998). *Social Determinants of Health: The solid facts.* Copenhagen: World Health Organization Regional Office for Europe.

World Health Organization (1986). *Ottawa Charter for Health Promotion.* Geneva: World Health Organization.

8 The limits of lifestyle: re-assessing 'fatalism' in the popular culture of illness prevention*

Charlie Davison, Stephen Frankel and George Davey Smith

Introduction: fatalism and control in contemporary health promotion

One of the most important changes in twentieth-century medical culture in industrial societies has been the shift in emphasis from acute and infectious diseases to chronic and multi-factorial disorders as the major causes of morbidity and mortality. This transition has been paralleled by the development of a stronger emphasis on the prediction and prevention of disease in both policy and practice circles.[1] This tendency has led professional and lay discourse increasingly to adopt the notion of risk as a central, guiding concept in constructing responses to disease. The aspect of this cultural process which forms the background of the present discussion is the heightened profile of disease prophylaxis as an organising motive in the everyday activities of the healthy population.

The gradual shift towards prevention in the general medical culture has meant that the circumstances and attributes of those who suffer and die from chronic disease have taken on a particular importance in the construction of risk. The central role of scientific epidemiology in identifying associations between disease and the various individual conditions of sufferers has been matched by the attempt to prevent people developing these dangerous or risky attributes. Perhaps the most striking feature of this process has been the development of a strong, officially-sponsored ideological perspective which emphasizes the personal responsibility of the individual citizen in the maintenance of their own health and the avoidance of chronic disease.[2]

Informing the public of the risks associated with certain behaviour, and exhorting the adoption of a 'good' diet, regular exercise and abstention from society's two main legally sanctioned non-medical drugs has become an important part of both General Practice and the newer state sectors of Health Education and Health Promotion. The overall responsibility of the individual in these areas has crystallized into the somewhat amorphous idea of the importance of following a 'healthy lifestyle'.

* From *Social Science and Medicine*. 34(6) (1992), 675–85. Oxford: Pergamon Press. © Pergamon Press plc 1992.

The term 'lifestyle' has recently come to be used widely in many contexts, and a brief clarification of the use of the term here is in order. Aside from its direct association with health-related behaviour, the word (or words) have been used to denote general conditions of living, as a product brand name, and to describe a type of television programming. Here we concentrate on the idea of 'lifestyle' issues as the aspects of health-related behaviour and conditions which entail an element of personal action at the individual level. The main fields covered by the rubric are diet, leisure activities (especially those involving exercise), intake of drugs, and personal body maintenance (hygiene, sleep, etc.). Our aim in this usage is to limit the term to behaviour and conditions which official and commercial health promotion has associated strongly with the possibility of individual choice and the triumph of self-control over self indulgence.[3]

One of the major problems facing the professions and institutions involved at the behavioural end of contemporary preventive medicine is the apparent failure of many individuals to comply fully with healthy lifestyle advice. In the developing discourse of health education, this situation has been attributed to two major causes. In the first place, it was suggested that there was a lack of accurate knowledge among the general public concerning the potential harm associated with certain aspects of everyday behaviour.[4] An image was canvassed that saw people with heart disease as 'victims of their own ignorance'.[5] This perspective assumed that, if knowledge were increased (or ignorance dispelled), rational people would decide to change their daily habits. In recent years, this approach has been labelled as outmoded by those with an academic or quasi-academic interest in lifestyle modification. Data gathered during ethnographic fieldwork, however, showed that many of those involved in the concrete business of giving health advice to the general public still regard ignorance as an important barrier to the adoption of healthy behaviour.

A second, slightly more sophisticated, line of analysis suggests that a major cause of non-compliance is the existence of an attitude which sees health as being largely determined by forces outside the control of the individual, and thus denies the possible relevance of personal behavioural change. As previous research and critique in this field has pointed out, the 'locus of control' trend in psychology has operated within an ideological perspective which takes as axiomatic that belief in individual control is 'correct', while belief in other agencies requires some kind of rectification (usually education). This type of analysis has led to the production of the idea that health promotion is involved in a battle for the hearts and minds of the population, a struggle between a modern belief in lifestyle and an atavistic culture of "fatalism".[6]

Two recent definitions of fatalism from quite different ends of the academic literature on lifestyle and health illustrate the currency of the concept:

> some members of the public have a fatalistic attitude to health and therefore do not believe that they have much control over their health status.[7]

> [their] attitudes were fatalistic: health was, as a general principle, the consequence of behaviour, but this did not apply to them; health was extremely important, but they themselves had no control over it.[8]

The first definition is taken from a report of survey data analysed in the somewhat partial fashion all too common in health promotion research. Having already decided on the moral status of smokers (reprehensible), the researchers proceed to 'prove' that which they plainly believed already. Their 'finding' is that people who smoke tobacco are also 'fatalistic' – a term they use against the backdrop of a barely-concealed contempt for a group of their informants they see as ignorant and/or culturally defective. We cite this paper as an extreme, though not unusual, example of the uncritical acceptance of the 'locus of control/fatalism' complex which pervades much British research and practice in the field of illness prevention.

The second definition, while coming from a study informed by a more proper scientific detachment, also includes the key notion that lies at the heart of the fatalism label – the idea that the individual feels that he/she cannot necessarily exercise control over his/her health . . .

Lifestyle and coronary heart disease

Our examination of the construction of personal control in the realm of CHD (coronary heart disease) prevention is based on extensive survey and ethnographic research in three communities in South Wales: Plasnewydd (a socially mixed ward of the City of Cardiff), Porth (an industrial and service town in the Rhondda Borough) and Llangammarch Wells (a village and rural district in the Borough of Brecknock). In total, extended semi-structured interviews were carried out with a randomly selected set of 180 adults of both sexes and a full range of socio-economic circumstances. The interviews covered general ideas of what 'health' might be, explanations of the causes of good and poor health, issues of control, prevention, illness avoidance, fault and blame, and a number of more specific topics concerning the heart and CHD . . .

The conceptual place of lifestyle

Aspects of life which, in the perception of our informants, have an effect on individual health status but cannot be individually controlled in any obvious way can be grouped, for the purposes of analysis, into three inter-locking fields:

- Fields involving the self-evident personal differences between individuals (e.g. heredity, upbringing, inherent traits).
- Fields involving the social environment (e.g. relative wealth and access to resources, risks and dangers associated with occupation, loneliness).
- Fields involving the physical environment (e.g. climate, natural dangers, environmental contamination).

To these three, a fourth conceptual area must be added. The fourth field exists, however, not as a substantive or concrete area in its own right, rather as a process or mechanism governing the first three. This fourth field concerns the operation of luck, chance, randomness and personal destiny. As the aspect of popular culture which gave its name to 'fatalism' itself, this fourth area is of obvious importance. But over and above this, our analysis indicates that, as a theoretical area involved with the explanation of the distribution of misfortune in an overall system based essentially on probability, these beliefs play a crucial role in the construction of culturally appropriate behaviour. We shall return to this area after examining the implications of the basic model.

While we have, thus far, followed the roughly orthodox path of placing an analytical or categorical division between lifestyle and these three sets of 'non-control' forces, the conceptual landscape we have observed during field research contains no such hard and fast barrier. Each of the three categories of areas outside personal control has a more complex relationship with individual health status and individual participation in healthy lifestyles than the fatalism/lifestyle dichotomy implies. In each case there is, on the one hand, a direct influence on health status, and on the other, an indirect influence, mediated through an effect on the possibility or ease of voluntary participation in healthy lifestyles.

The model can best be illustrated with an example. In the popular explanatory culture of CHD, being a 'worrier by nature' (a character trait widely recognized by our informants in Wales as being inherited via both genetic and social routes) can have various direct effects on the health of the individual. These are caused by the clenching of internal organs and muscles ('always being tensed up'), the disruption of normal blood chemistry ('too much adrenalin') and the consequent disruption of regular heart beat. Over and above these mechanisms, there exists the possibility of indirect health damage brought about through an effect of the condition on lifestyle. In the case of the 'worrier by nature' this occurs through combating worry with tobacco and alcohol and allowing worry to dictate inappropriate eating habits.

Lifestyle, then, as is the case with other elements of this model, did not really exist as an independent category for our informants. Rather it was only articulated in terms of its intimate but varied relationship with the other elements. As an issue concerning voluntarism and the possibility of individual choice and freedom, the relationship between health and lifestyle is of evident political importance. This political issue has resided at the centre of contemporary British debates concerning the social distribution of mortality and morbidity since the publication of the Black Report.[9]

If, as our simple model suggests, the entire lifestyle and health relationship is embedded in the wider operation of forces recognized as being outside individual control, there are strong implications for the construction of personal attitudes. Data from our three Welsh samples suggest that the key process involved is the assessment of the relevance of personal lifestyle change in the context of the unique position of the individual vis-à-vis the three substantial 'non-control' fields. Because diet, exercise, and drug consumption cannot be seen as being independent of the social and economic structures within which behaviour (and culture) are sited, they must also be involved with the realities of relative inequality in a stratified society . . .

General principles and individual events

Whether examined from the perspective of medical science or popular knowledge, prevention and control imply knowledge about cause. Attempts to exercise control over the timing and nature of events presuppose the existence of an explanation or set of explanations which account for the occurrence and distribution of the events themselves.[10] It has long been a commonplace observation in the discipline of social anthropology that cultural systems of explanation or accountability need to address two distinct issues. In the first place the general kind of misfortune requires explanation: how and why does it happen? In the second place, the site and time of particular misfortune require explanation: how and why did it happen to this person at this time?[11]

The healthy lifestyles movement within preventive medicine represents an attempt to reduce the second area of explanatory culture to a subset of the first. Indeed, as Gifford points out, the central concept of prevention (that of medical 'risk') is actually produced by the uncritical transposition of epidemiological associations derived from whole populations to the field of an individual life.[12]

The particular refinement of the healthy lifestyles movement as applied to heart disease has been to go to great lengths to place one set of general epidemiological principles (those involving behaviour open to personal control) at the centre of explanatory culture. Because the various 'non-control' mechanisms described here have been largely ignored in the publicity of the prevention movement, they have acquired an unofficial and even 'dissident' image.

A concomitant of this process is that these non-control areas have become somewhat marginalized in the explanatory culture associated with heart trouble. This marginalization is exhibited by the fact that they often enter public discussion as subsidiary agents in the onset of illness and death only after the assessment of the more scientifically mainstream and 'fashionable' lifestyle areas. Non-control areas in general, and the luck/fate field in particular, were observed to take centre stage most strikingly when illness and death struck individuals who 'should not have been victims' if the principles of lifestyle were always reliable . . .

An integral part of the modern prevention movement has been the public lowering of the threshold of risks concerning personal lifestyle. Although this process is ostensibly involved in extending the bounds of explicability and control, it has the paradoxical effect of highlighting anomalies. This has happened because aspects of life hitherto considered normal and safe (chip eating. lounging about, etc.) have become labelled as pathogenic. Because so many other factors are involved in illness causation and distribution, a result of this ideological development is that the number of people who survive dangerous lifestyles and do not get ill grows. Simultaneously, the cases of individuals who do all the 'correct' healthy things and yet still succumb to heart trouble become very well known.[13]

Because the everyday practice of lay epidemiology detects both anomalous deaths and unwarranted survivals, the tension or conflict between general principles and individual events is constantly made plain to members of society and has to be dealt with. An extremely common explanation of an anomaly thus becomes 'it was just one of those things', the full but unspoken version of which is 'it was just one of those things which violates general principles'.

Implications for health education and health promotion

Our investigation of the popular culture of illness avoidance and the protection of good health in three South Wales communities concentrated on the idea of control. By the very nature of the current social and political movements taking place in the public health field in all of Britain, we were led to focus on the interaction between popular culture and an intense official interest in promoting voluntary behavioural change.

In overall terms, we found that, by concentrating so heavily on the fields of diet, drug use and exercise, official health education messages and health promotion initiatives in the localities studied were quite seriously out of step with popular culture in those areas. We contend that this position is not unique to South Wales and that the same point could be made of the United Kingdom in general and quite possibly of other parts of the world. Our tentative recommendations for changes in health promotion practice are thus couched in relatively general terms.

If a greater cultural sensitivity could be achieved in health promotion practice, it is our view that some important areas of conflict could be eased. There are three specific areas in which health promotion could feasibly move towards a more culturally appropriate position.

First, the content of health education messages could be re-assessed. The effect of personal behaviour on health is apparently well understood by the vast majority of the population. While this does not necessarily imply that all individuals actually behave in concert with this knowledge, neither does it automatically indicate that repeated applications of the same propaganda would be beneficial. Indeed, a reassessment of the scientific epidemiology concerning lifestyle and the various non-control areas discussed in this chapter may be revealing. In our observation, popular belief and knowledge concerning the relationship of health to heredity, social conditions and the environment may be more in step with scientific epidemiology than the lifestyle-centred orientation of the health promotion world.

A second step towards a more culturally appropriate health promotion stance concerns the conceptual division between the controllable and the uncontrollable. At present, the official line is sharply drawn: lifestyle is controllable, everything else is not. Public concern with environmental matters, however, indicate that a willingness to attempt to control some aspects of these areas does exist within society at large. It is revealing, however, that local and national movements aimed at environmental improvements operate outside the health promotion sphere, and little institutional interest on the part of health promotion in bridging this gulf is in evidence. An easing of the stark official division between spheres open or closed to human control and a greater institutional interest in collective as well as individual action could be productive.

Finally, it is clear from our investigations that the existence of a random distribution of illness and death formed a central part of popular understanding in South Wales. Furthermore it is constantly and effectively re-affirmed by the workings of lay epidemiology. We believe that this finding from one small area of Europe will strike chords in many other places.

If a more effective collaboration between health promotion and the general public is to be achieved, a method of dealing with this area needs to be developed. In the branch of bio-medical culture concerned with individual diagnosis and cure, practitioners are satisfied to accept a certain level of mystery and use the label 'idiopathy'. The branch which focusses on prevention, however, is much more threatened by lacunae in the understanding either of causation or of distribution. This may have led to a counter-productive discourse in which exaggerated claims for predictability, regularity and certainty are made.

The fact remains, however, that, within the general statistical tendencies that can be observed within populations, there lies a more chaotic distribution of illness and death. Some fat smokers really do live till advanced old age, and some svelte joggers really do 'fall down dead'.

Falling back on the albeit honest defence that lifestyle advice is based on probability rather than certainty is plainly an inadequate response when the complexities of popular culture are properly taken into consideration. In this field more than any other, the fact that lay epidemiology is so firmly embedded in popular health culture poses a serious problem for health promotion. If the coronary prevention movement desires a good working relationship with society at large, both the true position of lifestyle and the real-life events addressed by fatalism need to be re-evaluated.

Notes

1. The conceptual conformity of British government policy spanning administrations run by both major political parties is illustrated in: Secretary of State for Health, *The Health of the Nation: A consultative document for health in England*, London: HMSO (1991), and in Department of Health and Social Security, *Prevention and Health: Everybody's Business*, London: HMSO (1976).
2. Crawford, R., You are dangerous to your health: the ideology and politics of victim blaming, *International Journal of Health Services*, 7(4), 663–80 (1977). Radical Statistics Health Group Health Education, Blaming the victim? In *Facing the Figures – What is really happening to the National Health Service?* London: Radical Statistics (1987).
3. Areas of life which have sometimes been described as 'involuntary lifestyle', which include behaviour and conditions routed in a collective field and therefore not directly open to change at the individual level. such as being exposed to industrial pollution, appear in our analysis as 'environmental' factors.
4. *Health Education News*, Heart disease risks ignored, London: HEC (September 1981).
5. A. Dillon, Director of the Coronary Prevention Group, speaking on BBC Radio 4 (October 1986).
6. Pill, R. and Stott, N. C. H., Development of a measure of potential behaviour: a Salience of Lifestyle Index, *Social Science Medicine*, 24(2), 125–34 (1987). Farrant W. and Russell J., The politics of health education, *Bedford Way Papers*, 28, University of London Institute of Education, 1986. Naidoo, J., Limits to individualism. In *The Politics of Health Education – Raising the issues* (edited by Watt, A. and Rodmell, S.). London: Routledge & Kegan Paul (1986).

7. Lewis, P. A., Charny, M., Lamber, D. and Coombes, J. A fatalistic attitude to health among smokers in Cardiff. *Health Education Research* 4(3), 361–5 (1989).
8. Blaxter, M., *Health and Lifestyles*. London: Tavistock/Routledge (1990).
9. Townsend, P. and Davidson, N., *Inequalities in Health: The Black Report*. Harmondsworth: Penguin (1982). Davey Smith, G., Bartley, M. and Blane, D. The Black Report on socio-economic inequalities in health 10 years on, *British Medical Journal* 301, 373–7 (1990).
10. In Social Anthropology this aspect of cultural life has generally been discussed in terms of 'accounting for misfortune'; in Social Psychology as 'attribution theory'.
11. Evans Pritchard, E., *Witchcraft, Oracles and Magic among the Azande of Anglo-Egyptian Sudan*. Oxford: Clarendon Press (1937).
12. Gifford, S. M. The meaning of lumps: a case study of the ambiguities of risk. In *Anthropology and Epidemiology* (edited by Janes, C. R. *et al.*), 213–46. The Hague: Reidel (1986).
13. Davison, C., Davey Smith, G. and Frankel, S. Lay, Epidemiology and the prevention paradox – the implications of coronary candidacy for health promotion, *Sociology of Health and Illness,* 13(1) (1991).

9 An *empowerment model* of health promotion*

Keith Tones and Sylvia Tilford

An empowerment model of health promotion

. . . An educational model and a preventive model of health promotion have been found lacking both ideologically and practically. A model is now proposed that seeks to remedy the deficiencies of these two alternative models. As the name suggests, particular emphasis is placed on the primacy of empowerment – and the synergism between education and policy. The model is shown in Figure 9.1.

Two major categories of 'input' are shown in Figure 9.1 as promoting health; the first of these is concerned with creating health public policy, the second with influencing individual choices. The policy dimension figures prominently and, is viewed as one of the major devices for managing the social, economic and material circumstances that have such an important influence on health. In short, there is a major 'upstream' focus in this particular model of health promotion.

As with the educational model and preventive model, the empowerment approach depicted in Figure 9.1 is also concerned to acknowledge the importance of influencing individual choices. After all, the most common health promotion work involves some kind of face-to-face encounter with individuals or small groups of individuals. However, whereas the preventive model seeks to persuade and coerce, and the educational model merely aims to provide information, the model favoured here seeks to empower choice by building individual capacity – as defined in an earlier reference to self-empowerment (Tones and Tilford, 2001). Additionally, of course, the measures defined in the model are designed to remove the broader environmental barriers militating against genuine freedom to choose.

Furthermore, whereas the opponents of the victim-blaming inherent in the narrow educational and preventive approaches to health promotion have emphasized the importance of achieving radical political action (principally through the processes of lobbying and advocacy) the present model argues forcefully for the inclusion of a 'radical-political' educational process having as its *raison d'être* a challenge to social rather

* From Tones, K. and Tilford, S. (2001) *Health Promotion: effectiveness, efficiency and equity*, 3rd edn, Cheltenham, Nelson Thornes Ltd, pp. 49–55.

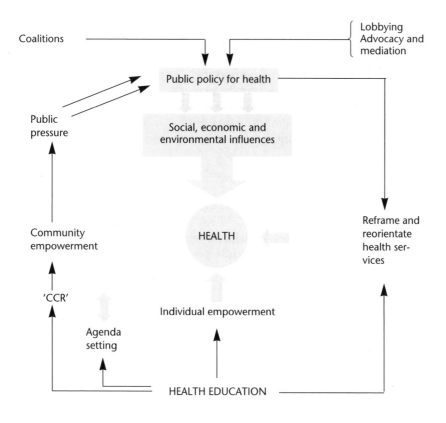

Figure 9.1   An empowerment model

than individual pathogens and the creation of public policy designed to counter these.

In short, the proposed characteristics for effective and ethical health education include the following principles:

- It makes a direct contribution to individual health by influencing health- and illness-related behaviour. It does not, however, operate in a discredited 'top-down' fashion; it does not seek to persuade, coerce and cajole, but rather contributes to self-empowerment. If successful, it enhances individuals' control over their lives and their health.
- It follows the preventive model's precedent in its concern to influence health services. Its function is, however, considerably different: it does not aim to promote the 'development and proper use of services' by, for example, persuading clients to use services in a medically approved fashion, but aims to reorientate those services by reducing barriers to access and making the services more 'user friendly'. More importantly, it contributes to 'reframing' perceptions of what health services should

be: for instance, it demonstrates how such diverse organizations as housing, transport and economic development corporations can make a significant contribution to health – or illness.

• Finally and, arguably most important, it seeks to mobilize community opinion and concentrate public pressure on government and other powerful agencies so that they are impelled to create policies designed to address the broad determinants of health. It does this by a process of 'critical consciousness raising' (CCR) and community empowerment . . .

Education for radical action: critical consciousness raising

The so-called 'new' public health has been associated with radical challenge. However. it is worth reminding ourselves of the role health education played in the 'old' public health, and there are indeed many interesting parallels between the first public health movement and the doctrine of health promotion. For instance, the sanitary reforms of the 19th century were associated with a general reforming zeal directed at the overall squalor, poverty and poor working conditions of the populace. Moreover, the reformers met with vigorous opposition and, as is the case at the time of writing, their demand for state intervention was seen as ideologically unsound . . .

Health education was not recognized as such, but health 'propagandism' and pamphleteering were in evidence – and greatly resented! Sutherland (1979) quotes a petulant article from *The Times* newspaper which declared that the people would 'prefer to take the chance of cholera and the rest than to be bullied into health' (p. 7). Incidentally, Sutherland also described a rather nice example of early-nineteenth-century victim-blaming when he referred to the Manchester and Salford Sanitary Association's employment of working-class women as indigenous health education aides to teach the 'laws of health' to the poor! We might also note the suggestion that one of the most significant influences on public health reforms was the perception by the wealthy that they themselves were at risk from the unrest and diseases of the underclass – a matter of some significance for contemporary predictions that the 'overclass' might well have to take refuge in fortified ghettos to keep the militant underclass at bay. Hopefully, appropriate consciousness raising will convince members of the 'overclass' to shrug off the 'culture of contentment' and recognize that the most comfortable solution all round is to tackle disadvantage and relative poverty. At all events, the pamphleteering of the nineteenth century would appear to have points in common with the radical health education process of modern times, and the most appropriate formulation for this is Freire's invention of 'critical consciousness raising'. The term critical consciousness raising is derived from the Brazilian-Portuguese term *conscientização* – translated as 'the development of the awakening of critical awareness' (Freire, 1974, p. 19).

Freire contrasts critical consciousness with 'magical consciousness', which apprehends facts and attributes them fatalistically to some superior power (the relationship with external locus of control will no doubt be self-evident). 'Naïve consciousness', on the other hand, involves a more realistic perception of causality but accepts it uncritically. In other words, it represents the 'false consciousness' of those who have accepted the rightful reality of a dominant ideology. The purpose of CCR is to help people break free of false consciousness and it does so by using the following four-step process.

- Fostering reflection on aspects of personal reality;.
- Encouraging a search for, and collective identification of, the root causes of that reality;
- Examination of implications;.and
- Development of a plan of action to alter reality.

This integral process of planning and action rooted in critical reflection was referred to as 'praxis' by Freire. The techniques and methods employed centred on group work ('culture circles') and used a 'dialectical' problem-solving approach to discussion. A more comprehensive discussion of Freire's radical strategy is beyond the scope of this chapter. However, Minkler and Cox (1980) provide a succinct analysis of the approach, with case studies of work in Honduras and San Francisco. Macdonald and Warren (1991) also offer a useful application of Freirean theory to primary health care.

The *quality* of the knowledge resulting from CCR is distinctly different from that of other educational approaches. Those who have participated in the group dialogue will have not only a deeper understanding of their circumstances (as opposed to their personal risk) but also some important beliefs about self, i.e. their capacity to influence their circumstances. Again, the implications of praxis are not at first glance dissimilar to the action planning built into the process of attitude change central to a preventive model. However, the commitment is to social rather than personal change and incorporates a powerful affective element: if CCR is effective, people will not only be aware of social issues, understand them and believe that it is possible to change their circumstances, they will also feel indignant and want to translate understanding into action.

The implication of what has been said so far about the Freirean approach might lead to the conclusion that, in challenging the dominant ideology and presenting an alternative meaning system, the radical model is in some way educating rather than persuading; it is providing a 'true' picture of reality. This is not necessarily the case and de Kadt (1982) strikes a cautionary note:

In post-revolutionary situations, in countries with Marxist governments, conscientization may be bound up with wider political activities and mobilization behind the party line . . . Freire insists that
people must be allowed to discover things for themselves, that
meanings must not be imposed for them on their world. Yet, of
course, the discussion leader cannot but make available certain
facts, give certain leads, encourage certain interpretations, which
effectively turn the perception of the 'learners' in certain directions.
This is above all true for the party militant, mobilizing the people
for a particular social transformation. One type of consciousness is
thereby replaced by another . . . the new consciousness will also be a
partial interpretation of reality. It may show little realism about the
obstacles that stand in the way of changing present structures, or
may provide little more than ringing generalizations and abstrac-
tions about the social arrangements to replace those at present stigmatized. (p. 743) . . .

There is a further limitation to Freire's philosophy and methods: an
empowered community – as depicted in Figure 9.1 – has not only been
elevated to a state of critical consciousness, it also has a sense of community and a high level of social capital together with a range of skills and
competences that can be used to convert consciousness into action.
Hopefully it will also have powerful allies!

   Again, although on occasions Freire would aim to provide some actual
skills to those whose consciousness had been raised (after all, his original
programme was concerned with adult literacy), there is no guarantee
that the learners will have been equipped to change social circumstances. Apart from any possible misrepresentations of reality created by
the teacher-activist, merely to raise consciousness in a general oppressive
environment is considerably more unethical than victim-blaming. In
short, CCR can be dangerous! A cartoon – ascribed to Morley –– illustrates the tightrope that political activists have to tread if they are to be
effective and remain alive. The health worker is depicted as an ostrich
confronting an authoritarian regime. (S)he is exhorted not to stick her
head over the parapet – or it might be blown off – but, on the other
hand, not to stick her head in the sand!

Agenda setting

Examination of Figure 9.1 will reveal an educational process paralleling
the 'mainstream' radical CCR/community empowerment function. It has
been labelled 'agenda setting', and it is superficially similar to CCR in its
concern to raise health issues for public consumption and in its potential effect on health policy. We can identify two main operations. The

first of these might merely consist of raising issues in order to facilitate decision making about policy matters. This function might be illustrated by the use of a television documentary to inform the public about any currently controversial issue. More typical, though, is the political use of agenda setting. In this latter mode, government may test the temperature of public opinion with a view to ascertaining the acceptability of new legislation. As we observed earlier, public policy measures are highly likely to result in some restriction of people's liberty or involve them in financial cost; psychological reactance (or, less technically, bloody-mindedness!) is a predictable outcome.

The government is, of course, reluctant to court electoral unpopularity and can therefore use agenda-setting tactics via mass media as a kind of 'softening up' process – an elaborated and extended version of policy 'leaks' to journalists. Agenda setting may well happen incidentally. For instance, a series of mass media campaigns in Britain set the scene for the introduction of legislation making the wearing of seat belts in cars compulsory. While the campaigns achieved only moderate success in persuading individual drivers and front seat passengers to voluntarily use seat belts, raising public consciousness about the problem of traffic accidents and the benefits of seat belts doubtless laid the foundations for legislation – despite the fact that it restricted individual liberty – without generating any serious electoral costs for the government of the day.

It could, of course, be argued that agenda setting and CCR are not qualitatively different processes. It could indeed be postulated that policy measures could be located on a spectrum of political acceptability. On the assumption that the government can afford to be only one small step ahead of public opinion, this spectrum would reflect the public's latitude of acceptance. For example, government might be favourably disposed to measures designed to alleviate inequalities in health, but consider that the increased cost in taxation would be met with furious opposition by taxpayers and therefore deemed to be electoral suicide. In short, the 'culture of contentment', – Galbraith's (1992) important notion, might prove too strong.

It is, in fact, possible to conceive of such a spectrum of acceptability. However, it is more useful to consider the agenda setting and CCR functions as being qualitatively rather than quantitatively distinct. As we have noted, CCR involves a *radical* challenge to dominant ideology, and should be reserved for situations where such a challenge can be demonstrated. Consider for instance the above-mentioned challenge to health inequalities. A left-wing government might be ideologically committed to remedying inequalities but be persuaded that the cost of the radical measures would be electorally unacceptable. Realpolitik might therefore dictate inaction plus some degree of agenda setting designed to produce a climate of public opinion conducive to some limited policy implementation. On the other hand, a right-wing government might be totally opposed ideologically to state intervention, irrespective of cost. Firm commitment to enterprise, the pursuit of profit and rampant individualism would be incompatible with radical healthy public policy. In this latter scenario more dramatic public pressure would be needed – perhaps in extreme cases leading to refusal to re-elect a recalcitrant government.

Consider the following, less politically challenging but none the less problematic, case of fluoridation of public water supplies. It is now firmly established that the fluoridation of public water supplies is the most effective public health strategy for reducing the incidence of dental caries – particularly in lower social groups. Clearly, any such policy constrains individuals' freedom to drink non-fluoridated water. The scene is therefore set for an ideological confrontation between, on the one hand, the values of dental and public health practitioners and, on the other, proponents of voluntaristic choice – possibly represented by members of the Pure Water League or a similar pressure group. Despite some qualms about accusations of fostering the 'nanny state', the ideological concerns of right-wing politicians – together with the conviction that money might be saved for the health service – may well be congruent with the wishes of the medical lobby. However, in the last analysis, perceptions of electoral gain may be the sole determinant of action. For instance, if agenda setting were to result in opinion surveys and focus groups revealing an increased level of acceptability for fluoridation, legislation would be enacted without further delay . . .

References

De Kadt. E. (1982). Ideology, social policy, health and health services: a field of complex interactions, *Social Science and Medicine*, 16, 741–52.

Freire, P. (1974). *Education and the Practice of Freedom*. London: Writers and Readers Publishing Cooperative (originally published in Portuguese, 1967).

Galbraith, J. K. (1997). *The Culture of Contentment*. Harmondsworth: Penguin.

Macdonald, J. J. and Warren, W. H. (1991). Primary health care as an educational process: a model and a Freirean perspective, *International Quarterly of Community Health Education*, 12(1), 35–50.

Minkler, M. and Cox, K. (1980). Creating critical consciousness in health: applications of Freire's philosophy and methods to the health care setting, *International Journal of Health Services*, 10(2), 311–22.

Sutherland, I. (1979). *Health Education: Perspectives and choices*. London: George Allen & Unwin.

Tones, B. K. and Tilford, S. (2001). *Health Promotion: Effectiveness, efficiency and equity*. Cheltenham: Nelson Thornes.

10 Counselling people living with HIV/AIDS*

Pete Connor

'Hope' is the thing with feathers
That perches in the soul
And sings the tune without the words
And never stops – at all . . .

Emily Dickinson (c. 1861)

Introduction

I felt very pleased to be asked to write this chapter on counselling people living with HIV (human immunodeficiency virus) as for at least 15 years, the work has been of great importance to me, both personally and professionally. Counselling in the HIV field has provided me with a career, friendships, personal development and a great sense of satisfaction. HIV infection as a condition, however, has also led to the deaths of my partner, David, in 1990 and, later, of two of my closest friends, Claire and Katie, as well as many other people for whom I felt affection. The work will always have special meaning to me.

AIDS (Acquired Immune Deficiency Syndrome) was first identified as a condition in 1981 and refers to the collection of infections, tumours and other illnesses that can develop when HIV damages the immune system of an infected person. Significant improvements in the medical treatments for HIV/AIDS have occurred since the early 1980s, and I aim to explore how the hope that these advances have brought has affected the counselling needs of people living with the virus. Also, through case examples and quotes, I aim to give a sense of the enormous diversity of people living with HIV in the UK, as well as to mention more general organisational issues connected to the HIV voluntary sector. Finally, I will explore my personal and professional reactions to the work.

I shall concentrate on the counselling needs of adults living with the virus and, to a lesser extent. the needs of partners and family members. since this is where most of my practice experience lies. Information specifically concerning children with HIV can be round in Sherr (1999), and Green and McCreaner (1996).

* From Etherington, K., (2002) (ed.) *Counsellors in Health settings*, Ch. 7, pp. 141–60, London, Jessica Kingsley Publishers Ltd.

I work from an integrative counselling perspective with person-centred theory informing my understanding of human beings. Excellent descriptions already exist of specific therapeutic approaches to HIV work, including analytic (Burgner, 1994), attachment-based (Purnell, 1996), existential (Milton, 1996) and systemic theory (Bor *et al.*, 1992). Here, however, I aim to explore issues faced by people with HIV in a way accessible to readers from any discipline or counselling approach . . .

Counselling issues

Initial diagnosis

> 'At that moment, when she said it was positive, I thought two things: that I was going to die and that my partner had been unfaithful.' (Woman living with HIV)

Despite some easing of the stigma associated with HIV and the increase in treatment options, initial HIV diagnosis, usually at a hospital genito-urinary department via an HIV antibody test, still frequently precipitates a period of emotional crisis. As a counsellor I attempt to offer a safe, supportive and empathic environment as the person begins to experience and explore waves or shock and numbness, despair and hopelessness, anger and depression.

In my experience, most newly diagnosed counselling clients have questions concerning medical facts, disease progression and the likelihood of death, as well as concerns regarding sharing their result with others. A double disclosure may be involved, with the person talking for the first time about their sexual orientation, sexual activity, or drug-use history. We often explore the impact of HIV on sexual relationships, body image and self-esteem, as well as working on any distress resulting from the resurfacing of past painful events, including abuse or bereavements. Clients frequently also need help to plan for the future, perhaps concerning drug treatments, employment, and having children, and to reflect on life's current meaning and purpose.

In initial sessions, we often spend time prioritizing concerns in order to prevent the sheer number and depth of the issues from overwhelming the client, and possibly me as counsellor. I am also watchful for factors that place clients at increased risk of severe anxiety, depression and suicidal thoughts as a result of their diagnosis. These factors include physical symptoms of HIV at the time of testing, low social support, and concurrent stress caused by bereavement or other losses of job, money and relationships. It is vital to explore the personal meaning of the diagnosis for each individual client.

Living successfully with HIV involves learning to live with uncertainty and the feelings of powerlessness that this can elicit. As a counsellor I can help clients to explore, release and understand their emotional reactions to a positive result, decide and prioritize goals, develop action plans, identify resources, and strengthen skills for coping with anxiety and depression. Just as important, however, are the times when I can simply be alongside a person as they struggle with their feelings of fear, hopelessness and isolation and eventually find the inner resources to manage those feelings. An obvious issue for me at these times is my own HIV status and personal experience of the virus, about which clients may have questions. I tend to answer these questions directly, while also using them to reflect on the meaning of having HIV for that individual.

Taking HAART

'I saw all those pills in front of me and I thought, "I'll never cope." But I have! It's still a real struggle sometimes, though.' (Man on combination therapies)

HAART (Highly Active Anti-Retroviral Therapy) treatments can reduce the amount of HIV (viral load) in the bloodstream to barely detectable levels and thereby inhibit its damaging action on the immune system. Many different drugs and drug combinations now exist, each having specific side-effects and regimes for taking. The decision to begin combination therapies is generally regarded as a lifetime commitment, since stopping or even missing doses may lead to the development of strains of HIV resistant to the drugs.

A significant portion of my counselling work now involves helping clients to make informed decisions concerning HAART, alongside advice from the prescribing consultants. We often explore strategies for coping with the recommended drug regimes, most of which require strict timing and/or dietary restrictions. We also usually make preparations for possible side-effects, which can range from unpleasant nausea, diarrhoea and tiredness to much less common but life-threatening side-effects such as pancreatitis.

Beginning combination therapies can be extremely stressful, especially until the individual develops confidence in the drugs. It can be a frightening time for the client and, I confess, sometimes for me as counsellor, as the person embarks on a new treatment, with the initial risks that can entail. A priority is to ensure that my own anxiety does not compromise the containment of client fears that counselling can provide.

Long-term adherence

'I skip a dose occasionally because I just can't face it. Day after day of pills and more side-effects and more pills and I just think, "What's the point, why bother?"' (Man on combination therapies)

Long-term, close adherence to the drug regime is vital for the effectiveness of treatments. However, some evidence, including Hecht *et al.* (1998), reflects my own experience of the difficulty that many clients have in maintaining drug regimes over the long term.

Having an accurate knowledge of their drugs and the importance of adherence certainly helps people to remain motivated, and I do see information-giving in this area as an important part of my counselling role. I can also offer clients support to cope with longer-term side-effects of treatments; such as peripheral neuropathy and lipodostrophy, which involves changes in fat distribution and body shape, and which can seriously affect self-image as well as physical well-being. The person's doctor may recommend diet changes or exercise, and again, counselling can support the person to adopt these measures. If side-effects prove to be intolerable, however, or if viral resistance to the drugs develops, a change of combination will be required and here again I can offer support to cope with possible new side-effects and adherence challenges.

Establishing confidence in and control of combination therapy is vital but difficult, especially since mood changes, including depression, anxiety and suicidal thoughts, have been reported by people taking HAART. Counselling can help people to manage these distressing psychological reactions, all of which will make adherence difficult. Clients also report that treatments act as continual reminders of their HIV status, and together we often need to revisit feelings concerning living with the virus as part of learning to manage HAART.

Julie, a 37-year-old Ugandan woman, was diagnosed four years ago. Her husband died of AIDS three years ago and she has been living with relatives in England for the past 18 months. She misses Uganda and the rest of her family but her health has not been good and she started combination therapies six weeks ago. Despite being well organized and having only minor side-effects, she has missed several doses.

In our initial sessions, Julie and I uncovered how profoundly depressed she has been feeling recently, and how she is torn between staying here and taking medication or returning to Uganda. She talked about her family back home, the hardships endured by those living with HIV, and the death of her husband. She felt guilty about friends who had no access to therapies and continued to become ill and die. Each time she took a tablet, Julie was reminded of her husband and friends.

Recognizing and relieving some of the grief and helplessness that Julie felt eased some of the emotional impact of the drugs and facilitated adherence, although this remained a daily struggle for her. Julie also decided to make more links with other African women with HIV via the Trust's women's group, and to use the Trust's treatment support project. This is a group of people already using HAART who offer information and advice for those just beginning or having difficulties with their treatments.

Working across gender, race and sexual orientation, as I did with Julie and with many other clients, demands that I confront my own sexism, racism and other preconceptions, prejudices and misinformation. I must also retain sensitivity concerning religious and cultural attitudes towards HIV, the family, relationships, health and medicine, death and bereavement, and towards the theory and practice of counselling and mental health generally . . .

Implications of a longer life

'I have been diagnosed for over ten years and, as time goes by, new issues arise. Knowing there is someone who will listen to my thoughts and feelings and not condemn me for them has helped to normalize my life. Counselling has helped me to come to terms with myself I am now living with my illness, not dying from it.' (Man living with HIV)

HAART has brought improvements in the health of many people, but adjusting to these can be difficult. Much of my work before HAART involved helping people to develop strategies for coping with a drastically reduced life expectancy. Decisions concerning relationships, finances, employment and housing tended to be made on the basis of having a much shorter time to live. Starting combination therapies, regaining good health and possibly having an extended life expectancy means revising these strategies and decisions.

It can be very moving for me now to explore with some clients the possibility of returning to work, further training or studies, when a few years ago ill health would have made this unrealistic. Those not in relationships may be considering looking for partners, and need support to do so, while clients already in partnerships may be reassessing their needs. An increasingly common counselling issue involves working with sexual problems, since improved health sometimes allows sexual desire to return, but drug side-effects or psychological problems may interfere with sexual functioning.

The long-term effectiveness of HAART drugs, however, is still unknown, and clients increasingly require help to cope with anxiety or depression resulting from this uncertainty. Also, existential issues may often become highlighted and explored as the person struggles to keep to drug regimes, manage side-effects and reinvest in life.

Simon, 45, was diagnosed eight years ago, at the same time as Jim, his partner. Jim died three years later after a slow decline into HIV-related dementia, Simon having given up work to look after him. Two years ago Simon became ill and reluctantly agreed to his consultant's advice to begin HAART, after which his health improved dramatically.

Having lived on sickness benefits for several years, Simon began to feel frustrated with his life and increasingly depressed. The intricacies of the benefits system made returning to work a difficult decision, and equally complex were the feelings Simon experienced resulting from his good health.

'I can carry on, can exist, without him but it's just so unfair that I'm here and he's not. He would still be here if only he'd got it later, if only he'd been more careful, if only . . . it does no good thinking that way but I can't seem to stop it.

I don't want to just exist. I want to live. But the better I feel physically, the worse I feel in my head. While I was ill, I could at least think that he was well out of it or that I would be dead soon too, but now . . . Now I Just wish he were here again. I seem to miss him more now than ever.'

Continuing good health robbed Simon of the possibility of an early death and an end to his separation from Jim. As Simon became physically healthier, his grief for Jim became more present and intense. Like many others diagnosed before the mid-1990s, Simon had seen HIV destroy his job, his own health and the life of his partner. Combination therapies gave him the opportunity to rebuild a life, but he felt ambivalent and confused.

In counselling, I supported and challenged Simon to mourn openly and deeply and to talk about his more difficult feelings, including his anger towards Jim at becoming infected and then infecting him. Gradually, as he expressed and managed his grief, Simon's desire for life began to return. He held on to his love for and memories of Jim but also took steps to involve himself in life again, including starting voluntary work. He knew that combination therapies held no guarantees but was prepared to take a risk.

Throughout my work with Simon, my thoughts and feelings would occasionally move towards my own partner, David, and my struggles to continue living without him. Today, ten years after his death, he is perhaps more solidly present in my heart and mind than at any time since his death. Having been lucky enough to be able to grieve openly for him and to have that grief acknowledged means that he truly does feel a part of me now and I no longer fear losing his presence, as I did soon after he died. It is a deeply comforting feeling.

Partners and families

'When my son, on a rare visit home, told me he was HIV-antibody positive, I was devastated and thought of all the years we had wasted. As well as lots of information about HIV and treatments, counselling has given me the chance to share my happiness and tears, my hopes and my fears. My relationship with my son is slowly improving and although my battle isn't over yet, I think I am getting there.' (Mother of man living with HIV)

As well as needing help to adjust to their loved one's diagnosis, partners and children of those with HIV may need to be tested, potentially leaving a family with more than one person with HIV. Several years ago, I worked with the father of a three-year-old HIV-positive boy, diagnosed following several bouts of ill health. Subsequent testing found that both the man and wife were also HIV-positive, and it was realized that the man had become infected through an earlier sexual relationship. He had passed the virus on to his wife, who later became pregnant with their son, who also became infected. The guilt, self-loathing and grief of this man were almost overwhelming, and much of our early work centred on looking at realistic alternatives to suicide.

Couples who experienced living with HIV before HAART may have difficulty adjusting to a better prognosis, with plans for the future and the carer and cared-for roles changing with the new situation. In particular, antiviral therapies and careful birthing procedures have meant a dramatic fall in mother-to-baby HIV transmission to around 2 per cent. This, and the increased life expectancy for adults, may mean that couples reconsider an earlier decision not to have children. The situation can be complex, however, depending on factors such as the woman's current immune functioning and any HAART combination being used, which may affect foetal development. If the man is HIV-positive, sperm washing (removing sperm cells from infected seminal fluid) is an option, but it is not 100 per cent safe for the woman and not easily available. Counselling can explore issues connected to starting a family, including looking at the possibility of one, or both of the couple, dying before the child is grown.

It is important for partners and family members to recognize the dual needs of supporting the person with HIV while also dealing with their own feelings. Families often gain from meeting others in the same situation, and partners' and families' support groups within the Terence Higgins Trust (THT), for example, are one way to assist this, encouraging peer support and information sharing . . .

The future

At the time of writing, the search for a vaccine against HIV slowly advances while the global situation continues to worsen at a terrifying rate. Reporting on the international Conference on AIDS in Durban, South Africa in 2000, the *Guardian* newspaper (8 July 2000) states that, in Africa as a whole, AIDS now kills two million people a year. Four million people were infected with HIV in 1999 alone, and without treatment most will die within ten to fifteen years. At the time of writing, around 34 million people around the world are living with HIV and an estimated 16 million have died so far from AIDS.

HIV transmission is preventable, but stigma, poverty and politics constantly undermine prevention programmes. HAART drugs remain too expensive for the majority of individuals and governments in developing countries to afford them, and even in the European Union (EU) alarm is being raised concerning the future financial burden of treatments.

As the number of people with HIV in the UK continues to rise, and as the estimated cost of drugs per person on HAART is now £10,000 per year resources will become ever more scarce. Treatments are continuing to improve, resulting in a wider range of drugs with decreased toxicity, fewer side-effects and simpler regimes, as well as specific drug formulations for children. Increasing numbers of men and women are now alive who were infected as children, and more information is becoming available concerning the emotional, neurological, cognitive and physical implications of the virus in babies and children.

Medical advances bring both hope and new dilemmas and choices. Improved life expectancy means a greater focus on quality of life issues, including housing, employment, economic security, relationships, sex and mental well-being. Those doing well on HAART will need psychological support to adhere to drug regimes and adapt to new lifestyles. Those not responding to treatments will continue to need regular support to cope with periods of ill health, possible physical decline and terminal illness.

HIV services, including counselling, will have the challenges of working in an uncertain and changing environment, with reduced resources, larger numbers of people living with the virus, and of working with an increasingly diverse group of people with differing needs.

The HIV voluntary sector is in a period of enormous change structurally, financially and culturally. For some, the process of agency closures, mergers and alliances is a necessary part of the maturing of the HIV field, ensuring the overall survival and effectiveness of services. For others, this process eventually will rob the sector of creativity and originality, with centralised control becoming more important than responsiveness to local needs.

The uncertainty of living with HIV is currently being mirrored in the uncertain future of many HIV organisations. Some workers in the sector report experiencing similar, although much less intense, feelings of loss, anxiety and powerlessness commonly associated with an HIV diagnosis. A phase of consolidation and stability within organisations will soon be vital, and the government's national strategy for HIV should assist in this. The strategy is badly needed in order to ensure equal access across the country to high quality HIV health promotion, treatment and care services . . .

Personal reflections

It has been important for me to be realistic concerning the limits of counselling. A person's needs for sufficient finances, adequate housing and accurate information have to be met alongside. emotional and psychological needs. Counselling is one of a series of THT West services, including a drop-in and meal service, support groups, buddying/befriending, complementary therapies, small grants, advice and advocacy. Users of the organisation are encouraged to draw on an integrated mix of services that suits their needs at a particular time.

Counselling can offer a safe and secure base (Purnell, 1996) as an individual attempts to manage the uncertainties of living with HIV. Boundary setting, including timing of sessions, contact with clients outside of sessions and physical contact, have traditionally offered containment and safety. Through visiting clients in hospital and at home, working with the same client from good health to the point of death, and through having close identification with many client issues, I have had the opportunity to confront and question these boundary issues many times.

Supervision has been a vital space for considering how a particular therapeutic boundary assists an individual client at a specific stage of his/her life, the aim being to ensure continuity while also recognizing practical and human needs. I agree with the psychoanalytic practitioner Burgner (1994) that there is no reason to behave differently as a therapist with clients with HIV than with any other clients, and so I would apply a questioning approach to boundaries, whatever the counselling issue. However, factors such as unpredictable health may increase the likelihood that questions concerning boundaries, including timing and setting, are raised when working with people with HIV.

Supervision with practitioners from a wide range of theoretical backgrounds has helped to keep my counselling focused, intentional and fresh. Personal therapy has given me the chance to explore, accept and challenge my own needs, fears, patterns and blindspots, as well as to identify my strengths and skills. Working as a counselling trainer and supervisor has allowed me to review regularly my personal theory and practice through the teaching of others, and exposed me to a range of counsellors working in very different settings. Supervision, personal therapy and work outside of HIV, therefore, have all increased my therapeutic effectiveness and been vital in preventing burnout, a common phenomenon in the HIV sector (Miller, 2000) . . .

Conclusion

HIV infection touches on the most crucial issues in society today. It connects with sex and sexuality, drug-use and addiction, racism, sexism and homophobia, the ethics of medical research and the power of drugs companies, the treatment and rights of the terminally ill and the bereaved, and with the status of the poor and the marginalized. It is a terrible medical condition for many and a vital social issue for all people. It is, for me, an intellectual, emotional, spiritual and constantly evolving challenge.

Along with intense joy, pride, sense of achievement and a great deal of laughter, I accept that grief and sadness form a significant part of this work. If I did not experience such feelings when a client dies, or another young person is newly diagnosed, or a mother is distraught with pain as she mourns her dead son, then it would mean that it was time for me to leave the work. The important need is to find ways to use those feelings for the therapeutic benefit of the client.

To be truly present with someone as they attempt to make sense of life and its meaning is a challenge and a privilege. It is healing for the client and, ultimately, healing also for me. Part of the meaning and purpose of my life has been derived from the work I have done with people living with HIV, complementing the fulfilment and love I have felt through my personal life. I have tried to learn from the strength and courage of so many clients and I know that my most important lesson is also the most obvious: to appreciate how precious and how delicate life and love can be and, as Emily Dickinson said, that hope is indeed a resilient bird with the sweetest of songs . . .

References

Barbour, R. (1995) The implications of HIV/AIDS for a range of workers in the Scottish context, *AIDS Care* 7(4), 521–35.

Bor, R., Miller, R. and Goldman, E. (1992) *Theory and Practice of HIV Counselling. A Systematic Approach*, London: Cassell.

Burgner M. (1994) Working with the HIV patient: a psychoanalytic approach, *Psychoanalytic Psychotherapy* 9(3), 201–13.

Davies, D. (1996) Towards a model of gay affirmative therapy. In Davies, D. and Neal, C. (eds), *Pink Therapy*. Buckingham: Open University Press.

Green, J. and McCreaner, A. (eds) (1996) *Counselling in HIV Infection and AIDS*, 2nd edn, Oxford: Blackwell.

Hecht, F., Colfax, G., Swanson, M. and Chesney, M. (1998) Adherence and effectiveness of protease inhibitors in clinical practice, Paper presented at the Fifth Conference on Retroviruses and Opportunistic Infections, Chicago, Ill., 2–6 February.

Kubler-Ross, E. (1969) *On Death and Dying*. New York: Macmillan.

Miller, D. (2000) *Dying to Care? Work, Stress and Burnout in HIV/AIDS*. London: Routledge.

Milton, M. (1996) An existential approach to HIV related psychotherapy. *Journal of the Society for Existential Analysis*, 9, 35–57.

Purnell, C. (1996) An attachment-based approach to working with clients affected by HIV and AIDS. *British Journal of Psychotherapy*, 12(4), 521–31.

Rogers, C. (1961) *On Becoming a Person*. London: Constable.

Sherr, L. (1999) HIV disease and its impact on the mental health of children. In Catalan J. (ed.), *Mental Health and HIV Infection*. London: UCL Press.

11 More than words: dialogue across difference*

Yasmin Gunaratnam

> Communication is another factor that influences the health service experience of black, Asian and other ethnic minority people. It has received a great deal of attention from researchers, although there is a strong tendency to think of communication solely in terms of interpretation and translation. Communication specialists would maintain that to be effective, 'communication must cover the way the organisation informs and listens to its staff, patients, carers, the broader community and other agencies',[1] but there is little available evidence relating these wider issues to the needs of black, Asian and other ethnic minority people. Nevertheless, the issue of language remains important. Individuals who use a spoken language other than English have a fundamental right to a correct diagnosis and appropriate treatment. This right can be seriously undermined when the quality of the interaction with a health care professional is compromised by language differences.
>
> (Alexander, 1999; p. 29)

In the quotation above, taken from a report on 'black, Asian and ethnic minority issues' commissioned by the Department of Health, ideas about the nature and the scope of communication in the provision of health care services are both questioned and broadened. At the same time, communication is seen as being fundamental to the experience of health care for organizations, service users, carers and communities.

I want to explore these issues further in this chapter, in relation to cross-cultural communication. Traditionally, the very term 'cross-cultural' has been seen as relating to communication across ethnic and national differences, in which debates have tended to pivot around the advantages and the disadvantages of what Ryen (2002) has called 'the insider–outsider problem'. What I want to do in this discussion is to problematize some of the underlying assumptions of current approaches to 'the insider–outsider problem' by drawing on the insights of Bakhtin's (1994) theory of dialogism. While the focus in this chapter is on ethnicity, I write with a broad interpretation of 'culture', in which I recognise that 'cultural' differences in communication can be experienced across a range

---

* Commissioned for this volume.

of intersecting social differences (Bradby, 2001), such as those relating to gender, class, age, disability, disease, sexuality or profession.

The chapter will address three main areas: first, it will provide a brief discussion of current approaches to 'race' and ethnicity; second, it will discuss practices of ethnic matching that are being advocated as strategies that enable 'ethnic sensitivity' in cross-cultural communication (Papadopolous and Lees, 2002); and third, it will explore how Bakhtin's theory of dialogism might be used to examine communication and meaning.

'Race' and ethnicity: entangled concepts

In broad terms, 'race' and ethnicity are now recognized as being social and political constructs, with 'race' being a category that signifies biological difference, and ethnicity as a category connoting cultural difference (for an overview of debates on the meanings of 'race' and ethnicity in relation to health, see Smaje 1996; Mulholland and Dyson, 2001). However, as Hall (2000) has noted, there are significant differences in how 'race' and ethnicity are theorized as concepts, and how they are given meaning in everyday life, particularly through racism:

> racism has its own 'logic' (Hall, 1990). It claims to ground the social and cultural differences which legitimize racialized exclusion in genetic and biological differences: i.e. in Nature. This 'naturalizing effect' appears to make racial difference a fixed, scientific 'fact', unresponsive to change or reformist social engineering.

> 'Ethnicity' by contrast, generates a discourse where difference is grounded in *cultural and religious* features. It is often, on these grounds, counter-posed to 'race'. But this binary opposition can be too simplistically drawn. Biological racism privileges markers like skin colour, but those signifiers have always also been used, by discursive extension, to connote social and cultural differences . . . The biological referent is therefore never wholly absent from discourses of ethnicity, though it is more indirect. The more 'ethnicity' matters, the more its characteristics are represented as relatively fixed, inherent within a group, transmitted from generation to generation, not just by culture and education, but by biological inheritance, stablilized above all my kinship and endogamous marriage rules that ensure that the ethnic group remains genetically, and therefore culturally 'pure'. (Hall, 2000, pp. 222–3; emphasis in original)

Following Hall, what I want to suggest is that approaches to cross-cultural communication in health care struggle with these fundamental tensions between recognizing 'race' and ethnicity as dynamic, socially constructed processes, yet treating them as, 'real', fixed and essential differences. What I mean by essentialism is that 'race' and/or ethnicity are seen as inherent, unchanging qualities that define the very being and experiences of different individuals and groups, and imply an 'internal sameness and external difference or otherness' (Werbner, 1997, p. 228). Although processes of essentializing 'race' and ethnicity can lead to oppressive practices and interventions, it is also the case that we can challenge racism and oppression by the development of approaches that recognize the dynamic and differentiated nature of experiences of 'race' and ethnicity, for those categorized as being in both 'majority' and in 'minority' positions.

What I want to do in the following sections is to examine ethnic matching as an approach that is being advocated to address some of the 'difficulties' of cross-cultural communication. Through this examination, I will show how essentialism can mark approaches that have been developed to enable 'ethnic sensitivity' and 'cultural competence' in health care. I will then go on to consider how we might develop approaches that are able to recognize the complex interactional, emotional and social dynamics of communicating across cultural differences.

Ethnic matching: from commonality to connectivity

Practices of ethnic matching, between practitioners and service users and/or local communities, occupy a central position in discussions about cross-cultural research and 'culturally competent' service provision and practice in health care (see Papadopoulos *et al.*, 1998; Alexander, 1999; Kai and Hedges, 1999; Papadopoulos and Lees, 2002 for examples). In a discussion of 'culturally competent' nurse research, Papadopoulos and Lees (2002) advocate ethnic matching as an example of 'ethnic sensitivity'. They suggest that matching should be practised 'whenever possible' because it:

> encourages a more equal context for interviewing which allows more sensitive and accurate information to be collected. A researcher with the same ethnic background as the participant will possess 'a rich fore understanding' (Ashworth, 1986) and 'an insider/emic view' (Leininger, 1991; Kauffman, 1994), will have more favourable access conditions and the co-operation of a large number of people (Hanson, 1994) and a genuine interest in the health and welfare of their community (Hillier and Rachman, 1996). (p. 261)

This statement by Papadopoulos and Lees encapsulates many of the assumptions that are made about commonality and difference in cross-cultural communication, in which ethnic correspondence is constructed as the best all-round solution to the complexities of communicating across difference. What is particularly striking and noteworthy in this example, is that ethnic commonalities are not just seen as a way of overcoming cultural and linguistic differences in research interactions, they are also promoted as reducing inter-subjective distances between the interviewer and the research participant (see also Bhopal, 2001; Dunbar *et al.*, 2002). That is, ethnicity is seen as a form of interactional and emotional capital that can be exploited to build rapport and co-operation, and to gain access to the subjectivity (processes of self and sense making) of minoritized research participants. This assumption about ethnic correspondence as enabling researchers/practitioners to move from being 'outsiders' to 'insiders' pervades a range of different approaches to health service provision and health promotion.

It is this assumption that is particularly dangerous in practices of ethnic matching, because it serves to essentialize 'race' and ethnicity as fixed, monolithic categories of difference, serving simultaneously to obscure other social differences and interactional and social power relations. There are three specific 'dangers' I wish to highlight. First, such strategies can serve to define the needs and the experiences of individuals and groups primarily in relation to their 'race' and or ethnicity. Second, experiences of ethnicity, but also language and its meanings, are treated as uncontested, rather than as multiple and shifting. And third, as Lewis (2000) has pointed out in relation to social work: 'no room is allowed for the possibility of shared understandings, correspondences of experiences or fluidity across group boundaries, nor indeed of heterogeneity within groups' (p. 127).

It is also important to point out that the claims made by Papadopoulos and Lees, in support of matching practices, need to be viewed with caution. We might ask, for example, how Papadopoulas and Lees know that ethnic matching 'encourages a more equal context for interviewing', leading to more 'sensitive and accurate' information? We have only to consider intra-ethnic violence and oppression, such as in Ireland, India and Zimbabwe to realise that shared ethnic and/or national identities can also be characterized by deep inequalities. Similarly, we might also ask how Papadopoulas and Lees can assume that the interest of 'matched' researchers will be any more 'genuine' than researchers from another ethnic group? In questioning such assumptions, and the rationale behind ethnic matching, my aim is not to deny the possibility or the value of points of connection across ethnicity and culture. Rather, I want to move away from essentialist discourses of 'commonality' that suggest an inherent, stable and naturalized affinity in communication, interpretation and understanding between members of the same ethnic/cultural group.

In moving away from essentialism, I want to move towards more dynamic notions of *'connectivity'* that are based upon both an active engagement with difference and a radical interrogation of 'sameness'. In other words, an approach in which all forms of communication are examined critically, enabling practitioners to engage with the spontaneous and unpredictable nature of connections, distances and differences in communication that are contingent on the unfolding dynamics of an interaction, and which can often involve multiple and even contradictory meanings.

I realize that my approach may sound feasible in theory, but much more problematic and fraught in practice. For instance, there are numerous examples from research on health care interactions of the critical importance of ethnic matching, and of the use of interpreters and advocates in enabling both linguistic and cultural interpretation (see Bradby, 2001). Where there are language differences between practitioners and service users or communities, I am not suggesting that such differences are insignificant, or that awareness of cultural patterns are not valuable. What I am suggesting is that we need to recognize that language, and ethnic and cultural identifications are just one part of the process of communicating across difference. My point is that ethnic matching does not by itself assure meaning and a quality of communication, and it can also serve to deflect attention away from the emotional, interactional, organizational and social dimensions of interactions.

In advocating a more complex, dynamic and multi-dimensional approach to cross-cultural communication, I want to use key themes from the social theorist Bakhtin's (1994) conceptualization of 'dialogism'. What I have found most valuable about these themes is that they displace the 'communication as communion' (Shields, 1996) model of ethnic matching, in which the practitioner's role can be transformed almost too readily from 'speaking with' to 'speaking as'. The focus of Bakhtin's work can be seen in terms of what Fine (1998) has called 'working the hyphen', where attention always questions and examines what is happening and what is not happening 'between', in the self/other encounter.

Within this framework, I want to suggest that there are no smooth surfaces of 'sameness' in which practitioners who are positioned as either the 'same' or as 'different' might take refuge. This is because such an approach is able to attend to the complex positioning of minoritized practitioners, where age, gender, class and health, for example, can disturb any easy sense of commonality along one axis of difference. At the same time, a practitioner, who, for example, might be working with an interpreter or advocate, is still implicated in a dialogic relationship with a service user/community, in which they need to account for their own positioning with the relationship and for the meanings that are generated through it.

Dialogism and creative understanding

> There exists a very strong, but one-sided and thus untrustworthy idea that in order to better understand a foreign culture, one must enter into it, forgetting one's own, and view the world through the eyes of the foreign culture . . . of course, a certain entry as a living being into a foreign culture, the possibility of seeing the world through its eyes is a necessary part of the process of understanding; but if this were the only aspect of this understanding it would merely be duplication and would not entail anything new or enriching. *Creative understanding* does not renounce itself, its own place in time, or its own culture; and it forgets nothing. (Bakhtin, 1994, pp. 6–7, emphasis added)

Bakhtin's formulation of 'creative understanding' when applied to health care interactions, challenges any sense of cross-cultural communication being about practitioners gaining full access to the meanings of 'others'. In this dialogic approach, meanings are always context related and multiple, constructed in the interaction and the engagement between participants, in which the aim is to enable differing points of view and experience to 'dialogue'. The 'other' is thus far from passive - someone who waits and hopes that they might be understood – rather, in any communication, there are always different levels of meaning and many 'voices' (Bakhtin's term is 'heteroglossia'), which problematize each other and which clamour for attention. As Shields (1996, p. 287) has argued: 'dialogical relationships are relationships between different judgements, positions and utterances'. Understanding within such an approach is more of an ethical than a technical act, in which the mutual nature of the production of meanings is recognized and explored.

In order to make this discussion less abstract, I want to use an example from my ethnographic research in a hospice (see Gunaratnam, 2001a and 2001b for examples) to look at how dialogic approaches to cross-cultural communication might challenge the essentialism of existing approaches. The example I want to use is taken from an interview with 'Frank' a black African-Caribbean man in his seventies with cancer of the prostate. In this part of the interview, which took place in Frank's home, I had asked him to tell me about his early life in Jamaica and the deaths of his mother and father. Frank had talked to me about these experiences during my participant observation work in the hospice day centre when he had asked me about my own parents, and I had told him that they were both dead. However, when I had asked Frank about his experiences in the interview some weeks later, Frank had told me that he did not want to talk about them:

Frank: . . . let me get that question you asked me . . . You see I don't want to bring that thing back here. Now as I told you that, I'm sorry to tell you, I but think I should stop you there because um, it brings back memories and, and I don't want it, it's $(1/2)^2$ poverty, poverty, I pass a lot (2). Well they say poverty is not a crime, but at times I say poverty is a crime really (1/2) so I don't like to talk about that anyway. *I don't want to bring back sore.*

Yasmin: Don't want to bring back . . . ?

Frank: Sore. You got sore on your body and so on, and that's what we say.

Yasmin: Oh, right. I've never heard of that before.

Frank: Ah, so you're never too old to learn.

Yasmin: Is, is that a Caribbean expression?

Frank: (1) Well, yes. (1/2) I don't know if it's, but that's where I learned it from anyway.

Yasmin: Yeah.

Frank: (2) And, very, very, very hard. It was very hard on me when I was a young boy growing up (1) through poverty. My mother was on her own (1) I was small, couldn't work. (5) But now this passed already and I don't want to talk about it (*Y*:   Sure) You know, I have to look for the (1/2) future (2), um, although, I doesn't really expects a future. Not really (3) mind you (5 taps of walking stick on floor, loud breath out) we don't know, I mean even another 2 years, 3 years, 4 years, 5 years or I may die at one time you cannot tell because only God knows.

There are many dimensions to this extract. However, what I want to concentrate on are the emotional and political meanings of the phrase 'bring back sore' (for a fuller interpretation of this extract, see Gunaratnam, forthcoming). You can see from the extract that I was unsure about the meaning of this term, and that I had asked Frank about its meaning in the interview. An ethnic matching approach might suggest that an interviewer of Jamaican descent may have had an 'insider' understanding of the term, enabling more 'accurate and sensitive' (Papadopoulos and Lees, 2002) interpretation of the meanings of this exchange. However, if we examine this extract using Bakhtin's approach of dialogism, that recognizes the co-production of meaning, interpretation of what at first sight looks like a cultural idiom, becomes more complex and layered, revealing something about the nature of the differences between Frank and myself in the interview.

For example, in my interpretation of dialogism, attention would be given to the psycho-social space of the interview, to changes in the research relationship between the hospice day centre and Frank's home, and how this might have had an effect on the interaction between Frank and myself. Attention would also be given to the shape of the whole interview, and to the exchanges that surround the term 'bring back sore'. However, what I want to highlight in this extract is how technical concerns with meaning can also act as emotional and political defences. For example, what I now feel is that I avoided the pain and the political implications of engaging with Frank's experiences of poverty, his lived experiences of a terminal illness, and the difficulties of talking about these experiences, by doing the work of trying to clarify meaning. Waddell (1989), in an article on social work, has suggested that the activity of 'doing the work' in many social care organizations is about a defence against the difficulties of thinking about, and tolerating, the psychic pain of 'clients'. Similarly, I would argue that technical preoccupations with meaning in cross-cultural encounters can serve as a defence against the anxiety of witnessing and holding emotional pain in health care interactions.

Such an interpretation is also made more complex in considering interactional and social power relations. For example, while I was in a more powerful research role in my interviews with Frank, he was also able to challenge these potentially authoritative forms of power by 'refusing' to talk about his experiences. I believe that Frank's comment to me that 'you're never too old to learn' invokes, resists and inflects elements of the differences in power and social location between us in the interview interaction. The effect of this comment was not simply patronising or ironic (in terms of the over 40 year age difference between Frank and myself). It can also be interpreted as a construction of Frank's authority and power in the interview, within the context of talk about his wounding experiences of poverty in the Caribbean, in which as a South-Asian woman and a middle-class researcher, I was positioned as having something to learn. The crucial point is that the extract is not simply about Frank's ethnic, gendered, class and illness-related experiences, it is also an interaction in which Frank and I *do* ethnicity, gender, class and health status (Wetherell and Edley, 1998). What I am talking about here is not simply a gap between experiences, but also Frank's challenge to me to learn, in which dialogism pushes me to interrogate the production and topography of my ignorance in this encounter.

Conclusion

Through the discussion in this chapter, I hope that I have been able to show some of the limitations of current approaches to cross-cultural communication. My approach to the production of meaning in intercultural encounters is not to assume the pre-determined existence and unchanging nature of meaning outside of interactions, that can be accessed and interpreted by cultural 'insiders'. Rather, by drawing upon themes in Bakhtin's (1994) theory of dialogism, I want to encourage a critical examination and exploration of the interactional, organizational and social contexts in which meanings are produced, negotiated and contested. There are two particular points to which I want to draw attention here. First, how an excessive concern with subjective and inter-subjective dynamics can obscure the construction, operation and effects of power relations throughout cross-cultural encounters. Second, how the 'activities' of technical preoccupations with meaning, can act as defences that can enable us to avoid emotional experiences of social difference. Through attention to the co-produced 'dialogue' between participants in a cross-cultural interaction, approaches to communication, meaning and interpretation become not only more challenging, but also more complex and interesting, in which Frank's assertion of the need for continual learning, has relevance to us all.

Notes

1 This is a reference to a report by the University of Central England (1998), entitled 'An Integrated Language and Communication Strategy for Birmingham (Stage 1).
2 The numbers throughout this transcript refer to the length of pauses in seconds.

References

Alexander, Z. (1999). *Study of Black, Asian and Ethnic Minority Issues*. London: Department of Health.
Ashworth, P. (ed.) (1986). *Qualitative Research in Psychology*. Pennsylvania: Duquesne University Press.
Bakhtin, M. (1994). Response to a question from the Novy Mir editorial staff. In Emerson, C. and Holquist, A. (eds), *Speech Genres and Other Late Essays*. Austin, Texas: University of Texas Press.
Bar-On, D. (1999). *The Indescribable and the Undiscussable: Reconstructing Human Discourse after Trauma*. Budapest: Central European University Press.
Bhopal, K. (2001). Researching South Asian Women: issues of sameness and difference in the research process, *Journal of Gender Studies*, 10(3); 279–86.
Bradby, H. (2001). Communication, interpretation and translation. In Culley, L. and Dyson, S. (eds). *Ethnicity and Nursing Practice*. London: Palgrave, 129–48.
Dunbar, C., Rodriguez, D. and Parker, L. (2002). 'Race, Subjectivity and the Interview Process' in Gubrium, J. and Holstein, J. (eds) *Handbook of Interview Research: Context and Method*. Thousand Oaks, California: Sage, 279–98.
Fine, M. (1998). Working the Hyphens: reinventing self and other in qualitative research. In Denzin, N. and Lincoln, Y. S. (eds), *The Landscape of Qualitative Research: Theories and Issues*. Thousand Oaks, Calif.: Sage, 130–55.
Gunaratnam, Y. (2001a). 'We mustn't judge people . . . but': staff dilemmas in dealing with racial harassment amongst hospice service users, *Sociology of Health and Illness*, 23(1), 65–83.
Gunaratnam, Y. (2001b). Eating into multi-culturalism: hospice staff and service users talk food, 'race', ethnicity and identities, *Critical Social Policy*, 21(3), 287–310.
Gunaratnam, Y. (forthcoming), *Researching 'Race' and Ethnicity: Methods, Knowledge and Power*. London: Sage.

Hall, S. (1990). 'Cultural Identity and Diaspora', in Rutherford, J. (ed) *Identity, Community, Culture and Difference*. London: Lawrence Wishart, pp. 222–37.

Hall, S. (2000) Conclusion: the multi-cultural question. In Hesse, B. (ed.), *Un/settled Multiculturalisms: Diasporas, Entanglements, Transruptions*. London: Zed Books, 209–41.

Hanson, E. (1994). Issues concerning the familiarity of researchers with the research setting, *Journal of Advanced Nursing*, 20(3), 940–2.

Hillier, S. and Rachman, S. (1996). Childhood development and behavioural and emotional problems as perceived by Bangladeshi parents in East London. In Kelleher, D. and Hillier, S. (eds), *Researching Cultural Differences in Health*. London: Routledge, 38–68.

Kai, J. and Hedges, C. (1999). Minority ethnic community participation in needs assessment and service development in primary care: perceptions of Pakistani and Bangladeshi people about psychological distress, *Health Expectations*, 2(1), pp. 7–20.

Kauffman, K. (1994). The insider/outsider dilemma: field experience of a white researcher 'getting in' a poor black community, *Nursing Research*, 43, 179–83.

Leininger, M. (ed.) (1991) *Culture Care, Diversity and Universality: A Theory of Nursing*. NLN Press: New York.

Leininger, M. (1995) *Transcultural Nursing: Concepts, Theories, Research and Practices*, 2nd edn. New York: McGraw-Hill.

Lewis, G. (2000) *'Race', Gender, Social Welfare: Encounters in a Postcolonial Society*. London: Polity Press.

Mulholland, J. and Dyson, S. (2001). Sociological theories of 'race' and ethnicity. In Culley, L. and Dyson, S. (eds), *Ethnicity and Nursing Practice*. London: Palgrave, 17–38.

Papadopoulos, I. and Lees, S. (2002). Developing culturally competent researchers, *Journal of Advanced Nursing*, 37(3), pp. 258–64.

Papadopoulos, I., Tilki, M. and Taylor, G. (1998). *Transcultural Care: A Guide for Health Care Professionals*. Wilts: Quay Books.

Ryen, A. (2002). Cross-cultural interviewing. In Gubrium, J. and Holstein, J. (eds), *Handbook of Interview Research: Context and method*. Thousand Oaks; Calif.: Sage, 335–54.

Shields, R. (1996). Meeting or mis-meeting? The dialogical challenge to Verstehen, *British Journal of Sociology*, 47(2), 275–94.

Smaje, C. (1996). The ethnic patterning of health: new directions for theory and research, *Sociology of Health and Illness*, 18, 139–71.

Waddell, M. (1989) Living in two worlds: psychodynamic theory and social work practice, *Free Associations*, 15, 11–35.

Werbner, P. (1997). Essentialising essentialism, essentialising silence: ambivalence and multiplicity in the constructions of racism and ethnicity. In Werbner, P. and Modood, T. (eds), *Debating Cultural Hybridity: Multi-Cultural Identities and the Politics of Anti-Racism*. London: Zed Books, 226–54.

Wetherell, M. and Edley, N. (1998). Gender practices: steps in the analysis of men and masculinities. In Henwood, K., Griffin, C. and Phoenix, A. (eds), *Standpoints and Differences: Essays in the Practice of Feminist Psychology*. London: Sage, 156–73.

12 The social marketing imbroglio in health promotion

Ralph C. Lefebvre

The article, by Hastings and Haywood (1991), coupled with conversations with a number of attendees at the WHO Seminar on Leadership Training in Health Promotion and the International Summer School on Health Promotion held in Cardiff in September 1991, caused me concern over how health promotion professionals think about, and use, social marketing in their work. Some of the key concerns I have about the present state of affairs, and what appear to be topics not being considered adequately by all of us, are presented to broaden the discussion, and roles, of social marketing in health promotion.

Concerns

Social marketing = health promotion

Because much of the focus of work and publications about social marketing occur within a 'health problem' context, there are, at times, interchangeable use of the terms (one 'socially markets' nutrition to patients with cardiovascular disease). At other times, the discussions of social marketing become so focused on individual health behaviour, or lifestyles, that professionals concerned with environmental and other social issues wonder if they are in the right conference room. We need to understand that social marketing is a tool that can be used for health promotion, but is not the exclusive province of health promoters. This brings me to a second issue.

Social marketing is a theory for health promotion

Without delving into the epistemological aspects of this concern, the recurring questions I receive about the 'theory of social marketing' give me pause. Often, it is University faculty and students who are 'exploring the theory' and advance these questions. What they are finding is that there 'is not much theory' to social marketing. Other groups, particularly those who fund research, are asking 'Does social marketing work?' as if

* From *Health Promotion International*, 7(1) (1992), 61–4. Oxford University Press. © Oxford University Press 1992.

it's different from other theoretical approaches to health promotion. What is clear to me is that social marketing is a framework, or structure (perhaps a paradigm?) in which to approach social and health problems. It is the theory of change which imbues this general approach and gives it a chance to succeed. Failures of social marketing programmes are failures to theory or implementation. Attributing lack of success with a programme to social marketing is, to me, akin to attributing failure of a group to solve a problem to an inherent problem with Robert's Rules of Order (which also highlights that just as some groups have never read Robert, some health promoters do not understand social marketing to effectively use it).

Social marketing targets people

I have become increasingly concerned that social marketing programmes continue to be presented in only an individual behaviour change context. In an early article, June Flora and I discussed the use of social marketing to target social institutions and structures (Lefebvre and Flora, 1988). While such efforts are being launched by various special interests and advocacy groups, we need to remind ourselves in health promotion that social marketing programmes not only have to be sensitive to their environment, but also be directed towards creating a healthier one.

Social marketing = mass communication

Perhaps the most difficult issue for me to understand is how social marketing has become equated with mass communication approaches to health promotion *only*. This issue arises for me when people ask 'How can we do social marketing programmes when community development approaches are what we are supposed to be doing?' Indeed, I have spent entire days working with health promotion offices to 'try to integrate the two'. For me, there is no reason why a 'social marketing programme' cannot *exclusively* take a community development approach to solving a problem. If programme *strategy* is based on identifying consumer needs, identifying priority audiences, knowing how to best reach these audiences, and structuring the project as a 'marketing mix' (though the terms may be different), then selecting the *tactics* of community development or mass communication is secondary. A marketing programme is constructed to target a social concern and reach certain objectives. Going back to the 'theory' concern, social marketing is a framework in which to address problems. It is not exclusive of any theoretical approach to solving problems. The interesting research question would be: Using a social marketing model, is community development theory or mass communications theory more effective in creating an intervention that leads to healthier lifestyles and environments?

Challenges

Environmental scanning

As noted by Hastings and Haywood (1991), health promoters need to be aware of their internal and external environments as they plan strategies and tactics. On-going SWOT analysis (strengths, weaknesses, opportunities, threats) is imperative for effective marketing efforts. A SWOT analysis can be used both within the organization and throughout the environment.

When doing this scanning key themes include (i) demographic and lifestyle trends, (ii) economic forecasts, (iii) business/industry activities, (iv) legislative/regulatory initiatives, and (v) potential partners, collaborators and intermediary groups for programme involvement. My scanning process includes reading marketing and business magazines, financial sections of newspapers, and professional newsletters. I also talk with many different types of people in order to 'take the pulse' of what people are thinking about, planning to do, or about to embark upon. It minimizes surprises, and can often lead to unique opportunities for programme expansion and increased activity. More focus needs to be given to analysing the context of our marketing efforts, and identifying how the context, and our response to it, shapes the intervention strategy and tactics.

Audiences

The central concern of social marketing is the consumer: we must stay in touch with them or risk creating programmes that are not responsive to their needs, issues and unique situations. An over-riding and continuing interest in the consumer is what differentiates social marketing from health information or health education campaigns. Empowering people, advocating for them, and using community development approaches (as already noted) should be included as part of the marketing planning and implementation process. Social marketing is often portrayed as a 'top-down' approach; yet, when we keep consumers in the centre of the programme, and have a continuing dialogue with them, a 'bottom-up' effect is inevitable. Modern marketing practice is looking to 'build relationships with consumers': it's a goal we in health promotion should set for ourselves as well.

Channel

How to reach our key audiences with our messages, products and services should be a constant question for us. Intersectoral action can be viewed as a way to open up numerous channels for health promotion.

However the nagging issue of so-called 'hard-to-reach' audiences is one that occupies much of our attention. We each have our particular 'hard-to-reach' groups. What I have noticed is that we can often characterize these groups quite well – down to the brand of cigarettes they smoke and the alcoholic beverage they consume. My question is, 'Why can tobacco and alcohol advertisers reach these people and we can't?' I do not believe the answer is simply they have more money and resources than we do! I think that health promotion professionals need to get smarter. We have to spend more time studying what these people do, learn from them and then use it to our advantage.

Process tracking

Many health promotion programmes are plagued by a lack of information on what they do and how effectively they do it. I do not mean by this that more programmes need outcome evaluation, but rather that *all* programmes need to understand whether they are reaching their intended audiences, whether these audiences understand that we are trying to communicate to them, and whether this understanding leads to attitudinal, and more importantly, behavioural change. Without process tracking systems, programme managers have little idea of how well they are progressing towards their objectives. It's somewhat akin to showing a person on a map a rather long, complicated and tortuous route to getting somewhere, and then sending them on their way without the map. Health promoters need to have their maps – not just to know where they are going, but to continually refer back so that they stay on the right path.

Exchanges

Marketing is a process of facilitating mutually rewarding exchanges between two or more parties – often referred to as 'creating win–win situations'. Making such exchanges tangible to consumers and health promoters occupies much of our time because, by virtue of our business, we are not always asking people for something tangible (e.g. money) in exchange for tangible goods (e.g. food, automobiles). What we do not understand very well is what I call the 'economics of health behaviour', that is, how and why people make decisions to adopt more healthful practices. In business marketing, consumer behaviour is an area of study in its own right. While health promoters have many theories from which to draw in developing their programmes, a critical part of the equation is missing. We need a good motivational theory for health behaviours, not just more rational ideas on how things should be. My question is always 'How do we motivate people?' The answer, when we stumble upon it, then defines how we structure the exchange process so we are successful (win) in improving the public's health (win).

Institutionalisation

Another shortcoming of many health promotion programmes is their transitory existence. As long as funding is available (usually from a single source), the programme thrives and is successful. Yet, as soon as funding is reduced, or cut altogether, the programme withers and dies. I have outlined elsewhere how institutionalization or the long-term maintenance, of health promotion programmes can be approached within a social marketing context (Lefebvre, 1990). What are important issues to consider include:

- Planning for institutionalization from the beginning of a programme or new initiative, not during its demise;
- Developing indigenous resources or secondary resources, to support the initiative; and
- Demonstrating success to both grass-roots opinion and the policy makers.

These issues need to be continually revisited by health promotion leaders if *our* long-term goals are to be met.

Management

The most critical variable for successful social marketing programmes is the management of the process. Among the issues I have touched upon, this is, to me, the weakest link in health promotion practice. We have to recognize that we will always be operating in a changing set of circumstances and, indeed, a changing world. The title of Tom Peter's book, *Thriving on Chaos*, needs to become our battle-cry – not our lament. Health promotion professionals must learn to manage change, not just in our sphere of health, but across the economic. social, business and political sectors of our world. This reticence to do so may be our Achilles heel. As Bill Novelli noted in a recent presentation, it is our unwillingness to earn our 'black belts' in marketing that limit the scope of what we can achieve.

Among the ideas touched upon by Peters that resonate with my view of health promotion management are the following:

- We need to *push* responsibility for programmes and initiatives *down* in our bureaucracies. We have to expect, and facilitate, excellence from our staffs.
- We need to 'fail forwards fast', to not be afraid of failure, but to encourage in our staffs an exhilaration for innovation. Failure needs to be viewed in the organization as an opportunity to learn, not to point fingers. But we also need to learn fast, and get on with it!

Finally, to be leaders in health promotion, we have to stop asking ourselves, our supervisors, and our staffs 'Why?' Rather, to end with a quote from George Bernard Shaw, we need to set the vision:

> You see things; and you say, 'Why?' but I dream things that never were; and I say, 'Why not?'

References

Hastings, G. and Haywood, A. (1991). Social marketing and communication in health promotion, *Health Promotion International*, 6, 135–45.

Lefebvre, R. C. (1990). Strategies to maintain and institutionalise successful programmes: a marketing framework. In Bracht, N. (ed.), *Health Promotion at the Community Level*. Calif.: Newburg Press, 209–28.

Lefebvre, R. C. and Flora, J. A. (1988). Social marketing and public health intervention, *Health Education Quarterly*, 15, 299–315.

Robert, S. C. (1990). *The Scott, Foresman Roberts's Rule of Order* (new revised). Glenview, IL: Scott, Foresman.

Peter, T. (1987). *Thriving on Chaos: Handbook for the management revolution*. New York: Knopf.

Novelli, W. D. (1990). Getting a 'black-belt' in social marketing. Presentation at the American Marketing Association (Washington, DC Chapter) Social Marketing Conference.

Questioning the evidence base of health promotion: introduction

Health promotion has sometimes been criticized for basing interventions on what might be viewed as insubstantial evidence and for a less than robust approach to evaluation. To justify its place in the purchaser-provider market, it is argued, health promotion must become more rigorous, self-critical and outcome-focused. This links to a broader endorsement of the concept of evidence-based health care, with the implication that much health practice hitherto was not based on research data but on clinical judgement. However, even when there is information which appears to be reliable, it may prove to be contradictory and provide more questions than answers. This Section seeks to lay out these issues and in particular unravels the question of what counts as evidence in health promotion. At a practical level, answering this question is important for clients who want advice about healthy choices, and for purchasers and policy makers seeking to use public money wisely. At a more philosophical level it relates to wider debates about the nature of evidence and whose views count, as well as important ethical implications.

The first chapter in Section Two takes up the issue of reliable evidence and the importance of understanding the methods used in collecting data before making assumptions about the relevance and reliability of conclusions reached. Joe Abramson argues in Chapter 13 that epidemiological studies need to be scrutinized in relation to a number of factors before using the results as the basis for interventions. He suggests that, despite methodological drawbacks, well conducted epidemiological research can collate evidence sufficiently reliably to enable informed decision making. However, conflicting evidence, as seen during the BSE (bovine spongiform encephalopathy) debacle, is as much part of epidemiological enquiry as is the replacing of old knowledge by new. Hence 'epidemiology should be taken with care'.

Examples of why epidemiology should be taken with care are to be found in the following two chapters. Michael Burr refers in Chapter 14 to the somewhat paradoxical situation in France, which has a comparatively low incidence of, and mortality rates from, ischaemic heart disease. These rates seem to be unexpectedly low given the high French intake of saturated fat, and the fact that serum cholesterol, blood pressure and smoking prevalence rates in France are similar to other countries. The role of wine drinking with meals is examined, to ascertain whether this confers protection against some of the effects of food. This 'paradox' is illustrative of the ways in which information is sometimes misconceived and presented. Norman Beale and Susan Nethercott, in Chapter 15, looked at GP consultation rates, comparing employees of a factory threatened with closure with other local residents. This study demonstrates that drawing conclusions about relationships between the threat of unemployment and consultation rates is rife with difficulties, but still can indicate certain patterns.

So what is to count as evidence, and who should decide this? This question is taken up in Chapter 16 by David McQueen and Laurie Anderson. In an increasingly market-based health system, purchasers are expected to ground their decisions in evidence of effectiveness and value for money. Yet in health promotion such evidence is often hard to come by, and evaluations and reviews of evaluation studies have for the most part failed to produce the kind of practical guidance called for by purchasers and policy makers. McQueen and Anderson take a critical stance in their review of the evidence base of health promotion, but conclude on a more optimistic note.

Christine Godfrey, in Chapter 17, also takes a largely optimistic and pragmatic view. Recognizing that much work remains to be done, she teases out the kinds of comparison that can be drawn and the tools that will help. Models such as PREVENT help to predict health gain, though most available models are limited to mortality measures. She also calls for ways of measuring changes in morbidity.

Echoing Godfrey's carefully analytic tone, but pointing to a very different conclusion, Roger Burrows and his colleagues argue in Chapter 18 that the hope of providing guidance for purchasers about the cost-effectiveness of health promotion initiatives is primarily a mirage. The project is essentially misconceived, they maintain, because health promotion does not lend itself to the kind of evaluation that has proved fruitful in biomedical research. Biomedicine and health promotion belong to different worlds (characterized respectively as modern and postmodern) and so require different kinds of evaluation. The object of study in the evaluation of health promotion (human interaction and behaviour) is an 'open system' subject to very complex patterns of determination at a number of levels. In short, no amount of technical and methodological refinement will provide solid evidence of cost effectiveness in health promotion, and it is pointless to keep trying.

What other forms of evaluation exist? Writing primarily from experience of the evaluation of social work, Angela Everitt and Pauline Hardiker sketch out in Chapter 19 an alternative 'critical' framework which, unlike rational-technical evaluation, acknowledges the significance of subjectivity, values and power. In so doing, they provide a powerful challenge to both medical and managerial assumptions about the nature of evidence and the meaning of success. It is important to be reminded that debates about the evidence base of health promotion need to be understood in the context of wider philosophical debates. This leads us, in the final chapter in Section Two, into an initial consideration of the ethical issues in health promotion through a case study by Alison Dines of mammography screening. In exploring the different ways in which health workers might respond to women's requests for advice, Dines highlights some of the dilemmas present in health promotion work. What are the boundaries of advice and information-giving? Where should professional intervention end and lay autonomy begin? We shall return to such questions in Sections Three and Four of the Reader.

13 Epidemiology – to be taken with care*

Joe H. Abramson

Epidemiology embraces not only the study of the distribution and determinants of health-related states and events in groups and populations, but also, according to the *Dictionary of Epidemiology* (Last, 1995), the application of this study to the control of health problems.

Epidemiological studies are not limited to diseases, deaths, disabilities, and other disorders. They encompass healthy growth and development, physical fitness, and other dimensions of positive health, as well as social, behavioural, environmental and other factors (including health attitudes and practices and the provision and use of health services) that influence health. This broad scope of interest and the wide range of methods (observational and experimental, quantitative and qualitative) available for the study of groups and populations enable epidemiology to supply much of the information required for the planning, implementation, monitoring and evaluation of health care, including health education and other intervention programmes aimed at enhancing the health status of a population or population sector. Epidemiology is the foundation science of public health (Detels, 1991).

But there is a need for caution – all that glitters is not gold. The results of epidemiological studies may sometimes be unhelpful or even misleading, and should never be utilized uncritically. Problems of various kinds may arise, singly or in combination. Ways of minimizing these problems when doing epidemiological studies, and of recognizing and handling them when interpreting findings, are central topics of all epidemiology teaching.

The main questions to be asked before using epidemiological results are:

1. Are the results accurately known?
2. How valid are the findings?
3. How valid are the inferences drawn from the findings?
4. How relevant is the information?
5. Is the information sufficient?

---

* Commissioned for this volume

Accurate knowledge of the results

An obvious precaution is that decisions should not be based on inaccurate reports or impressions. Press, radio and television reports, in particular, may be misleading. 'Journalism is an activity with no scientific methodology' (de Semir, 1996). In the hunt for 'news', prominence may be given not only to weak studies, but to 'the one positive result in a sea of negative data' (Mann, 1995). The blame for these distortions sometimes lies with investigators or research institutions, who may make exaggerated claims that go beyond what is said in the published study report (Mann, 1995; Pini, 1995). Where possible, reliance should be placed only on original study reports or experts who have read them.

Selective reporting or use of results is especially hazardous when vested interests or political issues are involved, as at the start of the furore concerning bovine spongiform encephalopathy (BSE–'mad cow disease') in Britain in 1996; the borderline between selective reporting and deliberate misinformation may then become tenuous. If (rather presumptuously) we refer to epidemiological results as 'the truth', the aim should be to know the truth, the whole truth, and nothing but the truth.

It is unwise to rely on a single study if others are available. 'What medical journals publish is not received wisdom, but rather working papers . . . Each study becomes a piece of a puzzle that, when assembled, will help either to confirm or to refute a hypothesis' (Angell and Kassirer, 1994). Different studies of the same topic often produce different information, as a result of chance variation or differences in study methods or circumstances or between study populations. Examples of contradictory findings abound (Angell and Kassirer, 1994; Taubes, 1995). But each new study is reported in isolation, as a new breakthrough, provoking the question:

'Why can't researchers get it straight the first time?' (Angell and Kassirer, 1994)

A single study should not be relied on, but obtaining a fuller picture is not always easy. If meta-analyses have been done, they are thus particularly useful. These are overviews of research on a specific topic, in which studies are systematically sought, methods are appraised, findings are compared, the reasons for differences are explored, and an endeavour is made (using appropriate statistical methods) to reach balanced overall conclusions. An important recent advance in this area is the development of the Cochrane Collaboration, an international network of individuals and institutions committed to preparing, maintaining, and disseminating systematic reviews of the effects of health care (Chalmers, 1993).

Validity of findings

No epidemiological study is perfect, and a critical appraisal of the design and methods is always advisable before deciding whether to use the findings.

The main consideration is the possibility that the findings may be biased, that is, that they may deviate from the truth. Ostensible findings may be artefacts. Bias is usually caused by shortcomings either in the selection of individuals or groups for study (selection bias) or in the collection, recording, coding or analysis of data (information bias). Both forms of bias may come about in many ways, some avoidable and some unavoidable, and it may or may not be possible to appraise their direction and magnitude, and compensate for their effects. The problems are generally methodological ones, although bias may also (rarely) result from conscious fraud or (more often) from lesser misdemeanours by scientists:

> Inventing data would clearly be wrong; suppression of inconvenient results would be less than honest. Yet they need not think too badly of themselves if they gloss over the study's methodological shortcomings, optimise the statistical analysis, cite published work selectively. (*Lancet*, 1995)

There may also be unconscious subjective processes whereby the investigator's preconceived opinions and preferences result in choices that lead to one-sided findings. Particular caution may be advisable with studies financed by tobacco firms or other manufacturers, or political or other bodies with vested interests; it is then prudent to be especially insistent on seeking confirmatory evidence elsewhere. A health worker with a grounding in basic epidemiological methods should have no difficulty in recognizing a study's main weak points with respect to sampling, selection of control groups, operational definitions of variables, methods of data-collection, etc. Checklists are available, e.g. for appraising case-control studies (Stolley and Schlesselman, 1982; Lichtenstein *et al.*, 1987) and trials (Chalmers *et al.*, 1990). Study methods and their impact on the validity of information are considered in more detail by (*inter alia*) Schlesselman (1982), Hulley and Cummings (1988), Vaughan and Morrow (1989), Abramson (1990, 1991), Berkelman and Buehler (1991), Feinleib *et al.* (1991), Greenberg and Ibrahim (1991) and Puska (1991).

A critical appraisal of study methods requires basic epidemiological know-how – which is of course one of the reasons why it is so important for all health workers to have some training in epidemiology. Lacking this, an assessment by someone more knowledgeable should be sought. Unfortunately there are no simple short-cuts. Reliance on the reputation of the researchers, the sponsoring agency, or the journal in which the results are published, for example, may be misleading. Nor is it enough to know what techniques were used, without considering the details of their use. Sampling that is random in name only, badly-chosen controls, unnecessary matching, injudicious statistical testing, confidence interval estimation in the absence of random processes or in the presence of bias or confounding variables and other abuses may yield deceptive findings.

Validity of inferences drawn from the findings

However valid the factual findings may be, the conclusions drawn from them may be questionable, particularly in analytic studies that try to explain associations between variables, where interpretation may require considerable skill and experience. It is obviously incorrect to conclude that there is a cause–effect relationship, just because an association has been found. A study of dog-bites showed that dogs kept chained were much likelier than unchained dogs to bite non-household members, but the conclusion that:

> owners may be able to . . . modify risk by . . . not keeping them chained. (Gershman, 1992)

was questionable, and was later toned down to:

> A dog may be chained as the result of having exhibited aggressive behavior which itself may be a risk factor for biting, rather than chaining somehow causing a dog to bite. (Gershman *et al.*, 1994)

Sometimes it is enough to know that a characteristic is associated with a disease, whatever the explanation. This may permit use of the characteristic as a screening test that identifies individuals or groups especially likely to have the disease, or as a risk marker that identifies those especially likely to contract the disease in the future. These uses do not require a causal relationship. As an example, a 10-year follow-up study of 90,000 American women showed that the risk of a hip fracture was more than twice as high for women at least 5'8" tall than for women under 5'2", after allowing for effects connected with age, obesity and other variables. This led to the suggestion that 'taller elderly women should be advised to consider preventive measures' (Hemenway *et al.*, 1995). This recommendation is based solely on the presence of the association; tallness is used as a risk marker, and whether or not it is a contributory cause (maybe because taller women fall from a greater height) is irrelevant.

But data interpretation becomes much more difficult if etiologic explanations are wanted. As an example, a study of 994 men and women born in Hertfordshire, UK, in 1920–30 showed that those who had sucked a dummy (pacifier) in their first year of life, according to health records maintained at that time, had a lower average IQ score as adults (Gale and Martyn, 1996). About 69 per cent of them had a lower score than the mean score of those who had not used dummies. This might mean that dummy-sucking impairs cognitive development (maybe because of drowsiness or because the baby is more placid and therefore receives less attention). In other words, the dummy may be a true risk factor (i.e. a *maker*, rather than only a *marker*, of risk). But other explanations must be explored and rejected before an etiologic inference can be accepted. First, the association may be a chance one; a significance test showed this to be very improbable ($P < 0.0001$). Also, a relationship may occur between variables even if they are not causally linked, if they share associations with other (confounding) variables. Appropriate analyses yielded no evidence that the dummy–IQ connection could be attributed in this way to links with mother's age, father's occupation, birth rank, method of feeding, or weight in infancy. But other possible explanations could not be tested; for example, maybe parents who used dummies had weaker parenting skills or were less intelligent (Feldman and Feldman, 1996) or less interested in their children's health, since dummies were at that time regarded as health hazards by child-care experts, and health workers in Hertfordshire specifically advised against their use. Nor was consideration given to differences in the presence or strength of the dummy–IQ association in different subgroups (e.g. males and females), reflecting possible modifying effects of other variables on the association; interactions of this sort often throw light on causal processes. Also, there might be a causal association in the other direction – 'perhaps babies who are willing to accept a dummy . . . are slightly less intelligent'. The association thus remained unexplained.

Even had there been findings pointing to the unlikeliness of all these other explanations, most epidemiologists would be inclined to consider the dummy–IQ association as causal only if there was additional positive evidence (Hill, 1965; Susser, 1973, 1986), such as a correlation with the time spent dummy-sucking (a dose–response relationship) and, especially, consistency of the finding in different studies.

The validity of inferences about causation can thus not be taken for granted. It depends on whether they are grounded on valid data, analytical procedures that allow for possible confounding and modifying effects, and a proper approach and sound judgement in data interpretation. The interpretation of evidence is a matter of judgement, and unfortunately judges may disagree. Usually no major problem arises; but sometimes the conclusions are debatable, or obviously flawed.

Weak associations are especially likely to be due to chance, bias or confounding variables (American Health Foundation, 1982), and unless the association has been confirmed repeatedly many epidemiologists demand at least a doubling (some say trebling or quadrupling) of risk before they will consider a cause-and-effect relationship, saying that 'it is so easy to be fooled that it is impossible to believe less-than-stunning results' (Taubes, 1995). But factors that increase risk only slightly can have a huge effect on the public's health if they are sufficiently widespread. This has been called 'the Catch-22 of modern epidemiology' (Taubes, 1995).

There is an extreme view, which most epidemiologists do not share, that epidemiological evidence alone, without laboratory and clinical studies that support and explain a causal relationship, can never be conclusive enough to warrant a preventive programme (Charlton, 1995). In this view, a preventive strategy at the population level is justified only if the 'black box' concealing the mysteries of causal mechanisms (Skrabanek, 1994) has been opened. Historical examples that refute this view include: the link between a dearth of fresh fruit and scurvy, demonstrated in 1753, long before vitamins were thought of (Lind, 1753); between exposure to soot and scrotal cancer, in 1775, when the carcinogenic role of polycyclic aromatic hydrocarbons was undreamt of (Pott, 1775); between polluted water and cholera, in 1855, before bacteria had been discovered (Snow, 1855); between a poor diet and pellagra in the second decade of the 20th century, when this was thought to be a communicable disease (Terris, 1964); and between smoking and lung cancer and other diseases before the pathogenetic mechanisms were understood (Doll and Hill, 1964; Hammond, 1966; Kahn, 1966). The link between smoking and cancer aroused a productive controversy (Gail, 1996), which culminated in the formulation of the criteria for drawing causal conclusions (Hill, 1965; Susser, 1973, 1986) – the 'rules of evidence' – now used by most epidemiologists.

A recent example is the finding that babies put to sleep on their stomachs have a higher risk of cot deaths (sudden infant death syndrome – SIDS). Although the reasons for this association are as yet unclear, the recommendation that healthy infants should be put to sleep on their backs or sides (Kattwinkel et al., 1992) has been applied in 'Back-to-Sleep' campaigns in the United Kingdom, New Zealand, Holland and other countries. These have been followed by appreciable reductions in cot deaths, without apparent decreases in other known risk factors (Hunt, 1994; Wigfield et al., 1994; Court, 1995; Willinger, 1995). Interactions discovered in epidemiological studies, such as an increase in the risk attached to prone sleeping if no adult sleeps in the room (Scragg et al. 1996) or if the baby has very warm clothes or covers (Williams et al., 1996) may, if confirmed, lead to a better understanding of the causal mechanisms.

There is often a need to decide whether to accept a specific causal explanation (knowing that this may later turn out to be incorrect) as a basis for action, whether to design a programme that caters for alternative etiologic possibilities, or whether to defer action.

Data interpretation and its problems are considered in more detail by
(*inter alia*) Susser (1973), Greenland (1991), Abramson (1994) and sym-
posia edited by Greenland (1987) and Rothman (1988), and most epidemiology textbooks. For statistical methods for use in analysing
epidemiological findings, see Kahn and Sempos (1989), Gahlinger and
Abramson (1995) and Selvin (1996).

How relevant is the information?

In a health care context, the epidemiological findings and inferences in
question may not be very relevant to the specific group or population
under consideration.

This problem does not arise if this group or population is the one that
was studied, which is of course why emphasis is placed on local epidemiological studies (community diagnosis, needs assessment) in commu-
nity-orientated primary health care (Kark, 1981; Abramson, 1988),
health care in schools and work-places, district health care (Vaughan
and Morrow, 1989), and other settings.

But the validity of generalizations from a study sample or population
to another population (the 'external validity' of the study) always
requires consideration. Populations differ in their health problems and
in the occurrence of risk and protective factors; causal processes that are
important in one population may be unimportant in another; and there
is wide variation in circumstances that may influence the effectiveness
of interventions. In planning a health promotion programme in a specific community, can use be made of information derived from a neigh-
bouring or similar community, or of information collected at a national
level? When planning a new programme, to what extent is it justifiable
to use the results of evaluative studies conducted elsewhere? Are the
results of studies of men applicable to women? Are results applicable
across ethnic or age categories? Such questions may be hard to answer.

Is the information sufficient?

However valid and relevant, the information may not suffice for the
purpose for which it is required, and there may be a need for more information about the population whose care is under consideration (i.e. a
fuller community diagnosis) or for information from epidemiological
studies elsewhere, as well as for information (e.g. on costs) from non-epi-
demiological sources.

The adequacy of the information will depend on the purpose for
which it is required. For example, to decide whether there is a sufficiently strong case to warrant intervention, it is not enough to know

that a problem exists, or even to have a quantitative measure of its occurrence. Three other main categories of information may be needed:

1. *Information about the importance of the problem* – e.g. its impact on mortality or the quality of life, and its relative importance compared with other problems competing for the same resources. A measure of impact may be more informative than a risk ratio; it is more helpful to know that 26–43 per cent of various asthma-like symptoms in young women in towns in East Anglia are attributable to the use of gas for cooking (Jarvis *et al.*, 1996; Brauer and Kennedy, 1996) than to know that the risk of these symptoms is elevated slightly in homes that use gas stoves.
2. *Facts relevant to the feasibility of intervention.* In the specific context, appraisal of feasibility may require information not only about costs and the availability of economic, professional and other resources, but about the community's felt needs and demands, its readiness and capacity to participate, prevalent attitudes and health practices, the nature and extent of the care presently available and given, the readiness of educational, welfare and other agencies to play their part, and so on.
3. *Information with a bearing on the predicted effectiveness and possible harmful effects of interventions*, taking account of biological, social, cultural and economic characteristics of the population (perceptions of the problem, probable compliance, etc.) and the results of evaluative studies elsewhere.

If it is intended to single out high-risk groups for special attention in a preventive programme, it is not enough to know that the probability that the disease or other problem will occur is higher – even many times so – when a given risk marker is present. Consideration must also be given to such features as the marker's estimated sensitivity and predictive value. The marker cannot be very helpful if it identifies only a small fraction of prospective cases; and if it identifies very many people who are not prospective cases this will impair the programme's cost-effectiveness and ethical justification. It may be helpful to know how many people must avoid exposure to a risk factor in order to prevent one case.

Similar considerations arise if screening tests are to be used to identify people with a high probability of currently having a particular disorder. Decisions may require such information as that 4,000 women had to be screened to prevent each death from breast cancer, and about 400,000 tests and 200 biopsies are required to prevent one case of cervical cancer (Wall, 1995).

If it is proposed to communicate information to members of the public, community leaders, or decision-makers in order to modify individual behaviour or public policy, it is important to have the right facts for this purpose, expressed in language (or pictures) that non-professionals will easily understand. Information about smoking hazards, for example, might include estimates of the percentages of deaths, cases and hospital admissions that are attributable to smoking, and the effect on average life expectancy. As a final illustration, when appraising the value of a programme it may not be enough to know that the objective e.g. a reduction in the prevalence of hypertension – has been achieved. However encouraging this may be, the outcome cannot (except in a well-controlled programme trial) be attributed to the programme unless other possible explanations have been explored and there is also supportive evidence from a process evaluation (a look into the 'black box' concealing the programme's mechanism) providing information on coverage, the performance of programme activities, utilisation of services, compliance with treatment, etc.

Conclusion

Information alone cannot modify health. Health educators have long abandoned the simplistic idea that the transfer of information will itself produce changes in individual health behaviour. At a public policy level, decision-makers are influenced by powerful factors other than the information at their disposal, which they sometimes reject or ignore.

But there is no doubt that if health care is to be planned rationally and provided effectively, appropriate information – especially from epidemiological sources – is essential; or that the communication of information is one of the tools that, used in unison, can modify behaviour and policy.

The availability of suitable information depends, ultimately, on epidemiologists' perception of their role in health promotion and on the development of epidemiological theory and methods to fulfil this function (Wall, 1995). The agenda for epidemiologists interested in applications to health promotion includes the following requirements:

1. A macrosocial view (Susser, 1987) – more attention to societal factors, such as economic, political and ideological processes and their interrelationships with health and health care.
2. Improved methods of community diagnosis and surveillance, and methods of monitoring health programmes in local communities, schools and work-places.
3. Development of methods of measuring and predicting the outcomes of interventions, in terms relevant to the interests of decision-makers and the public.
4. Development of rapid epidemiological methods (Scrimshaw and Hurtado, 1987; Smith, 1989) that can provide real-time answers to practical questions.

5. Improved techniques of meta-analysis for nonexperimental studies, especially the exploration of reasons for heterogeneous findings (Petitti, 1994).
6. Improved methods of communication with users of epidemiological information – health workers, decision-makers, mass media, and the public. Epidemiologists should make recommendations on whether and how their results should be applied in practice, and not just 'light the touch paper and then stand back' (Pharaoh, 1996).

The importance of epidemiology in health promotion is unquestioned. Even critics who say that epidemiology relies heavily on judgement, that 'epidemiological attribution of causation is not a science but an activity more akin to the arguing of a case in law: based on evidence but not dictated by the evidence', and that it cannot at present produce predictions as reliable as those produced by some other scientific disciplines (Charlton, 1996), do not question that it can bring together evidence in a way that permits decision-making in situations where there is no completely valid answer.

But the available information in a given study or at a given time may be defective, judgement may be variable or faulty, and external validity may be limited, so that it is not surprising that conflicting conclusions are often reached, or that reversals sometimes occur as new knowledge replaces old. Every review of controlled trials published by the Cochrane Collaboration is accompanied by a quotation from Xenophanes (c. 570–475 BC): 'Through seeking we may learn and know things better. But as for certain truth, no man hath known it, for all is but a woven web of guesses' (Chalmers, 1995).

Epidemiological information should never be accepted with undue haste or blind trust.

References

Abramson, J. H. (1988). Community-oriented primary care – strategy, approaches, and practice: a review, *Public Health Reviews*, 16, 35–98.

Abramson, J. H. (1990). *Survey Methods in Community Medicine: Epidemiological studies, programme evaluation, clinical trials*, 4th edn. Edinburgh: Churchill Livingstone.

Abramson, J. H. (1991). Cross-sectional studies. In Holland, W. W., Detels, R. and Knox, G. (eds), *Oxford Textbook of Public Health*, 2nd edn, 2, *Methods of Public Health*. Oxford University Press, 107–20.

Abramson, J. H. (1994). *Making Sense of Data: A self-instruction manual on the interpretation of epidemiologic data*, 2nd edn. New York: Oxford University Press.

American Health Foundation (1982). Conference report: weak associations in epidemiology and their interpretation, *Preventive Medicine*, 11, 464–76.

Angell, M. and Kassirer, J. P. (1994). Clinical research – what should the public believe?, *New England Journal of Medicine*, 331, 189–90.

Berkelman, R. L. and Buehler, J. W. (1991). Surveillance. In Holland, W. W., Detels, R. and Knox, G. (eds), *Oxford Textbook of Public Health*, 2nd edn, 2, *Methods of Public Health*. Oxford University Press, 161–76.

Brauer, M. and Kennedy, S. M. (1996). Gas stoves and respiratory health, *Lancet*, 347, 412.

Chalmers, I. (1993). The Cochrane Collaboration: preparing, maintaining and disseminating systematic reviews of the effects of health care, *Annals of the New York Academy of Sciences*, 703, 156–63.

Chalmers, I. (1995). What would Archie Cochrane have said? *Lancet*, 346, 1300.

Chalmers, I., Adams, M., Dickersin, K., Hetherington, J., Tarnow- Mordi, W., Meinert, C., Tonascia, S. and Chalmers, T. C. (1990). A cohort study of summary reports of clinical trials, JAMA, 263, 1401–5.

Charlton, B. G. (1995). A critique of Geoffrey Rose's 'population strategy' for preventive medicine, *Journal of the Royal Society of Medicine*, 88, 607–10.

Charlton, B. G. (1996). Attribution of causation in epidemiology: chain or mosaic?, *Journal of Clinical Epidemiology*, 49, 105–7.

Court, C. (1995). Britain: Incidence reduced by two thirds in five years, *British Medical Journal*, 310, 7–8.

de Semir, V. (1996). What is newsworthy?, *Lancet*, 347, 1163–6.

Detels, R. (1991). Epidemiology: the foundation of public health. In Holland, W. W., Detels, R. and Knox, G. (eds), *Oxford Textbook of Public Health*, 2nd edn, *2, Methods of Public Health*. Oxford University Press, 285–91.

Doll, R. and Hill, A. B. (1964). Mortality in relation to smoking: ten years' observations of British doctors, *British Medical Journal*, 1, 1399–410, 1460–7.

Feinleib, M., Breslow, N. E. and Detels, R. (1991). Cohort studies. In Holland, W. W., Detels, R. and Knox, G. (eds), *Oxford Textbook of Public Health*, 2nd edn, *2, Methods of Public Health*. Oxford University Press, 145–59.

Feldman, W. and Feldman, M. E. (1996). The intelligence on infant feeding, *Lancet*, 347, 1057.

Gahlinger, P. M. and Abramson, J. H. (1995). *Computer Programs for Epidemiologic Analysis: PEPI Version 2*. Stone Mountain, Georgia: USD.

Gail, M. H. (1996). Statistics in action, *Journal of the American Statistical Association*, 91, 1–13.

Gale, C. R. and Martyn, C. N. (1996). Breastfeeding, dummy use, and adult intelligence, *Lancet*, 347, 1072–5.

Gershman, K. (1992). Case-control study of which dogs bite (abstract), *American Journal of Epidemiology*, 138, 593.

Gershman, K. A., Sacks, J. J. and Wright, J. C. (1994). Which dogs bite? A case-control study of risk factors, *Pediatrics*, 93, 913–17.

Greenberg, R. S. and Ibrahim, M. A. (1991). The case-control study. In Holland, W. W., Detels, R. and Knox, G. (eds), *Oxford Textbook of Public Health*, 2nd edn, *2, Methods of Public Health*. Oxford University Press, 121–43.

Greenland, S. (ed.) (1987). *Evolution of Epidemiologic Ideas: Annotated readings on concepts and methods*, Chestnut Hill, Mass.: Epidemiology Resources.

Greenland, S. (1991). Concepts of validity in epidemiological research. In Holland, W. W., Detels, R. and Knox, G. (eds.), *Oxford Textbook of Public Health*, 2nd edn, *2, Methods of Public Health*. Oxford University Press, 254–70.

Hammond, E. C. (1966). Smoking in relation to the death rates on one million men and women. In Haenszel, W. (ed.), *Epidemiological Approaches to the Study of Cancer and Other Chronic Diseases*. Bethesda, Md.: Public Health Service, US Department of Health, Education and Welfare, National Cancer Institute Monograph, 19, 127–204.

Hemenway, D., Feskanich, D. and Colditz, D. A. (1995). Body height and risk fracture: a cohort study of 90,000 women, *International Journal of Epidemiology*, 24, 783–6.

Hill, A. B. (1965). The environment and disease: association or causation?, *Proceedings of the Royal Society of Medicine*, 58, 295–300, reprinted in Greenland, S. (ed.) (1987) *Evolution of Epidemiologic Ideas: Annotated readings on concepts and methods*. Chestnut Hill, Mass: Epidemiology Resources.

Hulley, S.P. and Cummings, S. R. (eds) (1988). *Designing Clinical Research*. Baltimore, Md: Williams & Wilkins.

Hunt, C. E. (1994). Infant sleep position and sudden infant death syndrome risk: a time for change, *Pediatrics*, 94, 105–7.

Jarvis, D., Chinn, S., Luczynska, C. and Burney, P. (1996). Association of respiratory symptoms and lung function in young adults with use of domestic gas appliances, *Lancet*, 347, 426–31.

Kahn, H. A. (1966). The Dorn study of smoking and mortality among US veterans: report on eight and one-half years of observation. In Haenszel, W. (ed.), *Epidemiological Approaches to the Study of Cancer and Other Chronic Diseases*. Bethesda, Md: Public Health Service, US Department of Health, Education and Welfare, National Cancer Institute Monograph, 19, 1–125.

Kahn, H. A. and Sempos, C. T. (1989). *Statistical Methods in Epidemiology*. New York: Oxford University Press.

Kark, S. L. (1981). *The Practice of Community-Oriented Primary Health Care*. New York: Appleton-Century-Crofts, reprinted (1989) Jerusalem: Akademon (Hebrew University).

Kattwinkel, J., Brooks, J. and Myerberg, D. (1992). Positioning and SIDS: AAP task force on infant positioning and SIDS, *Pediatrics*, 89, 1120–6.

Lancet (1995). Editorial: *Shall we nim a horse?*, *Lancet*, 345, 1585–6.

Last, J. M. (ed.), (1995). *A Dictionary of Epidemiology*, 3rd edn. New York: Oxford University Press.

Lichtenstein, M. J., Mulrow, C. D. and Elwood, P. C. (1987). Guidelines for reading case-control studies, *Journal of Chronic Diseases*, 40, 893–903.

Lind, J. (1753). *A Treatise of the Scurvy*. Edinburgh: Sands, Murray & Cochrane, reprinted (1953), Edinburgh: Edinburgh University Press.

Mann, C. C. (1995). Press coverage: leaving out the big picture, *Science*, 269, 166.

Petitti, D. B. (1994). *Meta-analysis, Decision Analysis and Cost-Effectiveness Analysis: Methods for quantitative synthesis in medicine*. New York: Oxford University Press.

Pharaoh, P. (1996). Bed-sharing and sudden infant death, *Lancet*, 347, 2.

Pini, P. (1995). Media wars, *Lancet*, 346, 1681–3.

Pott, P. (1775). *Percival Pott's Contribution to Cancer Research*. Reproduced in Potter, M. (1963). Washington, DC, National Cancer Institute Monograph, 10.

Puska, P. (1991). Intervention and experimental studies. In Holland, W. W., Detels, R. and Knox, G. (eds), *Oxford Textbook of Public Health*, 2nd edn, 2, *Methods of Public Health*. Oxford University Press, 177–87.

Rothman, K. J., (ed) (1988). *Causal Inference*. Chestnut Hill, Mass.: Epidemiology Resources.

Schlesselman, J. J. (1982). *Case-control Studies: Design, conduct, analysis*. New York: Oxford University Press.

Scragg, R. K. R., Mitchell, E. A., Stewart, A. W., Ford, R. P. K., Taylor, B. J., Hassall, I. B., Williams, S. M. and Thompson, J. M. D. (1996). Infant room-sharing and prone sleep position in sudden infant death syndrome, *Lancet*, 347, 7–11.

Scrimshaw, S. C. M. and Hurtado, E. (1987). *Rapid Assessment Procedures for Nutrition and Primary Health Care: Anthropological approaches to improving programme effectiveness*. Los Angeles: UCLA Latin American Center Publications.

Selvin, S. (1996). *Statistical Analysis of Epidemiologic Data*, 2nd edn. New York: Oxford University Press.

Skrabanek, P. (1994). The emptiness of the black box, *Epidemiology*, 5, 553–5.

Smith, G. S. (1989). Development of rapid epidemiologic assessment methods to evaluate health status and delivery of health services, *International Journal of Epidemiology*, 18, (Supp. 2), S1.

Snow, J. (1855). *On the Mode of Communication of Cholera*, 2nd edn. London: Churchill, reprinted in Frost, W. H. (ed.) (1936), *Snow on Cholera*. New York: Commonwealth Fund (reprinted 1965, New York: Hafner).

Stolley, P. D. and Schlesselman, J. J. (1982). Planning and conducting a study. In Schlesselman, J. J., *Case-Control Studies: Design, conduct, analysis*. New York: Oxford University Press, 101–4.

Susser, M. (1973). *Causal Thinking in the Health Sciences*. New York: Oxford University Press.

Susser, M. (1986). The logic of Sir Karl Popper and the practice of epidemiology, *American Journal of Epidemiology*, 124, 711–18.

Susser, M. (1987). *Epidemiology, Health, & Society: Selected papers*. New York: Oxford University Press, 171–232.

Swan, A. V. (1991). Statistical methods. In Holland, W. W., Detels, R. and Knox, G. (eds.), *Oxford Textbook of Public Health*, 2nd edn, *2, Methods of Public Health*. Oxford University Press, 189–223.

Taubes, G. (1995). Epidemiology faces its limits, *Science*, 269, 164–9.

Terris, M. (ed.) (1964). *Goldberger on Pellagra*. Baton Rouge: Louisiana State University Press.

Vaughan, J. P. and Morrow, R. H. (eds) (1989). *Manual of Epidemiology for District Health Management*. Geneva: World Health Organization.

Wall, S. (1995). Epidemiology for prevention, *International Journal of Epidemiology*, 24, 655–64.

Wigfield, R., Gilbert, R. and Fleming, P. J. (1994). SIDS: risk reduction measures, *Early Human Development*, 38, 161–4.

Williams, S. M., Taylor, B. J., Mitchell, E. A. and other members of the National Cot Death Study Group (1996). Sudden infant death syndrome: Insulation from bedding and clothing and its effect modifiers, *International Journal of Epidemiology*, 25, 366–75.

Willinger, M. (1995). SIDS Prevention, *Pediatric Annals*, 24, 358–64.

14 Explaining the French paradox*

Michael L. Burr

The French paradox

In many Western countries, including Britain, the biggest single cause of death is ischaemic heart disease (IHD). There are, however, some European countries where IHD mortality is much lower, and one of them is France, which has the second lowest IHD death-rate among developed countries, just above that of Japan. The differences are not trivial: the mean age-standardized IHD death rates for men and women in Austria, Germany and the Netherlands are twice the French rate, and those in the United Kingdom and Denmark are three times as high (Renaud and de Lorgeril, 1992). The question arises as to why the French are so fortunate.

Differences in fat intake are not the explanation: the average consumption of dairy fat is similar in all the above countries, although it is substantially lower in other Mediterranean countries that share France's low IHD mortality. The three classical IHD risk factors – blood pressure, serum cholesterol and cigarette smoking – are no lower in France than in other industrialized countries. These observations led Renaud and de Lorgeril (1992) to draw attention to 'the French paradox' of a low IHD mortality associated with a high intake of saturated fat and with other risk factors. A paper in the *Lancet* (Criqui and Ringel, 1994) examined data from 21 developed countries in an effort to resolve this paradox.

Is it an artefact?

Before we turn our attention to the various peculiarities of the French lifestyle as possible solutions, we should first ask whether the differences in death rates are real. Whenever the data from one country are markedly out of line with those from other areas, the possibility must be considered that there is some artefact of nomenclature or classification. Diagnosis is at best an inexact science, and when causes of death are entered on death certificates the wording may vary according to the certifying doctor's training, presuppositions and language as well as the actual pathology. Many deaths involve more than one disease process,

---

* From *Journal of the Royal Society of Health*, (August 1995), 217–19.

and the doctor has to decide which to select as the underlying cause of death; if several are mentioned on the death certificate the order in which they appear will determine how the death is ultimately classified. Fashions in terminology and certification are known to vary from one country to another, so that differences in disease-specific death rates should not necessarily be taken at face value.

The MONICA project set up by the World Health Organization has provided some information about the comparability of mortality and morbidity statistics from different countries. The results suggested that death certificate diagnoses are not the same in all populations, as there may be differential reporting of potential coronary deaths.

Three areas of France that participated in the study appeared to have very low IHD death rates, but on investigation it transpired that some deaths that elsewhere would be attributed to IHD were in France described in some other (usually vaguer) way. This appears to contribute to the French paradox, but it does not wholly explain it, since even when the French death rates were corrected for this low bias they still remained relatively low (Tunstall-Pedoe *et al.*, 1994).

Is it the wine?

It seems, then, that the French really do have lower IHD death rates than might be expected from their fat intake, serum cholesterol levels, blood pressures and smoking habits. Something about the French way of life must give them some protection from this disease.

France is famous for its wines, and the hypothesis that wine is the protective agent seems to have gained wide acceptance among the public at large. It certainly is an attractive idea. It also has some support from the evidence, particularly when different countries are compared with respect to their wine intakes and IHD death rates. St Leger *et al.*, (1979) examined various data from eighteen developed countries and found that IHD mortality was related positively to intakes of total and saturated fats, and negatively to alcohol consumption. When alcohol intake was classified as wine, beers and spirits, the alcohol effect appeared to be entirely accounted for by the wine intake. The wine effect was undiminished whatever other variables (such as gross national product, cigarettes, or diet) were taken into account. The analysis was repeated with France excluded (because of the possibility that France under-reports IHD deaths), but the results were not substantially altered. The authors concluded that a protective effect of wine is likely to be due to constituents other than alcohol. They regretted that they were unable to advise their friends about the relative advantages of red, white or rosé wine.

Some evidence on this latter point has been supplied by work on the

anti-oxidant properties of red wine. There are certain phenolic compounds in red wine with properties that powerfully counteract the oxidation of low-density lipoprotein (LDL) in the blood, a process which
contributes to the arterial damage underlying IHD (Frankel *et al.*, 1993).
The authors considered that their results provided a plausible explanation of the French paradox. Furthermore, a study in healthy volunteers
showed that the consumption of red (but not white) wine with meals
reduces the susceptibility of plasma and LDL to lipid peroxidation
(Fuhrman *et al.*, 1995).

Is it the alcohol?

The evidence pointing specifically to wine as the protective agent is
drawn largely from comparisons between countries, in terms of their
IHD death rates and *per capita* wine consumption. Another approach is
to record the drinking habits of a large number of individuals, follow
them up over time, and relate their initial intakes to their subsequent
development of (or death from) IHD. There have been numerous studies
of this kind, in different countries. and the results have been remarkably
consistent in showing that the incidence and mortality of IHD are
higher among moderate drinkers than among, non-drinkers (Burr, 1994).
A follow-up of British doctors confirmed previous studies in this regard
(Doll *et al.*, 1994). The relationship between alcohol consumption, and
all-cause mortality is U-shaped – i.e. the protection afforded by a moderate intake against IHD is not offset by increased deaths from other
causes, although at higher intakes this is certainly the case. Two recent
studies suggest that alcohol may protect against non-insulin-dependent
diabetes, a condition related to IHD (Perry *et al.*, 1995; Rimm *et al.*,
1995).

In most of these studies of individuals (as distinct from between-
country comparisons) any alcoholic drinks appear to be protective. In an
American study, wine and beer appeared to be similarly protective, but
'liquor' (spirits) was not associated with any reduction in risk (Klatsky
and Armstrong, 1993). Preference for red wine did not confer any advantage – indeed, those who preferred other types of wine had a marginally
lower risk. A Danish study found that mortality from cardiovascular and
cerebrovascular disease appeared to be reduced by beer-drinking and
(especially) wine-drinking, but not by drinking spirits; wine-drinkers had
the further advantage of a lower all-cause mortality (Grønbaek *et al.*,
1995). People who chose different types of alcohol may differ in other
ways, however; those who drink spirits tend to have unfavourable characteristics that may outweigh any protection derived from the alcohol.

Some of the physiological effects of alcohol could account for its
apparent effect on IHD. It raises the blood concentration of high-density

lipoprotein, which is negatively associated with IHD risk (Burr *et al.*, 1986). A negative (favourable) association with plasma insulin has been reported in women (Razay *et al.*, 1992). Alcohol has favourable associations with plasma fibrinogen (negative) and blood fibrinolytic activity (positive), which affect the formation of blood clots (Meade *et al.*, 1979). The French custom of drinking wine with the meal may confer extra benefit in that the alcohol is absorbed slowly and thus has a prolonged effect on clotting factors at a time when they are adversely affected by dietary fat: this protection has been detected experimentally 13 hours later (Hendriks *et al.*, 1994). Alcohol reduces platelet aggregation, another component of the clotting mechanism that operates in heart attacks, and this action presumably accounts for the observation that platelet aggregation was 55 per cent lower in French farmers than in Scottish farmers (Renaud and de Lorgeril, 1992). These observations have led to the conclusion that the French paradox is soluble – it can be explained by the fact that the French have the highest intake of alcohol in the world (Criqui and Ringel, 1994).

Is it the diet?

The authors just quoted considered the possibility of a dietary explanation, but dismissed it because of inconsistencies when data from different years were compared. A more detailed analysis examined the consumption of various nutrients in seventeen European countries (Bellizzi *et al.*, 1994). This analysis showed that IHD mortality was positively related to dairy products and their characteristic fatty acids, and negatively related to wine, vegetables, vegetable oils, vitamin C, β-carotene. and α-tocopherol (a component of vitamin E): the strongest relationships were with α-tocopherol, wine and vegetables. Mean blood levels of α-tocopherol, vitamin C and carotene show a similar inverse association with national IHD death rates, the α-tocopherol being the most important (Gey *et al.*, 1993). Each of these nutrients has antioxidant properties that may be relevant to IHD risk

A randomized trial of a 'Mediterranean diet' has been conducted in France and showed a significant reduction in IHD mortality in men who had recently recovered from a heart attack (de Lorgeril *et al.*, 1994). Although the authors laid special emphasis on the fatty acid composition of the diet it involved a higher intake of fruit and vegetables and produced higher blood levels of vitamins C and E. Follow-up studies of individuals showed that people with a higher vitamin E intake had a lower risk of IHD death (Rimm *et al.*, 1993: Stampfer *et al.*, 1993). These and other considerations led Bellizzi *et al.* (1994) to conclude that the 'European paradox' (as they prefer to call it) is explained by vitamin E, derived from various sources of which wine is only one.

What can we conclude?

The French paradox is exaggerated by under-reporting of IHD deaths but not entirely explained by it. Something about the French (and southern European) lifestyle seems to protect against IHD, despite unfavourable factors such as fat intake, blood cholesterol, blood pressure and smoking habit.

Two main explanations have emerged: alcohol and anti-oxidants. Both are known to affect physiological processes in ways that could reduce IHD risk. Both are characteristic of France, being found together in wine though not restricted to it. It is perhaps noteworthy that Criqui and Ringel (1994) found the negative association between IHD and wine ethanol to be stronger than the associations with total ethanol (as would be expected if alcohol were the only factor) or with wine volume (as would occur if something specific to wine were responsible). Maybe the French habit of drinking with the meal rather than at some later time confers additional benefit.

What are the practical implications? Criqui and Ringel point out that the cardioprotective effect of alcohol in France is cancelled out by increases in other causes of death. The U-shaped curve relating alcohol to all-cause mortality suggests that a moderate intake (say two drinks daily) may confer benefits which are not outweighed by other risks. Maybe if we eat more fruit and vegetables and drink wine with our meals we can be less worried about our blood cholesterol and so share the benefits of the French paradox.

References

Bellizzi, M. C., Franklin, D. E., Duthie, G. G. and James, W. P. T. (1994). Vitamin E and coronary heart disease: the European paradox, *European Journal of Clinical Nutrition*, 48, 822–31.

Burr, M. L. (1994). Alcohol and ischaemic heart disease, *Journal of the Royal Society of Health*, 114, 216–18.

Burr, M. L. Fehily, A. M., Butland B. K., Bolton, C. H. and Eastham, R. D. (1986). Alcohol and high density lipoprotein cholesterol: a randomised controlled trial, *British Journal of Nutrition*, 56, 81–6.

Criqui, M. H. and Ringel, B. L. (1994). Does diet or alcohol explain the French paradox? *Lancet*, 344, 1719–23.

de Lorgeril, M., Renaud, S., Mamelle, N., Salen, P., Martin, J.-L., Manjaud, I., Guidollet, J., Touboul, P. and Delaye, J. (1994). Mediterranean alpha-linolenic acid-rich diet in secondary prevention of coronary heart disease, *Lancet*, 343, 1454–9.

Doll, R., Peto, R., Hall, E., Wheatley, K. and Gray, R. (1994). Mortality in relation to consumption of alcohol: 13 years observations on male British doctors, *British Medical Journal*, 309, 911–18.

Frankel, E. N., Kanner, J., German, J. B., Parks, E. and Kinsella, J. E. (1993). Inhibition of oxidation of human low-density lipoprotein by phenolic substances in red wine, *Lancet*, 341, 454–7.

Fuhrman, B., Lavy, A. and Aviram, M. (1995). Consumption of red wine with meals reduces the susceptibilities of human plasma and low-density lipoprotein to lipid peroxidation. *American Journal of Clinical Nutrition*, 61, 549–54.

Gey, K. F., Moser, U. K., Jordan, P., Stahelin, H. B., Eichholzer, M. and Lüdin, E. (1993). Increased risk of cardio-vascular disease at suboptimal plasma concentrations of essential antioxidants: an epidemiological update with special attention to carotene and vitamin C, *American Journal of Clinical Nutrition*, 57, 787S–975.

Grønbaek, M., Deis, A., Sorensen, T. I. A., Becker, U., Schnohr, P. and Jensen, G. (1995). Mortality associated with moderate intakes of wine, beer and spirits, *British Medical Journal*, 310, 1163–9.

Hendriks, H. F. J., Veenstra, J., Wierik, E. J. M. V-te., Schaafsma, G. and Kluft, C. (1994). Effect of moderate dose of alcohol with evening meal on fibrinolytic factors, *British Medical Journal*, 308, 1003–6.

Klatsky, A. L. and Armstrong, M. A. (1993). Alcoholic beverage choice and risk of coronary artery disease mortality: do red wine drinkers fare best?, *American Journal of Cardiology*, 71, 467–9.

Meade, T. W., Chakrebarti, R., Haines, A. P., North, W. R. S. and Stirling, Y. (1979). Characteristics affecting fibrinolytic activity and plasma fibrinogen concentrations, *British Medical Journal*, 1, 153–6.

Perry, I. J., Wannamethee, S. G., Walker, M. K., Thomson, A. G., Whincup, P. H. and Shaper, A. G. (1995). Prospective study of risk factors for development of non-insulin dependent diabetes in middle aged British men, *British Medical Journal*, 310, 560–4.

Razay, G., Heaton, K. W., Bolton, C. H. and Hughes, A. O. (1992) Alcohol consumption and its relation to cardiovascular risk factors in British women, *British Medical Journal*, 304, 80–3.

Renaud, S. and De Lorgeril, M. (1992). Wine, alcohol, platelets, and the French paradox for coronary heart disease, *Lancet*, 339, 1523–6.

Rimm, E. B., Chan, J., Stampfer, M. J., Colditz, G. A. and Willett, W. C. (1995). Prospective study of cigarette smoking, alcohol use, and the risk of diabetes in men, *British Medical Journal*, 310, 555–9.

Rimm, E. B., Stampfer, M. J., Ascherio, A., Giovannucci, E., Colditz, A. and Willett, W. C. (1993). Vitamin E consumption and the risk of coronary heart disease in men, *New England Journal of Medicine*, 328, 1450–6.

St Leger, A. S., Cochrane, A. L. and Moore, F. (1979). Factors associated with cardiac mortality in developed countries with particular reference to the consumption of wine, *Lancet*, 1, 1017–20.

Stampfer, M. J., Hennekens, C. H., Manson, J. E., Colditz, G. A., Rosner, B. and Willett, W. C. (1993). Vitamin E consumption and the risk of coronary disease in women, *New England Journal of Medicine*, 328, 1444–9.

Tunstall-Pedoe, H., Kuulasmaa, K., Amouyel, P., Arveiler, D., Rajakangas, A-m. and Pajak, A. (1994). Myocardial infarction and coronary deaths in the World Health Organization MONICA Project. Registration procedures, event rates, and case fatality rates in 38 populations from 21 countries in four continents, *Circulation*, 90, 583–612.

15 Job-loss and family morbidity: a study of a factory closure*

Norman Beale and Susan Nethercott

Introduction

There can be little doubt that losing one's job is likely to be a traumatic experience. However, work itself is often stressful – many people are paid poorly for jobs which are tedious, grimy and sometimes dangerous. Nevertheless, despite the economic support provided by social security, most unemployed people repeatedly look for a job, at least while there remains any prospect of obtaining one. Clearly there must be incentives to work over and above any financial gain. These 'latent functions' of work were first described in the 1930s (Jahoda *et al.*, 1973) and later classified by Jahoda (1979) as follows:

- the imposition of a time structure on the day;
- regularly shared experiences;
- the linking of an individual to goals and purposes which transcend his own;
- the donation of personal status and identity;
- the enforcement of activity;

If work can gratify so many needs, the effects on the individual losing his job must be substantial. Childbirth, marriage and retirement are other examples of important psycho-social transitions (Murray Parkes, 1971) but the event for which increases in morbidity and even mortality have been most clearly demonstrated is bereavement (Dewi-Rees and Lutkins, 1967). The psychopathology of job-loss has been staged chronologically (as with bereavement); shock, optimism, pessimism, fatalism and eventual adaptation (Harrison, 1976). However, in the case of unemployment, there is little real evidence that these emotional upheavals result in increased psychiatric and/or physical morbidity. Watkins has summarized the problem of studying the health of the unemployed:

> Comparisons of the health of employed people with that of the unemployed are confounded by the fact that unemployment falls disproportionately on groups who would be expected to have worse

---

* From *Journal of the Royal College of General Practitioners*, 35 (November 1985), 510–14.

health, such as the lower social classes, people who live in deprived areas, people who work in declining industries, and people whose ability to work has been affected by their health. (Watkins, 1984)

It is possible to overcome this problem by studying a group of workers who have stable work records and subsequently lose their jobs because of the closure of their place of work. This type of investigation can demonstrate a causal relationship between unemployment and health; for example, that job-loss results in a decline in health.

Few studies of this type have been performed. Of the five studies reported in the literature (Jacobsen, 1972), none studied families, and none were carried out by British general practitioners. Comparative review of these studies is difficult, since all the groups used different criteria to measure morbidity. The longest (three and a half years) study was carried out by Iverson and Klausen (1981). Fisher (1965) and Westin and Norum (1977) studied women as well as men but did not distinguish between them. The only large, controlled study was that of Kasl and colleagues who examined 105 men before and after job-loss in two factories in the USA in the early 1960s (Kasl *et al.*, 1968; Kasl *et al.*, 1975). This particular study, and also that of Jacobsen (1972) detected an increase in morbidity on anticipation of unemployment.

None of these workers was able to use sequential long-term records, such as are available in general practices in this country, to establish a baseline of morbidity for their study subjects. Moreover, as Kasl has reported (1983), many of the findings may not now be applicable with the increase in unemployment rates in the 1990s. If unemployment does influence health this is likely to be of increasing significance, particularly for general practice as family doctors in Britain manage over 90 per cent of all reported illness without referral to specialist facilities.

Redundancies in Calne

In the first six months of 1982, the unemployment rate in the Calne area was 8.1 per cent – 9.3 per cent for men and 6.4 per cent for women (local Department of Employment statistics). Then, on 1 July 1982, the factory of C. and T. Harris (Calne) Ltd (manufacturers of bacon, sausages and pies) established in Calne in 1770, finally closed. For over two centuries the factory had been the most important work-place in the town and, until the mid-1960s, the only significant industrial concern.

The slaughterhouse and bacon-curing departments had closed, with little warning, in June 1979 – 86 men had lost their jobs leaving a workforce of approximately 800 in the factory. In January 1980, a further mass redundancy of 411 employees was announced. The workforce remaining after March 1980 were then given to understand that the company had a year in which to 'break even' and this veiled threat of complete closure took two years to realize.

Health care in Calne

Calne is a small market town with a population of 11,000. It is surrounded by numerous sparsely populated rural communities with a further 4,000 people. The main employment within the town is now light industry.

Primary care in Calne is provided by two long-established practices. One group of four doctors (on which this study is based) works from a purpose-built heath centre which was opened in 1970; 11,500 patients are registered there. The other practice is two handed and serves the remainder of the population. There have been no substantial changes in the characteristics of the population in the ten years since the health centre opened, and patient turnover is below the national average.

The nearest district general hospital is 17 miles away and there is no community hospital in the town. Therefore, even when patients are emergencies or casualties, virtually all would first contact their own general practitioner or one of his partners.

Aims

This longitudinal study aimed to examine consultations, episodes of illness, referrals to hospital, and attendances at hospital out-patient departments in the families of workers made compulsorily redundant and in their control counterparts – families of other industrial workers who remained stably employed. As with other factory closure studies the null hypothesis for testing was that there would be no significant differences in these indices of morbidity in relation to job-loss. It was also hoped that the general practice records for these families (the only source of the data) would indicate our professional awareness of the employees' present occupational status.

Method

Subjects

A list of the names and addresses of all 302 employees made redundant from C. and T. Harris (Calne) Ltd between 18 June and 16 July 1982 was obtained from the personnel department of the firm. The company also supplied the following information for each employee: date of entry into the factory; hours of work; type of occupation – productive, clerical and so on; and department in the factory.

Identification of those employees who were registered with the practice proved to be quite simple using this information. Cross-reference with practice records and the local electoral roll allowed identification of dependent relatives – defined as spouses and, as at 30 June 1982, children aged 16 years and under who live at home.

The employees and their dependent relatives were incorporated into the study if:

1. The family were registered with the practice for the entire study period.
2. The employees were engaged by the company continuously for the entire study period (prior to redundancy).
3. The employees were engaged full-time, that is, 37 hours or more per week (there were insufficient part-time employees to form a separate group).
4. The employees were engaged in a productive or clerical capacity; that is, in Registrar General's social classes 3, 4 and 5 (there were insufficient managerial staff to examine separately).

After applying these criteria, men aged 61 years or over and women aged 56 years or over were omitted from the study as, in effect, they were experiencing early retirement.

C. and T. Harris (Calne) Ltd had been the largest employer in the practice area. Therefore, all the other local firms were approached in seeking control subjects. Seven firms, dealing in a variety of products and services, were each able to provide a minimum of 10 long-term employees who fulfilled criteria analogous to the employees at the Harris factory but they had not been subject to redundancy at any time during the study period.

Study period

The study period was taken to be 1 July 1976 to 30 June 1984. The eight years of the study period were denoted as years one to eight. The study period allowed observation of the study cohort during six years of continuous employment and during the two subsequent years after redundancy. Similarly it allowed observation of the control cohort for eight years, a period in which they remained continuously and fully employed.

Observations

Consultations, reported episodes of illness and referrals to specialists were recorded as defined in the instructions for the third national morbidity study (1981–2) (OPCS *et al.*, 1981). However, attendances at antenatal clinics and other similar patient-contacts were not recorded. The number of attendances at hospital casualty and out-patient departments and the number of admissions to, and number of days in hospital were also recorded for each year. At no stage were any of the subjects approached personally – all the information was obtained from their medical records.

A search was also made in the medical file of each employee for any written record of their place or type of occupation. For the group employed by Harris Ltd, it was also ascertained whether or not there were any comments intimating unemployment.

A data card was constructed for each individual and these were filed in family groups.

Statistical testing

In this study the Mann–Whitney U test was applied to the data concerning consultations and episodes of illness while the Wilcoxon rank sum test was used for the data concerning referrals to, and attendances at hospital out-patient departments.

Results

The study group originally consisted of 133 Harris employees. Four of these employees left Calne in the two years after redundancy and they were omitted from the study. The remaining 129 employees consisted of 80 men (62 per cent) and 49 women (38 per cent). Seventy-four of their spouses were registered with the practice and 72 of their children. During the study period a further 16 children were born, five spouses died, seven employees married and one employee divorced.

There were 99 employees in the control group – 77 men and 22 women. Sixty-six of their spouses were registered with the practice as were 55 children. A further 16 children were born during the eight years of the study. No deaths were recorded, three employees married and one employee divorced.

Consultations

The preliminary results showed an obvious change in the number of consultations made per annum by the Harris group between years four and five (Table 15.1). The findings were therefore aggregated and examined during three time periods: years one to four (representing 'jobs secure'); years five and six (representing, for the Harris workers, 'jobs insecure') and years seven and eight (representing, for the Harris workers, 'jobs lost'). No significant differences were found when testing years five and six against years seven and eight. Therefore all subsequent analyses were performed on data aggregated for years one to four inclusive and years five to eight inclusive.

Three sets of comparisons were made: (1) data for Harris employees in years one to four were compared with years five to eight, and the same

Table 15.1   Annual consultation and episode rates

	Year	Mean number of consultations per patient per annum		Mean number of episodes per patient per annum	
		Harris families (275 patients)	Control families (220 patients)	Harris families (275 patients)	Control families (220 patients)
Jobs secure	1	2.66	2.78	1.54	1.68
	2	2.44	2.48	1.58	1.58
	3	2.44	2.66	1.46	1.71
	4	2.32	2.28	1.30	1.38
Jobs insecure	5	2.87	2.11	1.54	1.34
	6	3.06	2.40	1.68	1.54
Jobs lost	7	2.86	2.53	1.66	1.40
	8	3.05	2.51	1.68	1.49

for the control subjects. (2) data for Harris employees in years one to four were compared with data for control subjects in these years. (3) data for Harris employees in years five to eight were compared with data for control subjects in these years.

For the purpose of analysis, families were studied as units and then subdivided so that employees, spouses and children could each be examined as separate groups.

Table 15.2 shows those groupings for which significant increases in consultation rates were found between the years when jobs were secure (years one to four) and the years when jobs were insecure or had been lost (years five to eight) for the Harris employees. The second part of Table 15.2 shows significant differences between Harris employees and controls in the number of consultations over years five to eight. No significant differences in consultation rates were found between Harris employees and controls in years one to four.

Episodes of illness

The same statistical comparisons were applied to episodes of illness as for consultations. There was a 10.6 per cent increase in episodes of illness reported by the Harris families in the period when jobs were insecure or lost compared with a 9.3 per cent decrease for the control families over the same period. Although neither of these changes were significant, a decrease from 419 episodes (years one to four) to 330 episodes (years five to eight) reported by the control employees ($n = 99$) was found to be significant ($P = 0.05$).

Table 15.2 Significant differences in consulting behaviour

Group	Number of families	Number of individuals	Number of consultations over four years		increase	Percentage level for years	Significance
			Years 1–4	Years 5–8			1–4 versus years 5–8
All Harris families	129	275	2,792	3,353		20.1	P < 0.01
All Harris employees	—	129	1,202	1,400		16.5	P < 0.05
Families of female Harris employees	49	81	748	1,000		33.7	P < 0.05
Female Harris employees	—	49	528	605		14.6	P < 0.05

Group		Number of individuals	Number of consultations over four years (years 5–8)	Mean number of consultations per individual	Significance levels for Harris versus control employees
Male Harris employees	)	80	807	10.1	
Male control employees	)	77	603	7.8	P < 0.05
Spouses of Harris employees	74)	930	12.6		
Spouses of control employees	66)	733	11.1		P < 0.05

Note: Years 1–4 = jobs secure; years 5–8 = jobs insecure or lost.

The female Harris employees ($n = 49$) had significantly fewer ($P = 0.05$) episodes of illness than their control counterparts ($n = 22$) in the first four years and subsequently caught up.

Hospital referrals

The number of referrals to and attendances at hospital out-patient departments also showed obvious changes around 1980 and not, as had been expected, in 1982 (Figure 15.1). About one patient in seven only attends hospital in any one year in Britain and this severely reduces the data from the sample populations studied here. Therefore, the Wilcoxon rank sum test was the most appropriate statistical test and the results for the comparison of Harris employees in years one to four with years five to eight and the same comparison for control employees are presented in Table 15.3. No other comparison could be examined statistically since the Wilcoxon rank sum test requires paired samples.

No clear trends were apparent in the rates of admission to hospital in-patient departments. The mean hospital admission rate was 3.5 per cent of patients per annum and a much larger study would be necessary to detect consistent changes.

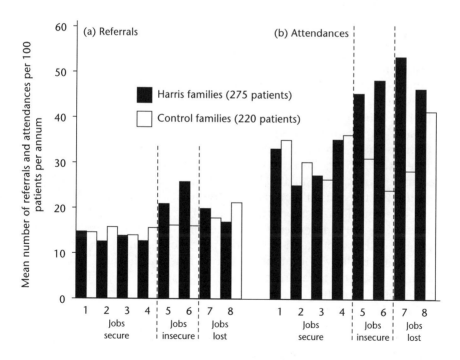

Figure 15.1 (a) Referrals to and (b) attendances at hospital outpatient departments

Notification of occupation and/or redundancy

The search of the records for details concerning the type or place of occupation of the patients revealed a written record for only 31 of the Harris employees (24 per cent) and 20 of the control employees (20 per cent). Details of redundancy had been recorded in the notes of only 18 Harris workers (14 per cent) by July 1984, that is, in the two years since they had been made redundant.

Discussion

This study demonstrates that unemployment results in a negative effect on health and not merely on welfare and morale. The results show a significant increase in the number of times that both men and women employees consult their doctors when subjected to compulsory redundancy. This increase is also shown by their spouses and when all the individuals studied are integrated into their family units.

The increase in stress exhibited was sufficient not only to provoke the Harris families into seeking the help of their doctors more often but also to give them symptoms which necessitate more frequent specialist advice. An equally important finding was quite unforeseen: the increase in morbidity began two years before redundancy – at the time when it became apparent to the Harris families that their economic futures were not secure. All other studies of factory closures have been performed over much shorter time periods and none were able to demonstrate the distinct importance of the threat of redundancy. However, one study has examined the psychiatric morbidity of the threat of unemployment and it was found that there was a decrease in symptoms when the threat was lifted (Jenkins et al., 1982). The majority of the working population probably experience concern that they may be made redundant when unemployment rates rise and perhaps there is now more evidence to suggest that, during an economic recession, those with a job may also feel under stress, as postulated by Brenner (1979).

Although the consultation rates for the Harris group rose by 20 per cent in the second four-year period, the number of new episodes of illness increased by only 11 per cent. Therefore, the number of consultations per episode of illness increased during the period of job insecurity and unemployment. Similarly, the number of attendances as hospital out-patients departments per referral increased for the Harris group while the same ratio dropped for the control group. The Harris families either developed an increased doctor-dependency or the symptoms with which they presented proved more difficult to diagnose and treat. It is possible that their problems were less clear-cut, their distresses more psychosomatic in type or their disorders less responsive to simple measures. These hypotheses are being tested at present by classifying the illnesses which were presented.

Table 15.3 Referrals to and attendances at hospital outpatient departments

Group	Number of individuals	Number of referrals per 100 patients		Significance levels for years 1–4 versus years 5–8	Attendances per 100 patients		Significance levels for years 1–4 versus years 5–8
		Years 1–4	Years 5–8		Years 1–4	Years 5–8	
All Harris employees	129	53	76	$P < 0.05$	84	145	$P < 0.05$
All control employees	99	65	82	NS	130	130	NS
Dependants of Harris employees	146	58	92	$P < 0.01$	147	230	$P < 0.01$
Dependants of control employees	121	58	69	NS	123	120	NS

Notes: NS = not significant. Years 1–4 = jobs secure; years 5–8 = jobs insecure or lost.

If the consultations with the Harris families were proving ineffective, were they also frustrating? Higgs (1984) has stated 'We do not always know what really brings a patient to the doctor'. Many consultations are unsatisfactory because the real reasons for the consultation do not emerge and there is an increased risk of chronicity. The results of this study lend credence to this for redundancy was only recorded in a minority of cases.

The reluctance of the unemployed to admit to their predicament is well-known – they see it as a stigma. Other major events such as marriage or divorce, changes of address and even foreign holidays more usually come to the notice of family doctors because of the necessary documentation. Fourteen per cent of the workforce in Britain were now suffering, together with their families, from what might correctly be called an epidemic, and for only a small minority is that fact recorded in their notes. Extrapolation of the observations made in this small study to the population at large is probably valid but several points could influence such projections. First, the rate of unemployment in the Calne area is lower than the national average. Secondly, the population of North Wiltshire is largely stable and closely-knit, has not been subject to any recent large migration and has no significant ethnic minorities. In addition, the employees themselves were a stable working group who were settled in their jobs (many for over 25 years) and worked in an unskilled or semiskilled capacity. However, it is interesting that the consultation and referral rates before 1980 for the Harris group and those for the controls throughout the study match closely the results of the second national morbidity study (OPCS et al., 1974).

At the time of writing it is not known how many of the ex-Harris workers have been successful in finding employment. It is hoped that a comparison of those remaining out of work for a long period with those who found a new job quickly will form the basis of a future study and that further analysis of the data might reveal other significant findings, such as the effect of the age of the employees. It had been expected that large numbers of the Harris families would have left the area in search of new work which would have complicated both the collection of data and the interpretation of the results. It is surprising that only four of the 133 Harris employees originally studied have moved away from the town in the two years since losing their jobs. This initial study shows that the information already stored in general practice records can provide useful facts about a population subjected to changes in its environment.

The organization of the National Health Service was an advantage in this study. When there is no cost to the patient at the point of service, those subject to financial hardship, such as unemployment, are not inhibited from seeking help. This would not be so in other countries where the inability to pay could obscure a real increase in morbidity or even result in an apparent decrease. On the other hand a 20 per cent increase in consultations (65 per cent of which generally end with a prescription) and a 60 per cent increase in visits to hospital out-patient departments by the families of the 3.3 million unemployed in Britain is a projection of startling economic consequences to the National Health Service.

Acknowledgements

This study was supported by a grant from the Scientific Foundation Board of the Royal College of General Practitioners and we are grateful for their support. We thank our families for their patience. Dr Ian Russell for his advice, all the staff at Calne Health Centre: in particular Miss Barbara Farquhar, Mrs Maureen Comley, Miss Beverly Earl and Miss Eloise Self, Dr Andrew Thornton for his critique of the manuscript and the whole partnership for their cooperation. Space does not permit us to thank, individually, all those who helped us in local industry but we must acknowledge the co-operation and hospitality of Mr Radford, Personnel Manager of Harris (Ipswich) Ltd. Finally we also acknowledge Miss Kate Clarke and her staff of the Medical Library, Postgraduate Centre at the Royal United Hospital, Bath.

References

Brenner, M. H. (1979). Mortality and the national economy, *Lancet*, 2, 568–73.

Dewi-Rees, W. and Lutkins, S. G. (1967). Mortality of bereavement, *British Medical Journal*, 4, 13–16.

Fisher, A. L. (1965). Psychiatric follow-up of long term industrial employees subsequent to plant closure, *International Journal of Neuropsychiatry*, 11, 267–74.

Harrison, R. (1976). The demoralising experience of prolonged unemployment, *Department of Employment Gazette* (April issue), 339–48.

Higgs, R. (1984). Life changes, *British Medical Journal*, 288, 1556–7.

Iverson, L. and Klausen, H. (1981). *Lukningen af Nordhavns (The closing of Nordhavns shipyard), 13*. Vaerflet: Institute for Social Medicine, University of Copenhagen, 199–207.

Jacobsen, K. (1972). Afskedigelse og sygelighed (Dismissal and morbidity), *Ugeskr Laeger*, 134, 352–4.

Jahoda, M. (1979). The impact of unemployment in the 1930s and the 1970s, *Bulletin of the British Psychological Society*, 32, 309–14.

Jahoda, M., Lazarfield, P. I. and Zeisel, H. (1973). *Marienthal – the sociography of an unemployed community*. London: Tavistock (first published 1933).

Jenkins, R., MacDonald, A., Murray, J. and Strathdee, G. (1982). Minor psychiatric morbidity and the threat of redundancy in a professional group, *Psychological Medicine*, 12, 799–807.

Kasl, S. V. (1983). Strategies of research on economic instability and health. In John, J., Schwefel, D. and Zouner, H. (eds) (1983), *Influence of Economic Instability on Health*. Berlin: Springer-Verlag.

Kasl, S. V., Cobb, S. and Brooks, G. W. (1968). Changes in serum uric acid and cholesterol levels in men undergoing job-loss, *Journal of the American Medical Association*, 206, 1500–7.

Kasl, S. V., Gore, S. and Cobb, S. (1975). Reported changes in health, symptoms and illness behaviour, *Psychosomatic Medicine*, 37, 106–22.

Murray Parkes, C. (1971). Psycho-social transitions, *Social Science Medicine*, 5, 101–15.

Office of Population Censuses and Surveys (OPCS), Royal College of General Practitioners and Department of Health and Social Security (1974). *Studies on medical and population subjects, 26. Morbidity statistics from general practice. Second national study, 1970–71.* London: HMSO.

Office of Population Census and Survey (OPCS), Royal College of General Practitioners and Department of Health and Social Security (1981). *Morbidity Statistics from General Practice: 3rd study (1981–82). Manual of definitions and procedures.* London: HMSO.

Watkins, S. J. (1984). Unemployment and health, *Lancet*, 2, 1464.

Westin, S. and Norum, D. (1977). *Nar sardinfabrikken nedlegees (When the sardine factory is shut down).* Bergen: Institute for Hygiene and Social Medicine, University of Bergen.

16 What counts as evidence: issues and debates*

David V. McQueen and Laurie M. Anderson[†]

The rise of the evidence discussion

. . . Today, in both medicine and public health, practitioners are urged to base their decisions on evidence. In health promotion, an inter-disciplinary field that overlaps substantially with public health, the issue of evidence has recently received considerable attention. in May 1998, for example, the Fifty-first World Health Assembly (World Health Organization, 1998a) urged all Member States 'to adopt an evidence-based approach to health promotion policy and practice, using the full range of quantitative and qualitative methodologies' . . .

At first glance, the discussion of evidence might appear to be merely an academic problem, one that turns on questions of epistemology and logic, a subject for debating halls and philosophers of science. Sober reflection, however, shows that the idea of evidence is intimately tied to very pragmatic issues. One wants evidence to take action, spend money, solve problems and make informed decisions. The use of the word *evidence* is at the very heart of current discussions in public health (Butcher, 1998):

> A piece of evidence is a fact or datum that is used, or could be used, in making a decision or judgement or in solving a problem. The evidence, when used with the canons of good reasoning and principles of valuation, answers the question why when asked of a judgement, decision, or action.

This chapter explores the discourse on evidence in health promotion and the evaluation of interventions. It does not provide a set of tools or principles on how to establish evidence for health promotion. This task is taken up in numerous documents and is the subject of many work-

* From Rootman, I., Goodstadt, M., Hyndman, B., McQueen, D., Potvin, L., Springett, J., and Ziglio, E. (eds) *Evaluation in Health promotion: principle and perspectives*, WHO Regional Publications, European Series, No. 92.
† For their sage advice, editorial comments and reflections on earlier drafts of this chapter, we are especially indebted to Michael Hennessey, Matt McKenna and Marguerite Pappaioanou, CDC. USA; Don Nutbeam, University of Sydney, Australia; and Alfred Rütten, Technical University of Chemnitz, Germany. The opinions expressed are ours.

shops and presentation at professional meetings (Nutbeam and Vincent, 1998). Here we examine some of the many assumptions underlying the nature of evidence . . .

Defining evidence

Evidence commonly denotes something that makes another thing evident: for example, the fact that a lake is frozen solid is an indication or sign of low temperatures. Words such as *apparent, manifest, obvious, palpable, clear* or *plain* may also be used when describing evident things or events, and all share the characteristic of certainty. In many ways this is a very strict definition. No one can fail to perceive what is evident. In brief, the everyday use of the word *evidence* carries very high expectations. If one has evidence, can there be any doubt?

In legal terms, evidence has a different meaning. In a criminal trial, for example, evidence is introduced to prove, beyond a reasonable doubt, that something has occurred. Juries and judges weigh the strength of evidence before a finding of guilt or innocence. Evidence is said to be overwhelming, to convince beyond the shadow of a doubt. Such language seems foreign to the field of health promotion, but this is exactly the framework espoused by Tones (Tones, 1997) in a recent editorial:

> Accordingly, I would argue that we should assemble evidence of success using a kind of *'Judicial principle'* – by which I mean providing evidence which would lead to a jury committing themselves to take action even when 100% proof is not available.

Evidence presented in a Western legal setting, however, is often a mixture of stories: witness accounts, police testimony and expert opinions, including those of forensic scientists. In short, it frequently comes from multiple sources and people of widely varying expertise. In this sense, determining the value of evidence requires the interpretation of accounts.

Evidence can also be understood as the product of observation or experiment, sometimes over a long period. Such evidence may be described as empirical. In some cases, observation has an underlying theoretical perspective, as with Darwin's observations leading to a theory of evolution. Observation as evidence is often tied to the notion of data as evidence. and this usage is quite common in public health.

A book by Weiner (Weiner, 1995), winner of a Pulitzer prize, explores the notion of observation as evidence in great depth; it uses research on the beak of the finch to tell the story of evolution. Weiner illustrates how modern observational techniques and data collection can reveal the operational mechanism of natural selection. He shows how years of careful, repeated measurement built the evidence base to show that the process of selection is both measurable and observable.

Two critical points might be inferred from this. First, there is no implied hierarchy of sources of evidence; evidence is convincing, whether it comes from forensic pathology or witness accounts. Second, evidence is often the result of a complex mixture of observation, experiment and theoretical argument . . .

Health promotion and the discussion on evidence

While defining health promotion is difficult, listing its characteristics is relatively easy. The field includes a wide range of research, programmes and interventions, and it has a profound ideological component. It also has a broad theoretical underpinning, which includes contextualism, dynamism, participation and an inter-disciplinary approach. Further, it is assumed that relevant theory would arise from multiple disciplines and represent research from diverse traditions. Finally, it is often argued that health promotion theory, research and practice should reflect the expressed needs of communities, groups and consumers (McQueen, 1993).

A recent view holds that practice should depend less on quantitative analyses and more on qualitative approaches. Sophisticated data analysis, it is argued, may provide too much unnecessary detail for policy makers, who may not be sufficiently familiar with the complexity of multivariate analyses and how they should be interpreted. Paradoxically, in a multi-disciplinary field such as health promotion, analyses often need to be complex, and a qualitative analysis may be as difficult to grasp as a quantitative one. In fact, complexity is a strong theme in the realm of population health research (Dean *et al.*, 1993); it reflects much of the current work in health promotion interventions that consider the combined effects of educational, political and social action on the health of individuals, groups and communities. How the debates over qualitative versus quantitative approaches and simple versus complex analyses are resolved should have important implications for the use of evidence in health promotion.

A major viewpoint incorporates the definition of the Ottawa Charter for Health Promotion (Ottawa Charter for Health Promotion, 1986). How exactly the specified control and improvement of health are to be obtained remains a subject of considerable research. A key factor, however, is the role of the context for action and, for many in the field, the appropriate setting is the community. Indeed, Green & Kreuter (Green and Kreuter, 1991) call the community the 'center of gravity' for health promotion and cite an extensive literature to support their assertion. This notion has been sustained during the 1990s. It appears to

derive from the convergence of sources including health promotion ideology, theory, policy and practice. In addition, the idea is tied into the
notions of control and empowerment, thus leading to community participation as a fundamental principle of health promotion. The active,
participating community is not a new idea in public health (Winslow,
1923), but it is a core principle for health promotion.

The concept of community comes with much ideological baggage,
but, if one accepts its centrality in health promotion, what does one
need as evidence that the community has been engaged appropriately?
In answering this question, one must understand that communities
cannot be conceptualized as individuals, and should not be reified as
such. While members of a community vary in attitudes, opinions and
behaviour, communities have collective behaviour. Communal behaviour has to be seen as the outcome of collective decision making
processes, which have a theoretical basis that is largely distinct from that
of individual decision making (Winslow, 1923; Coleman, 1964). It
follows that many evaluation considerations, including the role and
nature of evidence, need to be conceptualized accordingly.

Though health promotion is characterized by its complicated socio-
environmental setting, theories of health promotion have seldom started
with phenomena. They have started with ideology disguised as theory:
ideologies based on beliefs and cognitive understandings of the world
(McQueen, 1996), ideologies derived from the behavioural and social sciences that make up part of the ethos of health promotion. This heritage
has come from the belief that knowledge is a product of social, historical, cultural and political processes. Similarly, a notion such as evidence
cannot be separated from the processes in which it developed.

Health promotion is widely assumed to be based on science and a scientific basis for human behaviour. One could assert, however, that a
strictly scientific paradigm does not underlie this scientific basis. In
other words, the view that human behaviour is simply a response to
physiological and neural processes is largely rejected in flavour of characterizing human beings as organisms that live and operate within a
society that is a product of human behaviour. Further, a strong case
would be made that cognition is important, and that human behaviour
operates under a general concept of free will. Thus, if this behaviour is to
be understood in terms of an underlying scientific paradigm, this paradigm would not be deterministic but probabilistic, in which statistical
approaches to methods would be appropriate.

Given the diversity of research and practice in health promotion,
another issue to consider is who asks the question: 'What do we mean
by evidence?'. In many sciences the question is moot. The answer refers
to established researchers in the discipline, carrying out research in a
paradigmatic fashion. Further, the answer is the same for similar audiences. For example, the answer to the question of the type and amount

of fuel needed to get a spacecraft from the earth to the moon would be the same for all engineers and advocates of space programmes. The most efficacious way to get funding for this space mission, however, is a very different question, highly contextual and specific to the characteristics of the politics of the country in question.

One could further explore the above example in the light of health promotion concerns. The role of disagreement, difference and dialogue would be critical. In the first part of the example, disagreement and difference are not essential elements. While there might be probabilistic arguments on the fuel type and tonnage necessary to obtain escape velocity, engineers from different countries would be relatively close in their estimates. They would use the same calculating equations, address the same gravitational forces and consider the same propellant alternatives. Differences, if they arose, would be explained as errors of calculation; consensus would be the most likely outcome. In short, disagreement, difference and dialogue would be minimal. In sharp contrast, similar strategies to seek funds are difficult to imagine, and there would undoubtedly be disagreement, difference and dialogue among many different groups and people unconnected with the science of the voyage . . .

Problems with evidence in health promotion

The underlying epistemological basis for health promotion is not experimental science but the social and behavioural sciences. To a degree, some subgroups of the latter (such as clinical psychology) model their research and practice on the former. Nevertheless, most social science is non-experimental. Even in the very quantitative domains of sociology and economics, researchers' manipulation of variables is not characteristic, and experiment is largely absent in disciplines such as anthropology and political science. One could argue that most of the social and behavioural sciences are highly empirical: characterized by observation and classification, rather than any effort to manipulate the subject of study.

When intervention is intended to manipulate variables (to change knowledge, attitudes and behaviour, for example), the design can rarely possess the rigorous structure of an experiment. As pointed out elsewhere, researchers cannot control all the relevant variables or have a control group for comparison. The most that can be obtained is the oft-cited quasi-experimental design.

As participation is the chief characteristic of health promotion interventions, an ideal design would involve the collapse of the artificial dichotomy between researchers and the researched. This characterization and the attendant assumptions would make a rigorous experimental design totally inappropriate. Because evidence is so closely associated with rigorous experimental designs, the use of the term in health promotion becomes highly questionable.

For all the reasons given above, it is time to assert that the careless application of this term will deflect health promotion practice from concentrating on how best to design and evaluate interventions. It may mislead those who are not familiar with the epistemological base of health promotion into expectations deriving from a clinical science base. People in biomedicine are often criticized for having inappropriate expectations for health promotion research, but one could argue that these expectations result from the failure of those in health promotion to provide an understanding of the theoretical foundation and epistemology of the field.

Three critical and unresolved issues

Rules of evidence

Three critical issues await resolution. The first is establishing a basis for the rules of evidence. To begin with, the rules of evidence appear to be tied to disciplines, not projects. Over the years, scientific disciplines have developed their standards for what constitutes proof in observation and experiment. Thus the appropriate scientific method is both a product of historical development and the characteristic observables in the discipline, and rules of evidence differ between disciplines. Many community-based disease prevention and health promotion projects are not based on a discipline, but represent a field of action. No discipline-based epistemological structure therefore underlies the evaluation of effort. Underlying rules of evidence needed to be distinguished for the disciplines of public health that are related to community-based research and intervention: specifically, epidemiology, social psychology, sociology, anthropology and health education. Similarities and differences should be specified, and rules for fields of action should be considered.

Part of the problem of developing a basis for rules of evidence is the unresolved issue of a hierarchy of evidence. Within the general area of community research, intervention and evaluation, great debate focuses on what constitutes knowledge in the field, what evidence is, and even whether the notion of evidence is applicable to the evaluation of interventions in communities. Researchers and practitioners have not reached consensus on any hierarchy of evidence, and international groups have asserted that it is premature to prioritize types of evidence in a linear hierarchy (World Health Organization, 1998b). There remains a need to document this lack of consensus, to consider the pros and cons of consensus in the context of community intervention and to suggest directions for the future.

Finally, the complexity of multi-disciplinary, compound interventions makes simple universal rules of evidence untenable. Rules of evidence are often based on interventions that have relatively simple, demonstrable chains of causation, where the manipulation of single factors produces single, easily measured outcomes. Many community-based health interventions include a complex mixture of many disciplines, varying degrees of measurement difficulty and dynamically changing settings. In short, understanding multi-variate fields of action may require a mixture of complex methodologies and considerable time to unravel any causal relationships. New analyses may reveal some critical outcomes years after an intervention. Thus there is a need to recognize the complexity of community interventions and to suggest areas needing development to reach a better understanding of the analytical challenges. More appropriate analytical methods and evaluation designs should be developed and supported.

Indicators

The second unresolved issue is the search for, and identification of, indicators in health promotion. Despite years of what might be called indicator scepticism by positivists and indicator bashing by anti-positivists (McQueen and Norvak, 1998), two salient factors remain: decision-makers expect and often demand numbers derived from indicators, and most public health and health promotion practitioners and researchers have been trained to produce quantitative data and to respect them and the value of the associated indicators. Indicators and reports based on them often seem to galvanize interest and resources. An example is the strong interest at the time of writing in general health indicators such as QALYs (Quality Adjusted Life Years) and DALYs (Disability Adjusted Life Years). The World Health Organization is undertaking and supporting a large-scale project using DALYs to measure the global burden of disease (World Health Organization and World Bank, 1996). Individual countries are also taking up this task.

Appropriate theoretical basis

The third issue is the development of an appropriate theoretical basis for health promotion. This chapter has highlighted only a few of the many thorny theoretical issues that influence practice and the evaluation of initiatives. Lively discussion since the 1980s has not led to a general theory of health promotion. Theory provides the foundation for the research and practice paradigms of the field, and one could assert that the more substantial and coherent the theory base, the more credible research and practice will be, for the simple reason that the theoretical base establishes the parameters for what constitutes evidence.

Health promotion initiatives draw on a variety of disciplines and employ a broad range of ways to accumulate data. Since the field uses mixed methods to deliver interventions, it should develop a number of design strategies for evaluation. Health promotion is a relatively young approach, which has not had time to establish a deep theoretical base (McQueen, 1996) or the accompanying methodology. This forms a marked contrast to the history of clinical medicine, with hundreds of years of development accompanied by a century of experimental rigour. Even the social sciences forming the base for health promotion (sociology, anthropology, etc.) are relatively new, arising mainly in the middle of the nineteenth century and developing strong interest in methodology only since the 1950s. Thus the lack of a widely accepted paradigm for the conduct of health promotion research and therefore of consensus on the best evaluation strategies is not surprising.

Conclusions: optimism and the way forward

Despite its apparently critical tone, this chapter is much more a discussion of the issues than a condemnation of the current state of methodology in health promotion evaluation.

There is reason for optimism. First, the recognition of the complexity of the evidence debate reveals that researchers and practitioners cannot apply standard evaluation approaches to population-based community interventions. A need is now recognized for the careful design of evaluation strategies that take account of diversity, multi-disciplinary and local contexts. Thus the emerging theoretical perspective of health promotion, which embraces participation, context and dynamism, is being brought into the thinking on evaluation design.

Rigour in health promotion research requires the use of methods appropriate to the theoretical issues at hand, which may well mean avoiding one-shot studies in order to emphasize systematic replication in the appropriate setting. The result may be more integrated and productive studies, and less fragmented and irrelevant research. Scientific disciplines and the theories upon which they are built require epistemologies and accompanying methodologies that open the doors to new knowledge, rather than barring them.

A second reason for optimism is that the continuing search for appropriate indicators for health promotion success is now better informed, and only naive practitioners would believe that there are simple, single solutions to developing appropriate indicators. Further, the recognition of the need for appropriate indicators has reinforced the awareness that health promotion efforts affect the basic infrastructure of public health. For example, the tracking of behavioural risk factors, the number of health promotion surveys and the general concern with monitoring lifestyles have developed markedly in recent years in the Western indus-trialized world. This development is coupled with the desire that these surveillance systems extend beyond traditional concerns with etiology to address public awareness and expectations. There is an increasing desire to use these systems to assist the evaluation of population-based pro-grammes and changes resulting from health promotion interventions. The positive aspect of this is the shift of focus towards population health and away from the individual.

Most significant, the debate on evidence has led to a broadening of the base of appropriate evaluation in health promotion, and particularly community based programmes. This debate has always recognized that health promotion interventions could not be separated from issues of policy, resources, community interests, ideologies and other difficult-to-measure parameters, and that many interventions succeeded or failed owing to intangible factors that were known anecdotally but were diffi-cult to document. Thus, researchers and practitioners were often forced to rely on traditional evaluation approaches that stressed inappropriate design strategies. The current debate recognizes the many possible direc-tions in which to seek appropriate evidence. Although no perfect designs have yet been found, the accumulating scientific literature promises to identify the best of them.

References

Anderson, R. et al., (eds) (1998). *Health Behaviour Research and Health Promotion*. Oxford University Press.

Butcher, R. B. (1998). Foundations for evidence-based decision making. In *Canada Health Action: Building on the legacy. 5. Evidence and information*. Quebec: Editions Multimondes, 259–90.

Coleman, J. S. (1964). Collective decisions,. *Sociological Inquiry*, 34, 166–81.

Coleman, J. S. (1966). Foundations for a theory of collective decisions, *American Journal of Sociology*, 71; 615–27.

Dean, K., et al. (1993). Researching population health: new directions. In Dean, K. (ed.), *Population Health Research: linking theory and methods*. London: Sage, 227–37.

Green, L. W. and Kreuter, M. M. (1991). *Health Promotion Planning: An educational and environmental approach*, 2nd edn. Mountain View: Mayfield.

McQueen, D. V. (1993). A methodological approach for assessing the stability of vari-ables used in population research on health. In Dean, K. (ed.), *Population Health Research: Linking theory and methods*. London: Sage, 95–115.

McQueen, D. V. (1996). The search for theory in health behaviour and health promo-tion. *Health Promotion International*, 11(l); 27–32.

McQueen, D. V. and Novak, H. (1998). Health promotion indicators, *Health Promotion*, 3(1), 73–8.

Nutbeam, D. and Vincent, N. (1998). *Evidence-based Health Promotion: Methods, mea-sures and application*. 16th World Conference on Health Promotion and Health Education, San Juan, Puerto Rico, 23–26 June.

Ottawa Charter for Health Promotion (1986), *Health Promotion*, 1(4), iii–v.

Tones, K. (1997). Beyond the randomized controlled trial: a case for 'judicial review'. *Health Education Research*, 12(2), 1–4.

Weiner, J. (1995). *The Beak of the Finch: A story of evolution in our time*. New York: Random House.

Winslow, C. E. A. *The Evolution and Significance of the Modern Public Health Campaign*. New Haven, Conn.: Yale University Press.

World Health Organization and World Bank. *The Global Burden of Disease: A comprehensive assessment of mortality and disability from diseases, injuries and risk factors in 1990 and projected to 2020: a summary edited by Christopher J. L. Murray, Alan D. Lopez*. Cambridge, Mass.: Harvard School of Public Health (Global Burden of Disease and Injury Series, Vol. 1).

World Health Organization (1998a). *World Health Assembly resolution WHA51.12 on health promotion* (http://www.who.int/hpr/docs/index.html). Geneva: World Health Organization (accessed 8 December 2000).

World Health Organization (1998b). *Health Promotion Evaluation: recommendations to policy-makers: report of the WHO European Working Group on Health Promotion Evaluation*. Copenhagen: WHO Regional Office for Europe (document EUR/ICP/IVST 05 01 03).

17 Is prevention better than cure?*

Christine Godfrey

Introduction

Most health-care systems have been focused on illness services. Preventive health interventions have been far less developed than those for acute care. Is prevention better than cure? Which prevention strategies are cost-effective? What incentives are needed within health services to ensure that the correct balance of preventive and curative services is achieved?

Purchasers require answers to these questions if they are to maximize the health of their populations, given finite resources. However, many treatments remain to be evaluated and economic studies of prevention, especially health promotion interventions, are even rarer (Drummond *et al.*, 1987). Decisions are made based on limited information. An economic approach can give some guidance to setting priorities . . .

Future mortality and morbidity – the potential for prevention

To examine future changes in mortality, morbidity and costs accruing from current prevention activities requires sophisticated epidemiological techniques.

PREVENT is a simple simulation model which predicts changing patterns of deaths likely to occur if risk factors such as smoking, drinking, high blood-cholesterol or hypertension are reduced (Gunning-Schepers, 1989; Godfrey *et al.*, 1993). Figure 17.1 shows some results from the model using English and Welsh data. The prevention simulation was based on the *Health of the Nation* (HON) smoking targets: that prevalence of smoking should be reduced to 20 per cent, by the year 2000 and overall consumption of cigarettes should be reduced by 40 per cent over the same period.

It can be seen from Figure 17.1 that, although the interventions to achieve these targets would take place between the early 1990s and the year 2000, the peak reduction in the number of deaths is well after this

---

* From M. Drummond and A. Maynard (eds) (1993). *Purchasing and Providing Cost Effective Health Care*, ch. 13, 183–97 ©Edinburgh: Churchill Livingstone.

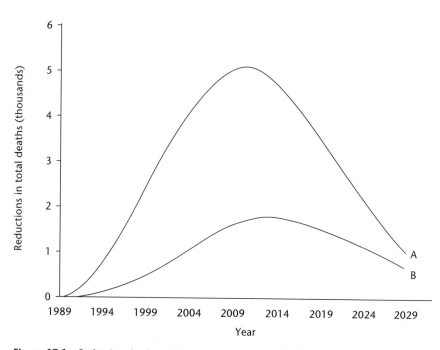

Figure 17.1   Reductions in the total number of deaths in England and Wales associated with achieving HON smoking targets: A for men; B for women

period and reductions in mortality are predicted over the whole period. If the results are expressed in terms of life years gained, then the risk factor reduction is predicted to lead to the saving of more than 54,000 life years between now and the year 2000, and a cumulative total of nearly three million life years by the year 2029. These simulations are based on all age groups, not just the under-65s.

Results from epidemiological models such as PREVENT (Gunning-Schepers, 1989) indicate that there are large potential health gains from reducing risk factors such as smoking. However, in terms of life years, gains occur over a long time period.

Considerable analyses can be undertaken to examine the potential benefits from prevention in terms of gains in the quantity of life. Far less information is available, however, about other indicators of ill-health and the potential gain in positive health if risk factors are reduced. Consideration of these potential benefits are likely to change the ranking between conditions. It should also be noted that these health gains to the quality of life may be realized in a shorter time period than those extending the quantity of life.

Identifying the options for prevention

Given the information on the potential for health gain, what are the means available to reduce risk factors and prevent disease? Health-care treatments are generally concerned with the consequences of disease or infirmity and are intended to restore some of the lost health status. Prevention activities are concerned with both preventing ill-health and with enhancing positive health, i.e. increasing current health status.

Examining the full range of prevention options can be an important component of a purchasing strategy. Prevention can be directed at the population as a whole – for example, media campaigns – or patients in the early stages of disease. There are many different prevention activities ranging from education through to legislation which can be undertaken and targeted at different groups in the population.

Defining prevention activities

There are a number of different levels of prevention activity but few common definitions. In this chapter, these levels are defined following Downie *et al.* (1992). Primary-level health promotion – exercised before the onset of any disease – includes activities such as health education on smoking for children and drug therapy for hypertension or high blood-cholesterol. Health promotion directed at halting the progression of disease or health deterioration would be considered secondary level prevention and would include screening for disease symptoms and any subsequent intervention. Tertiary level prevention consists of measures to help prevent the recurrence of an illness, and would include rehabilitation for heart attack patients.

The domains of health promotion

Most of the policy statements, in the United Kingdom and elsewhere, have concerned primary level health promotion and, in particular, the prevalence of certain risk factors, such as smoking, drinking, obesity, lack of exercise and poor diet. While secondary and tertiary level activities tend to be disease specific, some primary level activities overlap. Also behavioural change could be affected by many different interventions, not only from the health-care sector.

Tannahill (1985) developed a model in which health promotion activities are divided into three overlapping domains: health protection measures, comprising legal, fiscal or workplace controls, prevention activities (for example, immunization) which reduce the risk of occurrence; and health education activities.

Further divisions can be made by disease (or condition) and lifestyle behaviours. Such divisions are not mutually exclusive. A heart pro-

gramme could cover smoking, diet and exercise and a smoking programme cover cancer and heart disease. Health promotion, particularly
health education, can also be given in a number of settings.

The range of options that could be considered by a purchaser wishing
to reduce coronary heart disease through health education is illustrated
in Table 17.1. The choices include programmes with several elements
directed at a single risk factor, such as smoking or exercise, and multi-
risk, multi-element programmes, such as the Look After Your Heart initiatives.

Targeting health promotion

The final set of options available is whether health promotion or prevention is targeted at the whole population or at certain sub-groups. The
subgroups considered could be selected by age, sex, ethnic group or
socio-economic circumstance. The reasons for choosing different groups
may be due to disease and illness patterns, or the prevalence of adverse
lifestyles. Another form of targeting can take place if health promotion
activities are concentrated on those at highest risk of disease.

The options for prevention for any disease or risk behaviour are considerable. Some activities will be controlled by purchasers or providers
but many, such as tax levels or advertising restrictions, are not. Agenda-
setting activities may, however, help to influence policy.

Is prevention cost effective?

There are few economic evaluations of health promotion activities in
which comparisons to treatments have been made and results are mixed.
For example, opportunistic advice from general practitioners to stop
smoking frequently heads QALY or well year league tables. Other activi-

Table 17.1   Options for coronary heart disease health promotion

Main health promotion interventions	Intervention influences	
	Several risk factors	One risk factor
Workplace	Option A1	Option B1
School	Option A2	Option B2
Community based	Option A3	Option B3
Primary healthcare	Option A4	Option B4
Mass media/public education	Option A5	Option B5
	Programme A (e.g. HEA Look After Your Heart Programme)	Programme B (e.g HEA Smoking Programme)

ties, such as breast cancer screening, have been found to be less cost-effective. What determines the cost-effectiveness of different types of prevention activities?

The factors influencing both costs and benefits can be considered in two ways: in relation to whether prevention is more cost-effective than cure, and in relation to which mixture of prevention activities (for example, which of the options set out in Table 17.1) represents the best buy.

Treatment or prevention: numbers and time

Treatment only involves those who contract the disease or condition, whereas prevention can involve large numbers who may or may not develop the disease. Hence, the cost per individual for treatment can be much higher than the cost per individual for prevention, producing the same total cost for either option (Russell, 1986).

For some conditions, such as lung cancer, which are associated with adverse lifestyles, the survival rates may be poor and in other instances treatment may not restore the individuals to full quality of life.

A further issue is the time lapse before prevention results in health gains. In economic evaluations it is usual to discount future sums to a lower present value. However, if a discount rate is applied to future health benefits from prevention, the 'present' value of the health gains is reduced. Using the PREVENT simulation, a cumulative health gain of 2.8 million life years over the period 1989 to 2029 was predicted to result from achieving the *Health of the Nation* smoking targets. Discounting these health gains at 5 per cent to a present value for 1989, however, reduces the health gain to 720 000 life years.

Health economists continue to debate which discount rate should be used for health benefits. It has been suggested that all studies of health-care programmes should include the undiscounted figures, i.e. a zero discount rate (Parsonage and Neuburger, 1992). Purchasers face a considerable dilemma when, at the same time as current (and often identified) cases are waiting for treatment, they are being urged to commit resources to prevention where the health gains are anonymous and way in the future. It is likely that some discounting of future health benefits occurs in practice.

The timing of future health benefits also affects calculations about the potential for resource saving from prevention activities. This is an issue raised especially in areas where treatment is unlikely to prolong life. The avoidance of future treatment has been seen as a way of 'financing' prevention. However, such savings are often difficult to realize, due partly to the costs of prevention. Also, especially when considering behavioural changes, a decline in disease – and hence fewer patients requiring treatment often occurs with a time lag. Where the prevention activity involves screening for early signs of disease, which require some treatment, health-care costs may rise in the short term.

Treatment versus prevention – indirect costs

One of the indirect costs associated with prevention is the possibility of higher expenditure from increased longevity. These types of consequences can form part of a cost-effectiveness analysis where the value of the health benefits of a longer and healthier life and the indirect benefits from increased productivity would also be assessed. Such costs may also be less than predicted from the current pattern of health-care costs among the elderly. It has been argued that, for those who adopt healthy lifestyles in their older age, morbidity may be compressed and health-care expenditures reduced (Fries, 1989).

For many secondary prevention activities there may be some risk of side-effects. Although the risk is small per individual, the total cost of these adverse effects could be sizeable. There are also costs associated with screening procedures. The intangible costs through worry and anxiety can be extremely high for conditions such as HIV/AIDS (Godfrey et al., 1992).

The balance between preventive measures and treatment, or non-treatment, is likely to change over time. For example, immunization may become less cost-effective if previous activities have reduced the overall risk of disease.

Choices and costs and benefits of prevention activities

Other factors may influence the choice between different types of prevention activity. Secondary prevention will generally involve lower numbers than primary prevention. The costs of identifying a disease at an early stage, especially when it is asymptomatic, can be high. Also screening for disease precursors can only be worthwhile if early treatment is effective in enhancing quality and/or quantity of life. A further problem in screening (and health promotion clinics) is the difficulty of getting some of the population at highest risk to attend (Holland and Stewart, 1990).

Some health education campaigns may have adverse effects in creating a 'worried' well group. Early campaigns directed at raising awareness of HIV and AIDS, for example, were thought to have caused anxiety among those at low risk. However, the receipt of health information may have benefits as well as costs (Cohen and Henderson, 1988).

Another factor affecting the costs of different prevention activities is the frequency with which they have to be administered. Screening may need to be repeated. One question which may be addressed using cost-effectiveness techniques is the optimum timing of repeat screening.

Repetition may also be a factor in achieving behavioural change. For example, many smokers try quitting several times before finally succeeding and interventions at each attempt may influence the outcome.

Cost-effectiveness of targeting health promotion activities

The economics of targeting health promotion activities depend on the cost consequences of targeting and the effectiveness of a population approach. For example, screening the population to identify those with elevated blood-cholesterol levels, to give them either dietary advice or drug therapy, will be expensive but the health gain per individual could be high. In contrast, population approaches such as mass media campaigns or work with food companies to produce healthier products are likely to give a lower gain per individual but because of their coverage could give a higher overall gain. Most research in this area has concerned the most cost-effective strategy for lowering risk factors such as high blood pressure and cholesterol levels through primary care. Calculations by the Standing Medical Advice Committee (1990) suggested that population screening for elevated blood-cholesterol levels would not be cost-effective and that drug therapy should be considered as a last resort for the older age group with high cholesterol levels.

There are only a limited number of studies which can be used to illustrate the different factors influencing policy choice. Many studies of primary prevention have been based on assumptions about costs and benefits, rather than actual policy evaluations, to make conclusions about cost effectiveness (Williams, 1987; Hall *et al.*, 1988; Cummings *et al.*, 1989). Extensions of this type of work may be a first step in determining health promotion priorities.

The economic evaluation of health promotion activities presents a number of challenges, especially in designing studies to give robust results as not all initiatives are suitable for randomized controlled trials. There is also great difficulty in measuring the health outcomes from health promotion activities (Tolley, 1993). Models such as PREVENT (Gunning-Schepers, 1989) are a useful tool in providing predictions of health gains occurring over a time period. Most available models are, however, limited to mortality measures and it is important to attempt to measure changes in morbidity, especially those changes which may occur in the short term from different prevention activities.

Rosen and Lindholm (1992) list the factors often ignored when considering the cost-effectiveness of lifestyle interventions. This list includes intangible costs and benefits from different prevention strategies, the morbidity as well as the mortality effects, and the effects of a lifestyle change on the full range of diseases. They also consider how changes in behaviour by one person may also influence others (social diffusion).

Conclusions

Whether prevention is better than cure or lifestyle change is better than other prevention activities remains to be fully investigated. All ineffective interventions are a waste of scarce resources. This raises problems for both purchasers and providers, especially when some prevention activities, such as those directed at HIV/AIDS, involve diseases with devastating consequences. Systematic reviews are suggesting some effective prevention strategies while others have little value (Fisher, 1989; Holland and Stewart, 1990). Russell (1990) illustrates that cost-effectiveness criteria may alter some of the recommendations arising from such reviews. An economic approach as outlined has the potential for giving some initial guidance for purchasers. There is, however, a need to improve the monitoring and evaluation of prevention activities to ensure resources are being used cost-effectively.

It is clear that cost-effectiveness criteria have not been a primary concern at the initial policy planning stage of many recent reforms designed to encourage more health promotion. Scott and Maynard (1991) suggest for example, that the services that general practitioners were required to provide after a new contract was negotiated in 1990 were not proven cost-effective. They conclude 'examining the contractual obligations for health checks, it can be seen that the evidence points to the fact that such activities provide little or no benefit to the patient in terms of reducing mortality and morbidity, and incur substantial costs'. New arrangements have been proposed for the reimbursement of general practitioners for health promotion work. These should allow the encouragement of more opportunistic screening and advice, but initially requirements for health checks are to remain for the present.

Similar problems could occur as the *Health of the Nation* initiative is implemented (Akehurst *et al.*, 1991). The selection of areas to target and the level at which they were set were not driven by cost-effective criteria. Local circumstances may suggest different priorities than those given as national targets. There is, therefore, a danger that the pursuit of targets may neither maximize health gain nor use resources efficiently.

While there is widespread support for prevention, there are still many barriers to its implementation. A number of steps can be taken to identify activities which purchasers may consider have the best evidence for being good buys but change cannot be implemented without the right incentives. More attention is needed to provide both evidence of the cost-effectiveness of different prevention activities and the structures needed to ensure that where evidence is strong change takes place.

Acknowledgements

The author gratefully acknowledges the support of the Health Education

Authority for funding some of the research used in this chapter and the ESRC Data Archive and the OPCS for the provision of data used with the PREVENT model. The views expressed are those of the author alone.

References

Akehurst, R., Godfrey, C., Hutton, J. and Robertson, E. (1991). 'The Health of the Nation': an economic perspective on target setting, *Discussion Paper 92*. York: Centre for Health Economics.

Cohen, D. B. and Henderson, J. B. (1988). *Health, Prevention and Economics*. Oxford: Oxford Medical Publications.

Cummings, S. R., Rubin, S. M. and Oster, G. (1989). The cost effectiveness of counselling smokers to quit, *Journal of the American Medical Association*, 261, 75–9.

Department of Health (1992). *The Health of the Nation*, Cm 1986. London: HMSO.

Downie, R. S., Fyfe, C. and Tannhill, A. (1992). *Health promotion models and values*. Oxford: Oxford Medical Publications.

Drummond, M. F., Ludbrook, A., Lowson, K. and Steele, A. (1987). *Studies in Economic Appraisal in Health Care*, Vol. 2. Oxford University Press.

Fisher, M. (ed.) (1989). *Guide to Clinical Preventive Services*. Baltimore, Md.: Williams & Wilkins.

Fries, J. F. (1989). Health promotion and the compression of morbidity, *British Medical Journal*, 289, 481–3.

Godfrey, C., Tolley, K. and Drummond, M. (1992). The economics of promoting sexual health. In Curtis, H. (ed). *Promoting Sexual Health*. London: British Medical Association.

Godfrey, C., Hardman, G. and Tolley K. (1993). *Cost Effectiveness of Health Promotion: Application to coronary heart disease*. London: Health Education Authority.

Gunning-Schepers, I. (1989). The health benefits of prevention – a simulation approach, *Health Policy*, 12 (special issue).

Hall, J. P., Heller, R. F., Dobson, A. J. *et al.* (1988). A cost-effectiveness analysis of alternative strategies for the prevention of coronary heart disease, *Medical Journal of Australia*, 148, 272–7.

Holland, W. W. and Stewart, S. (1990). *Screening in Health Care – Benefit or Bane?* London: Nuffield Hospital Trust.

Parsonage, M. and Neuburger, H. (1992). Discounting and health benefits, *Health Economics*, 1, 71–6.

Rosen, M. and Lindholm, I. (1992). The neglected effects of lifestyle interventions in cost-effectiveness analysis, *Health Promotion International*, 7, 163–9.

Russell, L. B. (1986). *Is Prevention Better than Cure?* Washington, DC: The Brookings Institution.

Russell, L. B. (1990). The cost effectiveness of preventative services. In Goldbloom, R. B. and Lawrence, R. S. (eds), *Preventing Disease: Beyond the Rhetoric*. New York: Springer-Verlag, 433–7.

Scott, T. and Maynard, A. (1991). Will the new GP contract lead to cost effective medical practice?, *Discussion Paper 82*. York: Centre for Health Economics.

Standing Medical Advisory Committee (1990). *Blood Cholesterol Testing: The cost-effectiveness of opportunistic cholesterol testing*. London: Department of Health.

Tannahill, A. (1985). What is health promotion?, *Health Education Journal*, 44, 167–8.

Tolley, K. (1993). *Evaluating the Cost-effectiveness of Health Promotion*. London: Health Education Authority.

Williams, K. (1985). Screening for syphilis in pregnancy: an assessment of the costs and the benefits, *Community Medicine*, 7, 37–42.

Williams, A. (1987). Screening for risk of CHD: is it a wise use of resources? In Oliver, M. (ed), *Screening for Risk of Coronary Heart Disease*. Chichester: John Wiley.

18 The efficacy of health promotion, health economics and late modernism*

Roger Burrows, Robin Bunton, Steven Muncer and
Kate Gillen

Introduction[1]

All contemporary health care systems are interested in the efficacy and cost-efficiency of different modes of intervention Although there are various philosophies of evaluation it has become apparent that the discourse of health economics is increasingly being turned to. More and more the organisation and delivery of health care is being framed and articulated in terms of 'value for money' rather than any alternative moral discourses . . .

In reviewing the literature on this topic it became apparent that a variety of economic analyses had recently been carried out. However, despite their level of technical sophistication the nature of the conclusions reached were, without exception, lacking in specificity, and thus practically were of little use to policy makers and/or purchasers of health care. In this chapter we argue that the inability of health economics to deliver practical guidance highlights important epistemological issues concerning both the nature and evaluation of health promotion that no amount of technical advance in health economics will solve . . .

[U]ntil the 1990s there had been very few major published studies on the cost-effectiveness of either health promotion or health education activities (Drummond *et al.*, 1987; Cohen and Henderson, 1990). However, in the 1990s things changed in this respect, as the language of health economics entered ever more deeply into considerations of health care efficacy. Just as had happened in other organisational contexts (Burrows, 1991), the discourses of business, enterprise and efficiency have, despite resistances, increasingly become codified as *the* legitimating articulating principles of the British health service. This codification finds its most sophisticated expression in the frameworks and models of health economics.

There is an irony here, because although the language of organiza-

* From *Health Education Research, Theory and Practice*, 10(2) (1995), 241–9. © Oxford University Press 1995.

tional calculus is increasingly a rational one the 'reality' of contemporary organizational life is anything but. The process of socio-economic restructuring experienced by almost all (what used to be) public sector organisations (Burrows and Loader, 1994) since the 1980s has resulted in a chaos and confusion within organisational life with which most of us are familiar. However, this has been accompanied by a language of legitimation based upon economic *prioritization* and systematic *evaluation*. Our argument is that the emergence of this language in this context has little to do with modernist rationality and much to do with a desperate search for some form of [what the influential social theorist Anthony Giddens (1990) calls] *'ontological security'*. At just the point when, as Marx would have it, '[a]ll that is solid melts into air, all that is holy is profaned' the late modern subject searches for the apparent surety, rationality and solidity that the discourse of economics provides. The rise of health economics in the context of health care has then, in the end, more to do with the power of rhetoric than it has to do with rational decision-making (Ashmore *et al.*, 1987). In short, the indeterminant, complex and contradictory world of late modern health care has found in economics a touchstone with which to ease its aching head.

In summary our argument is that the procedures designed for the economic evaluation of modernist clinical and experimental work are often not appropriate for the evaluation of much non-clinical public health work, emblematic of late modern medicine, where data is more often than not based upon non- or, at best, quasi-experimental social survey research designs where there is no, or very little, possibility of using control groups. Further, unlike much biomedical research where statistical and causal relations are often more readily unravelled by experimental techniques, social survey-based research interested in environmental, sociological and psychological variables related to lifestyles and behavioural changes, are often more opaque, contingent and sometimes just simply impossible to relate to a causal view of the world.

The framework

The framework consists of seven elements (Tolley, 1993, pp. 53–5); defining the study problem; expressing the economic objectives; identifying the alternative options; choosing a study design; identifying and measuring costs; identifying and measuring outcomes; and calculating cost-effectiveness indicators.

Defining the study problem

This has two dimensions: the *level of analysis* and the *perspective* adopted.

There are four possible levels of analysis. First, the assessment of the cost-effectiveness of alternative, but analytically similar interventions, such as different health education programmes. Second, the assessment of the cost-effectiveness of one style of health promotion, such as health education, compared to alternative health promotion or prevention interventions. Third, the assessment of the cost-effectiveness of health promotion activities compared to treatment and curative interventions. For example, the economics of the new public health compared to more clinically-based medicine. Fourth, the assessment of the cost-effectiveness of health promotion compared to the allocation of additional resources to other areas of the public sector which, although beyond the domain of health policy as narrowly conceived, still have a considerable impact upon health outcomes: education, housing, transport, social security, environment and so on. These different levels of analysis can be viewed from three possible perspectives. First, that of a single agency such as a District Health Authority (DHA), a GP surgery, a Trust or even the Health Education Authority. Second, that of many agencies when health promotion strategies involve multi-agency collaborations such as community-based prevention programmes involving DHAs, Family Health Service Authorities, Social Services, Voluntary Organisations and so on. Third, that of society as a whole – the broadest perspective possible – where the costs and outcomes relevant to all agencies *and* members of the public are considered. Clearly, depending upon the perspective taken, one's economic conclusions can be dramatically different. Such a rational approach is, of course, in practice rarely possible. The messy world of health policy and resource allocation is only very infrequently articulated in terms of such alternatives.

Economic objectives

The stated objectives of *The Health of the Nation* (Department of Health, 1992) are the prevention of ill health and the promotion of good health and wellbeing. Thus, the economic objectives of health promotion can be viewed in terms of (1) the reduction of both mortality and morbidity levels, and (2) improvements in the quality of life at lowest cost. Thus, from the perspective of health economics health promotion strategies should be selected which produce the lowest cost per life year saved or, alternatively and perhaps more realistically, the greatest number of life years saved for a given cost. Thus, as has occurred in so many spheres of cultural, political and social life since the 1980s, it is the calculus of cost, rather than any other basis of decision making, which has come to predominate (Burrows, 1991). Under this regime the multiple and complex determinants of the 'irrationalities' of organizational life, i.e. tradition, morality, expert knowledge, culture, ecology, etc. are reduced to the supposed 'rationality' of economic calculation. Health economics promises an objective basis for the allocation of health care resources driven by a clear set of objectives (Ashmore *et al.*, 1987).

Health promotion options

There are a myriad of different health promotion strategies which can be followed. However, health economics demands a clear delineation of the different alternatives available if it is to be able to make rational comparisons of the costs and benefits of different approaches. Economics demands a systemic approach to health policy options. This involves the clarification of (1) the full range of different types of health promotion on offer, (2) a consideration of which 'risk factor strategy' to follow within each type of health promotion, (3) a consideration of the most appropriate location or setting for the strategy and (4) consideration of whether a 'high risk' or 'population' approach is to be followed. This systemic approach has led to some clear analytic distinctions being made in the conceptualization of health promotion as a generic set of practices, which is to be welcomed. One of the clearest conceptualizations is that offered by Tannahill (1985) and Downie *et al.* (1991). This is based upon a typology, which in its most simple version (Tolley, 1993, p. 21), makes distinctions between the four broad health promotion options: *prevention* (e.g. immunization/screening), *health education* (e.g. empowering individuals to be able to influence their own health), *health protection and support* (e.g. the provision of exercise facilities, no-smoking policies, etc.) and *progressive health education* (e.g. community development strategies). These four basic approaches can, of course, be combined in various different ways in order to construct more complex strategies.

These different strategies also have to be considered within the context of another set of possible options. First, what *risk factor strategy* is to be followed? A single risk factor strategy focuses on just one issue – smoking, high blood pressure, lack of exercise and so on, whilst a *multi-risk factor strategy* involves a programme which simultaneously attempts to modify a range of risk factors associated with a particular cause of morbidity and/or mortality such as heart disease. Next, consideration has to be given to what setting or site is most appropriate for the health promotion activity selected. Possible settings might include workplaces, schools, the 'community', primary health care sites, the mass media or public education channels, etc. Finally, decisions need to be made on whether *high risk* or *population-based* strategies are to be followed. For example, whether GP advice on smoking should only be given to those patients already identified as being 'at risk' or whether it should be aimed at all patients.

Study designs

The most rigorous study design is one based upon *experimental procedures* using random control trials. However, there are great problems in applying such research designs in the context of the real social settings of health promotion activities. Much more common in actual settings are *quasi-experimental designs*. This approach usually relies upon the statistical 'matching' of participants in health promotion programmes with individuals with similar social characteristics from a site not involved in the programme. Obviously, although more practicable, such designs possess a much lower level of reliability in controlling for the influence of variables outside of the health promotion programme. Finally, *non-experimental* designs, although perhaps the most common in health promotion research, are the least rigorous and reliable method for establishing the efficacy of health promoting activities. They, most commonly, rely upon 'before and after' study designs in which, for example, patterns of diet are measured prior to and then following a 'healthy eating' campaign in order to ascertain the extent to which the desired changes in the pattern of diet have occurred.

Social research is very different to clinical research not because it is any better or any worse, but because the object of its attention – the social – is a very different phenomena to the human body. It is an 'open system' subject to highly complex patterns of determination and, crucially, it is the product, at least in part, of the meaningful actions of intentional agents who reflexively monitor their performances in a way in which purely biological and physical entities do not. Experimental methods in such a context are, in large part, simply not possible (Stacey, 1987). Thus, evaluations of the 'measurable' efficacy, or otherwise, of health promotion is difficult, perhaps impossible, to determine. The usual response to this is to argue that radical methodological developments in the evaluation of health promotion interventions are required. However, little in the way of practical guidance as to what these methodologies might look like is available. As things stand the efficacy, and so it must follow, the cost-effectiveness of health promotion, is difficult to determine because the methods associated with measuring social interventions orientated to health are so blunt.

Costs

The costs included in any analysis of cost-effectiveness will obviously be a function of the perspective the study takes (see above). If a single agency approach is taken only direct costs to the agency might be included. If a multi-agency approach is taken the costs to all the agencies should be included. Finally, if a society perspective is adopted then the costs of all provider agencies *and* the costs to all individuals receiving the intervention (such as travel costs, the cost of other activities foregone, etc.) should be included. In addition future cost savings (such as GP time saved in the future due to health promotion activity now) should, in theory at least, be included in any evaluation. This process of costing is, in practice, extremely difficult if not impossible to carry out. Further, the cost of collecting the cost data can itself be very high. Thus, it might be that the cost effectiveness of a given intervention could be undermined by the very process of economic evaluation. Further, the nature of the assumptions made about costs at this stage can, and do, have a dramatic impact upon the conclusions of any study.

Outcomes

There are three interrelated measures of outcome. First, necessary but of least overall importance, are *process indicators* which provide an indication of both the supply and demand of health promotion artefacts. An example of a supply indicator would be the number of smoking cessation leaflets distributed, and an example of a demand indicator would be the extent of public awareness of a mass media campaign on the risks associated with smoking. Second, *intermediate outcomes* relate to the influence that health promotion has on behaviours and lifestyles. For example, the impact a smoking cessation campaign has upon rates of smoking. These then are the mediating factors between health promotion interventions and changes in health status. Finally, and crucially, final outcomes relate to such measurable changes in health, if any, associated with the mediating changes in behaviour and/or lifestyle. These might be measured in terms of reductions in the prevalence of a given disease, life years saved or Quality Adjusted Life Years (QALYs) gained from changes in mortality and/or morbidity rates due to the original health promoting intervention.

However, the measurement of outcomes are, like costs, very difficult. First, as discussed above, research designs in health promotion tend, for good reason, to be non-experimental and thus efficacy is very difficult to quantify. Second, as is well known, the use of final outcome measures based upon QALYs and the various other scales available, originally designed for clinical settings, tend to be insensitive in the context of health promotion. Outcome measures of qualitative changes of subjective wellbeing amongst the population due to interventions are notoriously difficult to construct. Third, the health gains from health promotion tend to occur over the mid to long term and are thus difficult to quantify within short-term research designs.

The only 'solution' to some of these problems has been to use epidemiologically-based simulation models such as PREVENT (Gunner-Schepers, 1989; Godfrey, 1993) in order to provide crude estimates of the possible outcome measures associated with various health promotion interventions. Although problematic, such an approach may be the only really viable option available to agencies who have neither the time nor the resources to undertake large-scale, long-term research projects. PREVENT and similar simulations are statistical models which are able to estimate changing aggregate patterns of death given estimates of relevant risk factors such as smoking, drinking. high blood cholesterol, hypertension and so on. Such models are analogous to econometric simulations of the economy which attempt to estimate changes in variables such as growth, unemployment and inflation given changes in other variables such as taxation, interest rates, government expenditure and so on. Parameter estimates for the evaluations which constitute the model can be derived from the (few) long-term cohort studies which do exist and/or other sources of evidence.

The problems with such an approach to the estimation of outcomes are, however, numerous. Two problems in particular are important. First, there is only very limited evidence for the reliability of the strength of associations between both health promotion interventions and risk factor modification and between risk factor modification and disease outcomes. In short, evidence for the link between behavioural change and physiological impact is, to say the least, limited. Second, most models concentrate on mortality rather than morbidity and have great difficulties in dealing with changes in the rather opaque area of 'quality of life' which may be the only outcome of some styles of radical community based health promotion and education interventions Nevertheless despite these problems the development of such simulation models appear to be the only viable source of estimates of outcome data in most analyses short of the funding of large-scale cohort studies over two or more decades.

Cost-effectiveness indicators

The final stage of the framework is to bring together cost data and outcome data and, ideally, present it in such a manner as to inform rational decision making as to the most appropriate allocation of resources. This would normally be expressed in terms of a comparison between calculations of, for example, costs per life saved or costs per QALY. It will be clear from the discussion above that such calculations are rarely unproblematic. Even if reliable data is available on both costs and outcomes – and we have been unable to find any such studies (Bunton *et al.*, 1994) – a view still has to be taken on how best to deal with two other crucial issues.

First, consideration has to be given to what the most appropriate *discount rate* should be. This refers to the idea that people and/or organizations tend to prefer to delay costs but to obtain immediate benefits: hence, e.g.:

consumers . . . prefer to pay for a washing machine using interest-free credit or will only deposit their money in a restricted access savings account if a high rate of interest is paid on the sum. (Tolley, 1993, p. 53)

In relation to health, the Department of Health suggests that a 'zero' discount rate is appropriate, i.e. health benefits in the future are worth as much as they are in the present. However, this is unrealistic given the seemingly inherent 'short-termism' of much public sector funding. Whatever the rhetoric might be, at the time of writing at least, health service organizations are going to value measurable gains in health *now* more highly than any future gains. Given that the cycle of performance measures for individuals in such organizations tends to be annual as well, this also reinforces a favourable disposition towards policies aimed at short-term rather than long-term results. A discount rate of greater than 'zero' will clearly – if it can be measured – reduce cost-effectiveness. However, it is apparent from the literature that such discount rates are – and this despite the 'technical' character of much of the justifactory discourse which surround them – essentially subjective imputations, which tend to vary from between about 5 to 10 per cent.

Second, although not a priority for *The Health of The Nation*,[2] equity has been demonstrated to be an important correlate of national mortality rates (Wilkinson, 1992) and is, consequently, an important element of many local strategies for public health (e.g. NRHA, 1992). Considerations of cost-effectiveness should then perhaps include predefined equity objectives (McGuire *et al.*, 1988). This might result in the (possibly) higher costs of health promotion activities being justified in order to have an impact on socially deprived localities if equity objectives are explicitly built into the calculus of considerations. Indeed, unless equity objectives are explicitly considered in cost-effectiveness considerations they will be implicitly excluded on cost grounds. In short, it may be that the most effective strategies are not the most cost-effective.

Conclusion

The framework is the most sophisticated one available to health economists. It can be used, for both retrospective reviews of existing studies – a kind of ideal typical template against which any particular study might be 'deciphered – or in a prospective manner, in any future research and/or evaluation designs. However, as we have already indicated few, if any, of the studies which exist on the economics of health promotion can live up to the demands of this ideal type. In short, although conceptually coherent in terms of the paradigm of health economics it is, and we argue will remain, empirically unoperationalizable because of the nature of the phenomena to which it is being directed. In short, the problem is not one of methodological refinement, it is a problem inherent to life under late modernism . . .

Notes

1. This paper derives from work carried out for Bunton *et al.* (1994), a report commissioned by the (then) Northern Regional Health Authority (NRHA). We gratefully acknowledge the support of the NRHA. The views expressed here are, however, only those of the authors and do not in any way represent the views of the NRHA.
2. However, it is interesting to note that in November 1993 the Department of Health commissioned a review and evaluation of interventions which attempt to address the issue of health inequalities.

References

Ashmore, M., Mulkay, M. and Pinch, T. (1987). *Health and Efficiency*. Buckingham: Open University Press.

Bunton, R., Burrows, R., Gillen, K. and Muncer, S. (1994). *Interventions to Promote Health in Economically Deprived Areas: A critical review of the literature*. Northern Regional Health Authority.

Burrows, R. (ed.) (1991). *Deciphering the Enterprise Culture*. London: Routledge.

Burrows, R. and Loader, B. (eds) (1994). *Towards a Post-Fordist Welfare State?* London: Routledge.

Cohen, D. and Henderson, J. (1990). *Health Prevention and Economics*. Oxford: Oxford Medical Publications.

Department of Health (1992). *The Health of the Nation: A strategy for health in England*. London: HMSO.

Downie, R., Fyfe, C. and Tannahill, A. (1991). *Health Promotion: Models and Values*. Oxford University Press.

Drummond, M. F., Ludbrook, A., Lowson, K. and Steel, A. (1987). *Studies in Economic Appraisal in Health Care*, Vol. 2, Oxford: Oxford Medical Publications.

Fox, N. (1994). *Postmodernism, Sociology and Health*, Buckingham: Open University Press.

Giddens, A. (1990). *The Consequences of Modernity*. Cambridge: Polity Press.

Giddens, A. (1991). *Modernity and Self-Identity: Self and society in the late modern age*. Cambridge: Polity Press.

Godfrey, C. (1993). Is prevention better than cure? In Drummond, M. and Maynard, A. (eds), *Purchasing and Providing Cost-Effective Health Care*. Edinburgh: Churchill Livingstone.

Gunner-Schepers, L. (1989). The health benefits of prevention – a simulation approach, *Health Policy*, 12, 12–55.

Hall, S., Held, D. and McGrew, T. (eds) (1992). *Modernity and its Futures*, Cambridge: Polity Press.

Kelly, M. and Charlton, B. (1995). The modern and the postmodern in health promotion. In Bunton, R., Nettleton, S. and Burrows, R. (eds), *The Sociology of Health Promotion*. London: Routledge.

McGuire, A., Henderson, J. and Mooney, G. (1988). *The Economics of Health Care*. London: Routledge.

Northern Regional Health Authority (NRHA) (1992). *How Do We Create a Healthy North?* Northern Regional Health Authority.

Stacey, M. (1987). The role of information in the development of social policy. *Community Medicine*, 9, 216–25.

Tannahill, A. (1985). What is health promotion? *Health Promotion Journal*, 44, 167–8.

Tolley, K. (1993). *Health Promotion: How to measure cost-effectiveness*, London: Health Education Authority.

Wagner, P. (1994). *A Sociology of Modernity: Liberty and Discipline,* London: Routledge.

Wilkinson, R. (1992). National mortality rates: the impact of inequality? *American Journal of Public Health*, 82, 1982–1084.

19 Towards a critical approach to evaluation*

Angela Everitt and Pauline Hardiker

. . . In the market economy of social welfare, a rational–technical approach to performance measurement, underpinned by the notion of causality relating input and output, is being applied to such an extent that a form of managerial evaluation is emerging. Evaluation thus is rapidly becoming part of the repertoire of those controlling policy and resource allocation mechanisms . . .

In this chapter, we now explore evaluation approaches located within alternative paradigms, acknowledging the significance of subjectivity, values and power in the shaping of understandings of programmes, projects and practice . . .

Interpretivist evaluations

The first responses to the criticisms of rational–technical evaluations came from evaluators approaching understandings of the world within an interpretivist, sometimes called naturalistic, paradigm . . .

[This] assume[s] that the social world is fundamentally different from the physical and natural one in that it is made up of people with subjectivities. Subjectivity cannot be eliminated by controlling it. To pretend to such an endeavour is to fail to capture the richness and variety of people's subjective understandings. And to assert that values can be eliminated through control is to negate the inevitable influence of values on data collected and on their analysis: thus leaving such values intact and implicit. This applies to the subjectivities and values of all involved in the evaluation process. So, rather than knowledge of practices and programmes being generated through supposedly neutral and objective data collection and analysis processes, these are treated as being given meaning by the range of actors involved in the practice. It is these meanings that are sought by the evaluator. This position is clearly articulated by Smith and Cantley, for example, in proposing:

* From A. Everitt and P. Hardiker (1996). *Evaluating for Good Practice*, Ch. 5, 83–215. London: Macmillan, as part of BASW series Practical Social Work.

the need to develop a more pluralistic approach which could cope with diversity and conflict. A more subjectivist methodology would promote the collection of multiple perspectives on the programme (not necessarily in agreement with each other) and would incorporate them into the evaluation exercise. Ambiguity and lack of agreement in perception between parties of the policy-shaping community would then be a central feature of the research, rather than an embarrassment as is the case when the presumption of consensus fails. (Smith and Cantley, 1985, pp. 8–9)

These evaluations, then, reject the notion of value-free, neutral objectivity. Instead, evaluation:

- Seeks to capture people's understandings of what is going on and to what effect, recognizing that these will not be the same for all people;
- Reflects on the subjectivity of the evaluator, recognized as important to the development of understanding;
- Focuses on processes through which meanings are attached to practices and programmes;
- Reveals understandings rather than causal explanations;
- Tends to generate qualitative data and analyses these as such;
- Focuses on meanings ascribed by people;
- Does not control or pretend to eliminate values but treats them as fundamental to the meanings people attach to their experiences.

Having regard to equality, this approach is clearly an advance on the managerial, rational–technical model in that it accords all involved, including users, the right to know and be heard. And the evaluators must make their own subjective values explicit. The approach holds evaluators accountable for their values . . .

Towards a critical evaluation

Critical theorists criticize interpretivists for their failure to take account of the structures and processes through which subjectivities are shaped and maintained. There are theories of power which help locate people's views of their experiences and their expectations of, and aspirations for, social welfare projects and programmes. These theories, too, help to decide who to include on the list of stakeholders and, furthermore, to actively draw into the process those who otherwise might be excluded. In informing and facilitating the evaluation process, theories of power help to understand whose interests may be actively articulated, by themselves and others, at the expense of whom. Structural and interpersonal expressions of power render some as powerful and others as powerless. It is these forms of power that can provoke both conflict and consensus in the project or organization. If evaluation is to be effective in ensuring 'good' practice and revealing or inhibiting 'poor' and 'corrupt' practice, it needs to develop ways to puncture consensuses that produce taken-for-granted, uncontested ways of understanding and intervention that may not be in everyone's interests.

Critical social science can help in a number of ways in our search for such an evaluation model. It:

- Locates social welfare projects, programmes and practices, and people's understandings and evaluations of them, historically and in their social, political and economic contexts;
- Reveals how dimensions of oppression such as social class, gender, race, age, disability and sexuality generate and maintain certain practices and understandings;
- Deconstructs commonly accepted ways of doing things and understandings so that these are not taken-for-granted but are exposed for the extent to which they both influence and are influenced by prevailing ways of thinking; is informed by theories of democracy and social justice that help to guide both the processes of judgement making and the judgements to be made; is committed to provoking change in the direction of equality . . .

The evaluation process may be conceptualized in two phases, although in practice these are interrelated. First is the phase of generating evidence about the practice, the programme or project. Critical social science theorizes the ways in which people's views, experiences, aspirations and expectations are shaped through dimensions such as age, class, gender, race, sexuality and disability. Through their understanding of the ideological shaping of subjectivities, critical social scientists claim that they are able to generate a more true version of reality than interpretivists who accept subjectivity at face value. Rather than generate ideologically constructed versions of reality, through their methods of data collection and analysis, critical social scientists claim that they can take account of ideology in their search for truth.

The second interrelated phase of evaluation is that of making judgements about whether the practice is 'good', 'good enough' or 'poor' or 'corrupt'. Critical social science provides us with standards against which to make such judgements: standards of justice and equality.

Case example

The evaluation of the young women's project based in an area of social and economic disadvantage did not only involve stakeholders who could readily be identified as being associated with the project.

Certainly, there were such people who were involved in the evaluation from the beginning: the workers in the project; the local
authority personnel who were responsible for recommending to the
authority that it continue to grant-aid the project; members of the
voluntary management committee, there as professionals, feminists
and/or former and current users; volunteers; and workers in other
agencies such as a nearby family centre and the area office of the
social services department which refer young women to the project.
The project's aims included a commitment to making the project
accessible to all young women, black and white. The evaluation
adopted this commitment as a statement of equality and justice by
which the work of the project could be evaluated.

Generating evidence about the project revealed that the meaning
of this commitment was becoming increasingly contested as the
project employed black workers with different views about the
needs of young black women. Some workers, black and white, felt
that it was all right that black young women did not use the project.
They argued that the project was not appropriate for young Black
women, who would be better served by developing their own activities, such as sewing groups. The project currently offered discussion
groups and activities that would facilitate discussion around issues
such as single parenting, child abuse and domestic violence. Other
workers, black and white, argued strongly that the project and all its
activities should be more accessible to black young women.
Additionally there should be some black-only groups to provide
space for Black women to share accounts of their experiences and
develop understandings of racism.

Taking a critical social science perspective, the evaluation did not
accept all the workers' views at face value, a process which would
have resulted in a plurality of perspectives being documented. It
theorized race and racism as influencing the views of white and
black workers. It engaged in a process of data generation and debate
in the project to address more critically the processes that resulted
both in the de-politicizing of the lives of young black women and in
leaving invisible to the project young black women living in the
locality. The evaluation team was expanded to include a black
woman and data were collected to identify potential stakeholders,
potential users. The picture that emerged was of a predominantly
white locality with issues of racism being experienced directly by
women of mixed ethnicities who sometimes identified themselves
as white, sometimes as black. There were also issues of racism for
young white mothers with black children.

The black member of the evaluation team conducted a study day
with the project to facilitate informed debate about race and
ethnicity in the project. For debate, or critical dialogue, the project

had before it the data that had been generated in such a way as to take account of race and racism. The study day also was concerned to develop some agreed priorities for the future work of the project, (Everitt and Johnson, 1992).

This analysis of evaluation approaches and their development across positivist, interpretivist and critical paradigms shows a continuing struggle on the part of evaluators to refine their methodologies and methods to generate the truths of the practice, programme or project. What is going on? What is being achieved? Is it 'good', 'good enough', 'poor' or 'corrupt'? Who thinks so and who doesn't? Who decides?

These are the difficult questions that have troubled evaluators. However, for us, those evaluators who take account of subjectivity and have an understanding of relationships between subjectivity and power are more likely to generate sensitive and political understandings of practice and its value. A critical approach to evaluation that recognizes dimensions of power and treats evaluation, practice and the policy arena as political processes would seem to meet our conditions for effective evaluation.

At this stage it is useful to reflect . . . on those conditions to test the relevance of critical social science approaches:

- The importance of moral debate and everybody, irrespective of power, status and position, having the right to legitimate opinions.

Critical social science puts faith in what is called the process of emancipatory reasoning. Through reasoning and debate, the truth of practice and the extent to which it is moving in the direction of the 'good' would become evident.

- Scepticism of rational–technical modes of practice.

Critical evaluators understand the rational–technical mode for the ways in which, through supposed control of values, it fails to take them into account, leaving them unchallenged. It thus maintains the status quo and serves powerful interests.

- The recognition of power, powerlessness and empowerment.

Critical evaluators have an understanding of structural and interpersonal processes of power and engage in evaluation as a tool for empowerment, or, in other words, to achieve practice and policy change for equality.

- The development of genuine dialogue between users and those within the organization, and within the organization itself.

Critical evaluation engages with users in dialogical processes to provide opportunities for them to develop greater understandings, and through these, enhanced control of their lives. Consciousness-raising is valued as a process through which people lift the mantles of ideology to reveal their true experiences, feelings and views. Users of services within social welfare would be regarded as people likely to be discriminated against through dimensions of race, gender, disability, age and sexuality.

- Attention to be paid to the fundamental purpose of the organization, and caution about becoming diverted into demonstrating productivity.

The critical evaluator would pay attention to the purpose of the organization regarding this as a statement not only of goals and objectives but of values. This would be used by the critical evaluator to facilitate judgement-making about the programme, project or practice.

- The encouragement of openness, questioning, complaints and criticisms from outside and within the organization.

Critical evaluation is about opening up the influence of ideology. It questions what appears to be, scrutinizing the taken-for-granted, ensuring that people are not saying about a service, policy or organization what they think they are supposed to say. Evaluation within this paradigm would provide space so that people may feel free to be critical without fear of being penalized.

- The removal of 'otherness' that may be attributed to those lower in the hierarchy, to users and to those relatively powerless in the community.

Critical evaluators, having an awareness of power and powerful processes, would be alert to those who usually are excluded from meaningful decision-making about services, policies and their development. Critical evaluation would ensure that such people, particularly workers and users, have a say in judging the effectiveness of projects. It would ensure that people are not marginalized through racism and/or sexism or because of their social class, age, disabilities or sexual orientations.

We are still not sure however about claims that critical social scientists make to the effect that they are able to lift the mantle of ideology to discover the real views and experiences of people. This reliance on reasoning as a way of seeking out the truth does not fit with our experience of the ways in which such judgements are made in organizations. In our view, the social world of practice is such as to suggest that there are potentially many truths. There is no one answer. Processes of generating and debating evidence of practice in evaluation do not produce the truth of practice. They may produce an agreed version that will do for the moment. The processes of generating and scrutinizing evidence do not obviate the need, in the end, to make moral judgements about whether practice is 'good', 'good enough', 'poor' or 'corrupt' . . .

References

Everitt, A. and Johnson, C. (1992). *A Young Women's Project: An evaluation.* Social Welfare Research Unit, University of Northumbria at Newcastle.
Smith, G. and Cantley, C. (1985). *Assessing Health Care: A study in organisational evaluation.* Milton Keynes: Open University Press.

20 A case study of ethical issues in health promotion – mammography screening: the nurse's position*

Alison Dines

Introduction

All nurses in the United Kingdom may be called upon to play a part in the national mammography screening programme. This may involve anything from working in a screening centre to simply being ready to inform members of the public about breast cancer screening should their professional knowledge be called upon. The programme, which forms an important part of the government's health promotion strategy, poses complex ethical issues. No work has so far examined how nurses and other health promoters might respond to these. This chapter explores the nurse's position in the light of these moral dilemmas.

Background to mammography screening

Early detection of disease through screening is generally held to be one component of health promotion (see for example Tannahill, 1985). The United Kingdom now has a national mammography screening programme for the early detection of breast cancer as part of its health promotion strategy (Department of Health, 1992). This was originally recommended by the Forrest Report in 1986 (Department of Health and Social Security, 1986). Now women between 50 and 64 years are invited to be screened every three years. The rationale for this is that successful screening will detect the disease at a stage when there is scope for effective treatment, thereby reducing the overall mortality rate.

Mammography, however, is a contentious issue. Internationally, opinion differs considerably about its benefit. Thus Sir Patrick Forrest (1990, p. 104) concluded, 'There can be no doubt that screening by mammography benefits women who develop breast cancer'. In contrast,

* From Wilson-Barnett, J. and Macleod Clark, J. (eds) (1994) *Research in Health Promotion and Nursing*, London: Macmillan, ch. 6, 43–50.

Schmidt (1990, p. 223), an authority writing from Switzerland, believes, 'Breast cancer screening does likely more harm than good . . . to women of the 50–75 age group'. The uncertainty surrounding mammography is further complicated by the fact that the first reports from the UK trial (UK Trial of Early Detection of Breast Cancer Group, 1988), whilst demonstrating that the mortality rate *is* lower in the screened population by 15 per cent, did *not show this to be statistically significant*. The reasons for the absence of *statistical* benefit are complex, but it may be due to low attendance for mammography.

Mammography therefore raises complex ethical issues. This chapter explores the nurse's position in the light of these moral dilemmas. Two specific questions will be addressed. What position should a nurse take in a position of such uncertainty? In addition, if as health promoters we are interested in participation and enablement, how can we offer women health education in this situation?

The nurse's position

The question 'what is an ethical response in a situation of such uncertainty?' may be approached by thinking about four positions a nurse might adopt. These are outlined below.

Position I
The nurse might assess the evidence and decide mammography is of benefit and therefore be fully involved with the programme.

Position II
The nurse might assess the evidence, decide mammography is harmful, have no involvement with the programme and endeavour to have it stopped.

Position III
The nurse might decide it is best not to be involved with a programme that is not proven and wait until the evidence is conclusive.

Position IV
The nurse might decide to maintain a 'healthy scepticism' about the programme, be involved with it, whilst at the same time observing the continued evaluation of the effectiveness of the programme and informing women about the uncertain situation.

Let us now examine these positions in greater depth. Each 'position' has been given a name to help capture something of the flavour of the ethical stance being adopted.

Position I 'Nurse Committed'

A nurse of this persuasion might say:

> The negative findings of various research reports into mammography screening can all be explained in terms of various methodological issues. Breast cancer is a huge problem and we must do something about it. I think time will show it to work.

It is interesting when examining each of these 'positions' to look at some of the assumptions being made. Nurse Committed assumes that 'doing something' in the face of a problem is better than doing nothing. This is an approach almost 'reinforced' at times by nursing itself. It has been challenged by some in recent years as not always appropriate. The advantages of Nurse Committed's approach is that women have a chance of being helped in the fight against breast cancer. In addition, mammography has the best chance of being tested as a new procedure because of high uptake. The disadvantages of her stance are that if mammography is subsequently found not to benefit women the public may be harmed through the perceived misuse of resources, a loss of confidence in health promoters and what may be viewed as an unnecessary intrusion into people's lives. The moral duties which are pertinent here are the duty of beneficence or doing good, the duty of veracity or truth telling and the duty of non-maleficence or not causing harm.

Position II 'Nurse Agin'

A nurse of this persuasion might say:

> There is enough evidence from the international trials to show that mammography is not working. We are raising false expectations to allow it to continue. It was only introduced because it was politically useful in an election year.

The advantage of Nurse Agin's position is that it avoids the possibility of harming the public, at least in the short term. The disadvantage, however, is that mammography remains untested and women continue to die with breast cancer. The same moral duties of non-maleficence, veracity and beneficence mentioned with Nurse Committed are also relevant here.

Position III 'Nurse Sidelines'

This nurse might say:

> It is unethical to offer untested remedies to members of the public. Until there is sufficient evidence to prove mammography works I cannot be involved.

Nurse Sidelines makes some interesting assumptions. First, that it is possible to 'prove' something. Many thinkers concerned with the philosophy of science would question this view of scientific knowledge. She also assumes it is possible to 'not be involved' and that inaction is a morally neutral position. Once again, many people would challenge this, seeing inaction as equivalent to a decision not to act and therefore not as neutral as we might first think. The advantage of Nurse Sidelines position is that she does not personally risk causing harm to members of the public through a new procedure. The disadvantage of the view is that if everyone adopted this position no advances in research would ever be made and in this case women would continue to die of breast cancer. Similar moral duties appear to be important here to those identified with Nurse Committed and Nurse Agin, in particular the tension between present and future beneficence.

Position IV 'Nurse Fence-Sitter'

This nurse might say:

> The only way to behave in such uncertainty is to try mammography out and see, but keeping a 'weather eye' on the programme monitoring and evaluation and keeping women aware of the uncertain position.

The advantages of Nurse Fence-Sitter's position are that she is being honest with the women thereby enhancing their autonomy and the women have a chance of being helped through the early diagnosis of breast cancer. The disadvantages are that the women she encounters may be confused and worried, they may not attend for breast screening and therefore have no opportunity of benefit. In addition, the programme is less likely to work due to poor attendance. There may also be a personal cost to the health promoter arising from her involvement with a programme that may not be working. The moral duties involved include veracity, respect for persons and non-maleficence.

Having looked more closely at the four nurses' views, the intriguing question is, who is behaving in the most ethical fashion? Is it Nurse Committed, Nurse Agin, Nurse Sidelines or Nurse Fence-Sitter?

Health education about mammography

Let us now leave this as food for thought for a moment and consider the question, how can we as health promoters educate women in this situation? Once again we shall examine how the various 'nurses' above would approach this.

Nurse Committed might say to the women she is working with, 'Finding breast cancer early gives the best chance of cure, do go when invited.'[1] Alternatively, she might suggest, 'The benefit of being screened for breast cancer far outweighs any risk of harm, make sure you take advantage of the service.'[2]

Nurse Agin might say in her work as a health promoter, 'Mammography does not offer women any benefit, I recommend you do not bother to go.' In a stronger fashion she might say, 'Mammography is harmful, it should be stopped.'

Nurse Sidelines might remain silent or say, 'I have no comment. I cannot advise you about breast cancer screening.'

Nurse Fence-Sitter might say, 'Mammography has possible benefits and drawbacks, it is very complex.' She could then ask the woman what she wishes to know about mammography and drawing upon her communication skills, she may try to convey some background facts in a manner appropriate to the individual woman. Nurse Fence-Sitter might draw on some of the following information for this discussion.

- Every year your chances of dying from breast cancer are 1 in 2,400, after screening they may be about 1 in 2,900 (Rodgers, 1990).
- Breast cancer screening offers the possibility of less radical treatment for breast cancer (Austoker, 1990).
- The woman's breast will need to be compressed to 4.5 cm (Forrest, 1990).
- 14,000 women will need to be screened to save one life (Rodgers, 1990).
- 142,000 women will be recalled with some false positives and some overdiagnosis (Rodgers, 1990).
- For every seven women found to have breast cancer, six will not live any longer as a result of early diagnosis (Rodgers, 1990)
- Some breast cancers will be missed at mammography (Rodgers, 1990; Skrabanek, 1989; Woods, 1991).
- Some cancers will develop in the three-year interval (Forrest, 1990).
- The cost of saving one life from screening is £80,000 (Rees, 1986).
- Treatment of breast cancer may include lumpectomy, mastectomy, radiotherapy, chemotherapy, hormone treatment.
- *Individual* benefit cannot be guaranteed (Skrabanek, 1989).

Having considered how the various 'nurses' above would approach health education, it is interesting to ask, what are the strengths and weaknesses of these various ways of informing women?

Nurse Committed's information is clear, simple and persuasive. It is based on a professional's paternalistic judgement about what is of benefit to women and advises on that basis. Women are given clear simple guidance about their health and are spared the burden of assessing complicated evidence for themselves. At the same time, however, they receive little information about which to make their own judgements and remain dependent upon the health promoter. The women are therefore denied the opportunity to assess mammography for themselves and make a free choice on that basis. They may be harmed if the paternalistic judgement of the health promoter proves to have been incorrect or differs from the judgement that the women themselves would have made had they been given the opportunity.

Nurse Agin's information is clear, simple and persuasive. It too is based upon a professional's paternalistic judgement about what is of benefit to women and advises on that basis. The strengths and weaknesses of Nurse Agin's stance are very similar to those of Nurse Committed, as once again women are given clear, simple guidance about their health but little information upon which to make their own judgements.

Nurse Sidelines' information is straightforward and non-committal, it provides little information and does not advise. Women are given an honest response by the professional but receive no guidance about their health and no information about which to make their own judgements. This approach might be harmful if adopted by all health promoters.

Nurse Fence-Sitter's information depends to some extent upon her communication skills and her ability to respond to and convey a message appropriate to the individual women whose health she is concerned to promote. The information at her disposal is detailed, somewhat complicated and non-committal. Attempting to share this knowledge is based upon a belief in the need to respect a person's autonomy through informed consent. The women are given no advice and may be confused or alarmed, in addition they may be less likely to attend for breast screening. The women do, however, have a lot of information about which to make their own judgements. In addition, the health promoter has been honest with the women.

Which then is the most ethically sound approach in health promotion? Is the paternalism of Nurse Committed and Nurse Agin most appropriate, the 'neutrality' of Nurse Sidelines or the respect for autonomy through informed consent of Nurse Fence-Sitter?

The answer to this question is complex, it is worth considering some other questions which might help us as we think about our own view. In health promotion we are concerned with encouraging people to work with us as partners in safeguarding their health, enhancing and regaining control over their health. Two interesting questions are therefore, which of these approaches allows the woman to *participate* in her own health to the greatest degree? Which of these approaches *enables* the woman to increase control over her health? In addition, we might note that we accept both paternalistic judgements and those respecting autonomy through informed consent in caring for *patients*. Does the fact that *healthy people* are involved in breast cancer screening make any difference? What if we view women attending for mammography screening as *research subjects*. How might this influence our health education as either paternalistic or respecting autonomy through informed consent? What if we view the women as *potential patients*, does this make any difference to health education? Does the question of whether the duty of the nurse is to the *individual* before her or to *society* as a whole have any relevance?

Conclusion

The ethical issues in mammography screening are paralleled in many other areas of health promotion. The evidence in this chapter suggests that nurses and other health promoters are placed in a difficult position in situations of such uncertainty. We need to debate the best way forward to be certain we are behaving in an ethical fashion.

This chapter has raised many questions and begun to answer only a few. These ideas are left as continuing food for thought and debate amongst nurses in their work as health promoters.

Acknowledgements

This chapter draws upon research being undertaken for Ph.D. studies. The research is being jointly supervised by Professor Jennifer Wilson-Barnett, Department of Nursing Studies, King's College, University of London, and Dr Alan Cribb, Lecturer in Ethics and Education, Centre for Educational Studies, King's College, University of London.

Notes

1. The phrases used here are adapted from the Women's National Cancer Control Campaign (1989) leaflet entitled, 'Breast screening by mammography. Your questions answered', and the poster entitled, 'Have you heard about free breast screening?'
2. The phrases used here are adapted from the Women's National Cancer Control Campaign (1989) leaflet entitled, 'Breast screening by mammography. Your questions answered', and a Cancer Research Campaign (1991) leaflet entitled, 'Be breast aware'.

References

Austoker, J. (1990). *Breast Cancer Screening: A practical guide for primary care teams* (rev. edn). Oxford: NHSBSP (National Health Breast Screening Programme).

Department of Health and Social Security (1986). *Breast Cancer Screening. Report to the Health Ministers of England, Wales, Scotland and Northern Ireland, by a working group chaired by Professor Sir Patrick Forrest.* London: HMSO.

Department of Health (1992). *The Health of the Nation.* London: HMSO.

Forrest, Sir P. (1990). *Breast Cancer: The decision to screen.* London: Nuffield Provincial Hospitals Trust.

Rees, G. (1986) Cost benefits of cancer services, *The Health Service Journal* (10 April), 490–1.

Rodgers. A. (1990). The UK breast cancer screening programme: an expensive mistake, *Journal of Public Health Medicine,* 12(3–4), 197–204.

Schmidt, J. G. (1990). The epidemiology of mass breast cancer screening – a plea for a valid measure of benefit, *Journal of Clinical Epidemiology,* 43(3), 215–25.

Skrabanek, P. (1989). Mass mammography: the time for reappraisal, *International Journal of Technology Assessment in Health Care,* 5, 423–30.

Tannahill, A. (1985). What is health promotion?, *Health Education Journal,* 44, 167–8.

UK Trial of Early Detection of Breast Cancer Group (1988). First results on mortality reduction in the UK trial of early detection of breast cancer, *Lancet,* ii, 411–16.

Woods, M. (1991). Behind a screen, *Nursing Times,* 87, (27 November), 48.

Promoting health in a wider context: introduction

Health promotion is a multi-layered activity and many of the contributions in Sections One and Two have argued that people's health is more than a matter of individual responsibility. The influence of physical, social, cultural and economic environments on the health chances of the individual have been emphasized many times. The focus of health promotion during the 1990s and beyond has been to take action within the domains identified in the Ottawa Charter of 1986: building healthy public policy; creating supportive environments; strengthening community action; developing personal skills; reorientating health services. The contributions in Section Three are concerned with the wider agenda that arises from these priority areas.

Anthony McMichael and Robert Beaglehole set the scene in 'The Changing Global Context of Public Health' (Chapter 21). They argue that aspects of globalization are jeopardizing health by eroding social and environmental conditions, exacerbating the rich–poor gap and disseminating consumerism. They suggest that contemporary public health must encompass the interrelated tasks of reducing social and health inequalities and achieving health-sustaining environments. The importance of community development approaches is addressed in extracts from the writings of Paulo Freire (Chapter 22) whose work inspired much of the community development movement in the 1960s and 1970s. Although written from the perspective of developing countries, these extracts from his influential book *Pedagogy of the Oppressed* remind us of the dangers of 'cultural invasion', where the ultimate seat of decision regarding the action of those who are invaded lies not with them but with the invaders. And when the power of decision is located outside rather than within the one who should decide.

The late Wendy Farrant, in Chapter 23, 'Addressing the Contradictions; Health Promotion and Community Health Action in the United Kingdom' explored the community development approach based on participation and community involvement. She argued that, in spite of the World Health Organization (WHO) global strategy, this was largely located outside the National Health Service (NHS). It was not until the late 1980s that the NHS began to embrace the principles of user involvement in health with initiatives such as 'Listening to Local Voices' and moves to make general practice more community orientated.

Wendy Farrant exposed some of the contradictions in the increased NHS support for community development approaches, and warned of the dangers of 'colonization'.

The empowerment of communities is a major part of the agenda of community action for health, and in Chapter 24 Alan Beattie asks how effective is community action, and poses the dilemma of evaluating such a diverse activity. He explores the changing discourses in evaluating community health projects. Marian Barnes takes up the issue of user involvement in Chapter 25, and argues that one of the challenges facing current locality based initiatives will be to ensure that locality-based action embraces difference and diversity and does not exclude the experiences of people who may be regarded as 'different'.

Jenny Douglas further explores the themes of difference and social inequalities in health in relation to black and minority ethnic groups. In Chapter 26, she analyses work at the local level which has identified key issues and concerns involved in trying to improve the health of people from black and minority ethnic groups. She concludes that, while work at the community level is vital, there is a need for health promotion to operate at the policy level on issues such as employment and immigration policy which are germane to the health of black and minority ethnic groups.

Building healthy public policy involves putting health on other agendas, especially those which have hitherto not focused on health. Chapters 27–29 discuss health in relation to environmental and transport policies as well as an innovative project which uses sport as a vehicle for health promotion. Ronald Labonté (Chapter 27) sets out principles for building a healthy environment. He suggests that health and environmental issues have converged, and that health promoters cannot afford to ignore issues such as pollution, global warming, species decline or excessive industrial development. Think globally – act locally is becoming a watchword for health promoters as well as environmentalists.

Billie Corti and her colleagues offer us in Chapter 28 a glimpse of an innovatory and potentially transformatory approach to health promotion. The notion of sponsorship raises important questions about effectiveness and the marketing of health messages.

Adrian Davis (Chapter 29) examines the politics and policy issues in relation to transport and health policy and asks the question 'Can the health sector influence transport planning for better health?' From research conducted in Copenhagen, Groningen and Sheffield, he examines the necessary pre-conditions of inter-sectoral collaboration on health and transport. The impact of crime on the health of individuals has received little attention until recently. In the final contribution in this section John Middleton (Chapter 30) concludes that crime, and the fear of crime remain a major threat to public health and quality of life, and is a public health problem.

21 The changing global context of public health*

A. J. McMichael and R. Beaglehole

Future health prospects depend increasingly on globalization processes and on the impact of global environmental change. Economic globalization – entailing deregulated trade and investment – is a mixed blessing for health. Economic growth and the dissemination of technologies have enhanced life expectancy widely. However, aspects of globalization are jeopardizing health by eroding social and environmental conditions, exacerbating the rich–poor gap, and disseminating consumerism. Global environmental changes reflect the growth of populations and the intensity of economic activity. These changes include altered composition of the atmosphere, land degradation, depletion of terrestrial aquifers and ocean fisheries, and loss of biodiversity. This weakening of life-supporting systems poses health risks. Contemporary public health must therefore encompass the inter-related tasks of reducing social and health inequalities and achieving health-sustaining environments.

We are living through what is, historically, a major transition in the health of populations. There have been broad gains in life expectancy since the 1950s. Fertility rates are declining. The profile of major causes of death and disease is being transformed; the pattern of infectious diseases has become much more labile (and antimicrobial resistance is rising widely); and health inequalities between rich and poor persist. Today, the prospects for future health depend to an increasing – but as yet uncertain – extent on the processes of globalization and on the emergence of global environmental changes occurring in response to the great weight of economic activity . . .

Improvements in the health profile of Western populations since the 1800s have resulted primarily from broad-based changes in the social, dietary and material environment, shaped in part by improved sanitation and other deliberate public health interventions. In less-developed countries, health gains have begun more recently in the wake of increased literacy, family spacing, improved nutrition and vector control, assisted by the transfer of knowledge about sanitation, inoculation and treatment of infectious diseases (Powles, 1992). These observations remind us that public-health researchers and practitioners, and

---

* From McMichael, A. J. and Beaglehole, R. 'The changing global context of public health' (2000) *The Lancet*, 356: 495–9, 5 August.

those in the political and public realms with whom they interact, must take a broad view of the determinants and, indeed the sustainability, of population health. This is an ecological view of health; an awareness that shifts in the ecology of human living, in relation to both the natural and social environments which account for much of the ebb and flow of diseases over time.

What, then, is to be the scope of 'Public health'? Broadly defined, public health is 'the art and science of preventing disease, promoting health, and extending life through the organised efforts of society' (Acheson, 1998). There is now a growing recognition of the importance of two fundamental dimensions to this public health task. First, because social and material inequalities within a society generate health inequalities, an important task is to elucidate, through research, the underlying determinants of these health inequalities (Leon and Walt, 2001) . . .

The advent of human-induced global environmental change – especially global climate change, depletion of freshwater supplies, loss of biodiversity, and the degradation of managed ecosystems (especially arable lands) – jeopardizes the life-supporting capacity of the biosphere (McMichael, 1993; Watson, 1998).

The scope of contemporary public health analysis must therefore encompass those two larger-scale dimensions: the reduction of social and health inequalities, and the striving for health-sustaining environments. In traditional, largely self-contained, agrarian-based societies that produce, consume and trade on a local basis and with low-impact technologies, the social and environmental determinants of health are predominantly local. However, the industrialization and modernization of the twentieth century altered the scale of contact, influence and exchange between societies, institutionalized hierarchical economic relations, exacerbated the rich–poor gap worldwide and increased the scale of human impact on the environment.

An important step towards addressing these two dimensions has been the recent affirmation that a population's health reflects more than a simple aggregation of the risk-factor profile and health status of its individual members. It is also a collective characteristic that reflects the population's social history and its cultural, material and ecological circumstances (Loomis and Wing, 1990; Pearce, 1996; McMichael, 1999).Epidemiological analysis that is confined to studying 'risk factor' differences between individuals gives little insight into variations in population health indices, either between populations or over time. For example, the effect on mortality of heatwaves and cold spells differs between European populations at low and high latitudes, reflecting differences in culture, housing design, and environmental conditioning . . .

Globalization and population health

From a public health perspective, globalization appears to be a mixed blessing (Kinnon, 1998).On the one hand, accelerated economic growth and technological advances have enhanced health and life expectancy in many populations. At least in the short-to-medium term, these material advances allied to social modernization and various health care and public health programmes yield gains in population health. On the other hand, aspects of globalization jeopardize population health via the erosion of social and environmental conditions, the global division of labour, the exacerbation of the rich–poor gap between and within countries, and the accelerating spread of consumerism (Kinnon, 1998; Stephens *et al.*, 1999; Yach and Bettcher, 1998; McMichael, 1996).

Examples of health risks posed by economic and other globalization processes

The primary health risks, a result of globalization on social and natural environments. Include:
- Perpetuation and exacerbation of income differentials, both within and among countries, thereby creating and maintaining the basic poverty-associated conditions for poor health.
- The fragmentation and weakening of labour markets as internationally mobile capital acquires greater relative power. The resultant job insecurity, sub-standard wages, and lowest-common denominator approach to occupational environmental conditions and safety can jeopardize the health of workers and their families.
- The consequences of global environmental changes (includes changes in atmospheric composition, land degradation, depletion of biodiversity, spread of 'invasive' species, and dispersal of persistent organic pollutants).

Other, more specific, examples of risks to health include:
- The spread of smoking-related diseases as the tobacco industry globalizes its markets.
- The diseases of dietary excesses as food production and food processing become intensified and as urban consumer preferences are shaped increasingly by globally promoted images.
- The diverse public health consequences of the proliferation of private car ownership, as car manufacturers extend their marketing.
- The continued widespread rise of urban obesity.

- Expansion of the international drug trade, exploiting the inner-urban underclass.
- Infectious diseases that now spread more easily because of increased worldwide travel.
- The apparent increasing prevalence of depression and mental health disorders in ageing and socially fragmented urban populations.

Economic 'globalization' has, in fact, been a long-evolving feature of a world dominated by Western society. For example, the start of the twentieth century was a time of vigorous free trade, subsequently curtailed in the aftermath of the First World War. However, contemporary globalization differs in both the scale and the comprehensiveness of change, and in the associated decline in a country's capacity to set social policy (Yach and Bettcher, 1998). Although the Western world's post-First World War international development project anticipated initially that countries everywhere would converge towards the Western model of national democratic capitalism, that project has latterly evolved towards the building of an integrated and deregulated free-market global economy (McMichael, 1996). These globalizing processes, in turn, have become a major determinant of national, social and economic policies (Gray, 1998; Navarro, 1998). Thus while responsibility for healthcare and the public health system remains with national governments, the fundamental social, economic and environmental determinants of population health are becoming increasingly supranational. It has become evident that this global combination of liberal economic structures and domestic policy constraint promotes socio-economic inequalities and political instability (Gray, 1998), each of which affects population health adversely. Unless the moderating role of the state or of international agencies is strengthened, increasing competition for the world's limited natural resources is likely to damage inter-country relations, local and global environments, and population health (Gray, 1998; UN Environment Programme, 1999).

One aspect of the growth in international trade with particularly deleterious public health consequences has been the escalation in the sales of weapons, much of it facilitated by Western governments. Sub-Saharan Africa provides many tragic examples of these effects as does the the 1999 Balkan crisis. The nature of modern conflict is such that most casualties are civilians, with women and children being particularly vulnerable (Levy and Sidel, 1997).

Global environmental change and health

A major manifestation of the increasing scale of the human enterprise is the advent of global environmental changes. While not being caused

directly by the globalization processes discussed above, global environmental change reflects the increasing magnitude of population numbers
and the intensity of modern consumer-driven economies (McMichael
and Powles, 1999). Humankind is now disrupting at a global level some
of the biosphere's life-support systems (Watson and Dixon, 1998; Daily,
1997), which provide environmental stabilization, replenishment, biological productivity, the cleansing of water and air, and the recycling of
nutrient elements. Our predecessors could take these environmental 'services' for granted in a less-populated world. However, human beings are
changing the gaseous composition of the lower and middle atmos-
pheres; there is a net loss of productive soils on all continents, depletion
of most ocean fisheries and many of the great aquifers upon which irri-
gated agriculture depends; and an unprecedented overall loss rate of
whole species and many local populations (McMichael 1993; Watson
and Dixon, 1998). An estimated third of the world's stocks of natural
ecological resources have been lost since 1970 (Loh *et al.*, 1998). These
changes to the earth's basic life-supporting processes pose long-term
risks to the health of populations (McMichael 1993; Last, 1992).

Global climate change

Climate scientists forecast that the continued accumulation of heat-trap-
ping greenhouse gases in the troposphere will change global patterns of
temperature, precipitation, and climatic variability in the coming
decades (Houghton *et al.*, 1996). A rise of 1–3°C by 2050, greater at high
than at low latitudes, would occur faster than any rise encountered by
man since the inception of agriculture around 10,000 years ago. The
UN's Intergovernmental Panel on Climate Change and various other
national scientific panels have assessed the potential health consequences of climate change (Houghton *et al.*, 1996; Climate Change
Impacts Review Group, 1996; McMichael *et al.*, 1996; McMichael and
Haines, 1997). These risks to human health will arise from increased
exposure to thermal extremes and from regional variable increases in
weather disasters. Other substantial risks may arise because of the disruption of complex ecological systems that determine the geography of
vector-borne infections (such as malaria, dengue fever and leishmani-
asis), and the range, seasonality and incidence of various food-borne and
water-borne infections, the yields of agricultural crops, the range of
plant and livestock pests and pathogens, the salination of coastal lands
and freshwater supplies because of rising sea-levels, and the climatically
related production of photochemical air pollutants, spores and pollens
(McMichael and Haines, 1996; McMichael and Haines 1997).

Public health scientists now face the task of estimating, via interdisciplinary collaborations, the future health impacts of these projected sce-

narios of climatic–environmental conditions. Mathematical models have been used, for example, to estimate how climatic changes would affect the potential geographic range of vector-borne infectious diseases (McMichael and Haines, 1996; Martens *et al.*, 2000).

Stratospheric ozone depletion

Depletion of stratospheric ozone by manufactured gases such as chloro-fluorocarbons has been occurring during the past few decades and is likely to peak by about 2020. Ambient ground-level ultraviolet irradiation is estimated to have increased by up to 10 per cent at mid-to-high latitudes since the 1980s (UN Environmental Programme, 1998). Scenario-based modelling, integrating the processes of emissions accrual, ozone destruction, ultraviolet irradiation flux and cancer induction indicates that European and US populations will have a 5–10 per cent rise in skin-cancer incidence during the middle decades of the twenty-first century (Slaper *et al.*, 1996).

Biodiversity loss and invasive species

As humankind's demand for space, materials and food increases, so populations and species of plants and animals are being extinguished increasingly rapidly. An important consequence for human beings is the disruption of ecosystems that provide 'nature's goods and services' (Daily, 1997).

Biodiversity loss also means that before discovery, many of nature's chemicals and genes, of the kind that have already conferred enormous medical and health benefits are being lost. Myers estimates that five-sixths of tropical vegetative nature's medicinal goods have yet to be recruited for human benefit (Myers, 1997).

Meanwhile, 'invasive' species are spreading worldwide into new non-natural environments via intensified food production, commerce, and mobility. The resultant changes in regional species composition have many consequences for human health. For example, the choking spread of water hyacinths in East Africa's Lake Victoria, introduced from Brazil as a decorative plant, is now a breeding ground for the water snail that transmits schistosomiasis and for the proliferation of diarrhoeal disease organisms (Epstein, 1998).

Impairment of food-producing ecosystems

Increasing pressures of agricultural and livestock production are stressing the world's arable lands and pastures. We enter the twenty-first century with an estimated one-third of the world's previously productive land seriously damaged by erosion, compaction, salination, waterlogging, and chemicalization that destroys organic content (UN Environment Programme, 1999; Pimentel *et al.*, 1995; Resources Institute, 1998). Similar pressures on the world's ocean fisheries have left most of them severely depleted or stressed (FAO, 1995). Almost certainly we must find an environmentally benign and socially acceptable way of using genetic engineering to increase food yields if we are to produce sufficient food for another 3 billion people (with higher expectations) by 2050.

Modelling studies, allowing for future trends in trade and economic development, have estimated that climate change will cause a slight decrease globally of around 2–4 per cent in cereal grain yields (which represent two-thirds of world food energy). The estimated decrease in yield will be considerably greater in the food-insecure regions in South Asia, the Middle East, North Africa, and Central America (Parry *et al.*, 1999; UK Meterology Office, 1998)

Other global environmental changes

Freshwater aquifers in all continents are being depleted of their ancient 'fossil water' supplies. Agricultural and industrial demand, amplified by population growth, often greatly exceeds the rate of natural recharge. Water-related political and public health crises are threats to some regions in the coming decades(UN Environment Programme, 1999).

Various semi-volatile organic chemicals (such as polychlorinated biphenyls) are now disseminated world wide via a sequential 'distillation' process in the cells of the lower atmosphere, thereby transferring chemicals from their usual origins in low-to-mid latitudes to high indeed polar, latitudes (Watson and Dixon, 1995; UN Environment Programme, 1999). Consequently, increasingly high concentrations are accumulating in polar mammals and fish and in traditional groups of people that eat them. Various chlorinated organic chemicals, butylytin and other compounds adversely affect the immune systems and reproductive systems of mammals, including human beings (World Resources Institute, 1998). Chemical pollution is no longer just an issue of local toxicity.

Conclusion

The mix of rapid processes of socio-economic change, demographic change and global environmental change requires a broad conception of the determinants of population health. A deficiency of social capital (social networks and civic institutions) adversely affects the prospects for health by predisposing to widened rich–poor gaps, inner-urban decay, increased drug trade, and weakened public health systems. The large-scale loss of natural environmental capital – manifested as climate change, stratospheric ozone depletion, degradation of food-producing systems, depicted fresh-water supplies, biodiversity loss, and spread of invasive species – is beginning to impair the biosphere's long-term capacity to sustain healthy human life.

Scientists and policy makers face unfamiliar challenges in addressing these broader contextual issues in population health. Koopman, recognizing the general challenge, states that 'epidemiology is in transition from a science that identifies risk factors for disease to one that analyses the systems that generate patterns of disease' (Koopman, 1996). Other public health sciences, too, will need to engage in this systems-orientated study of large-scale influences on health. We must, of course, continue to identify, quantify and reduce the risks to health that result from specific, often local, social, behavioural, and environmental factors. Meanwhile, we must anticipate the influences on population health of today's larger-scale socio-economic processes and systemic environmental disturbances. We should take heart from the now well-advanced integration of systems-based ideas and ecological ideas across other scientific domains, including physics, the neurosciences, and evolutionary biology (Capra, 1996; Wilson, 1998).

This human ecology perspective will broaden the theory and practice of public health, and will help to integrate the consideration of health outcomes into decision making in all policy sectors. The sustained good health of populations requires enlightened management of our social resources, economic relations and the natural world. There is a win–win opportunity in this situation: many current public health issues have their roots in the same socio-economic inequalities and imprudent consumption patterns that jeopardize the future sustainability of health. There are great challenges here for public-health practitioners and researchers.

References

Acheson, D. (1998). *Independent inquiry into inequalities in health*. London: HM Stationery Office.
Capra, F. (1996). *The web of life*. New York. Anchor.
Climate Change Impacts Review Group (UK) (1996). *The potential effects of climate change in the United Kingdom*. London: DETR.

Daily G., (ed.) *Nature's Services: societal dependence on natural ecosystems*. Washington, DC: Island Press.

Epstein, P. R., (1998). Weeds bring disease to the East African waterways. *Lancet*, 331, 577.

Food and Agriculture Organization (1995). *State of the world's fisheries 1995*, Rome: FAO.

Gray, J. (1998). *False Dawn: The delusions of global capitalism*. London: Granta.

Houghton, J. T., Meira Filho, L. G., Callander, B. A. *et al.* (1996). Intergovernmental Panel on Climate Change (WGI). Climate change, 1995 – The science of climate change: contribution of working group I to the second assessment report of the intergovernmental panel on climate change. Cambridge University Press.

Kinnon, C. M., (1998). World trade: bringing health into the picture, *World Health Forum*, 19, 397–406.

Koopman, J. S. (1996). Emerging objectives and methods in epidemiology. *American Journal of Public Health*, 86, 630–2.

Last, J. M. (1992). Global environment, health and health services. In Last J. M. and Wallace, R. B. (eds), *Public Health and Preventive Medicine*. Norwalk, Conn.: Appleton Lange, 677–86.

Lee, K. (2000). Globalisation and health policy: a review of the literature and proposed research and policy agenda. In Bambas, A., Casas, J. A., Drayton, H. and Valdes, A. (eds), *Health and Human Development in the New Global Economy*. Washington, DC: Pan American Health Organization, pp. 15–41.

Leon, D. A. and Walt, G. (eds), (2001). *Poverty, inequality and health*. Oxford University Press.

Levy B. S. and Sidel V. W. (eds) (1997). *War and public health*. New York: Oxford University Press.

Loh, J., Randers, J. and McGillivray, A. *et al.* (1998). *Living planet report, 1998*. Gland: WWF International.

Loomis, D. and Wing, S. (1990). Is molecular epidemiology a germ theory for the end of the twentieth century? *International Journal of Epidemiology*, 19, 1–3.

Martens W. J. M., Kovacs, R. S., Niihof, S. *et al.* (2000). Climate change and future populations at risk of malaria. *Global Environmental Change*.

McMichael A. J., (1993). *Planetary Overload: global environmental change and the health of the human species*. Cambridge University Press.

McMichael A. J. and Powles, J. W. (1999). Human numbers, environment, sustainability and health *British Medical Journal*, 319, 977–80

McMichael A. J., Haines, A., Slooff, R. and Kovacs, R. S. (eds) (1996). *Climate change and human health*. Geneva: WHO.

McMichael, A. J., Haines, A. (1997). Global climate change: the potential effects on health. *British Medical Journal*, 315, 805–9.

McMichael, P. D. (1996). *Development and social change: a global perspective*. Thousand Oaks, Calif.: Pine Forge Press.

Myers, N. (1997). Biodiversity's genetic library. In Daily, G. C. (ed.), *Nature's services: societal dependence on natural ecosystems*. Washington DC: Island Press.

Navarro, V. (1998). Comment: whose globalization?, *American Journal of Public Health*, 88, 742–3.

Parry, M., Rosenzweig, C., Iglesias, A., Fischer, G., Livermore, M. T. J. (1999) Climate change and global food security: a new assessment. *Global Environmental Change*, 9, 51–67.

Pearce N. (1996). Traditional epidemiology, modern epidemiology, and public health, *American Journal of Public Health*, 36, 678–83.

Pimentel, D., Harvey, C., Resosudarmo, P. *et al.* (1995). Environmental and economic costs of soil erosion and conservation benefits, *Science*, 267, 1117–22.

Powles, J. W. (1992). Changes in disease patterns and related social trends. *Social Science Medicine*, 35, 377–87.

Slaper, H., Velders G. J. M., Daniel, J. S., de Gruijl, F. R., van der Leun, J. C. (1996). Estimates of ozone depletion and skin cancer incidence to examine the Vienna Convention achievements, *Nature*, 384, 256–8.

Stephens, C., Leonardi, G., Lewin, S. and Chasco, M. S. S. (1999). The multilateral agreement on investment: public health threat for the twenty-first century, *European Journal of Public Health*, 9, 3–5.

UK Meteorology Office, UK Department of Environment, Transport and Regions (1998). *Climate change and its impacts*. London: Met Office Communications.

UN Environment Programme (1998). *Environmental effects of ozone depletion: 1998 Assessment*. Lausanne: Elsevier.

UN Environment Programme (1999). *Global Environment Outlook 2000*. Nairobi: UNEP.

Watson R. T., Dixon, J. A. and Hamburg S. P. *et al*. (1988). *Protecting our planet. Securing our future: linkages among global environmental issues and human needs*. Washington: UNEP/USNASA/World Bank.

Wilson, E. O. (1998). *Consilience: the unity of knowledge*. New York: Knopf.

World Resources Institute (1998). *World resources 1998–1999: Environment and health*. Oxford University Press.

Yach, D. and Bettcher, D. (1998). The globalization of public health, I: Threats and opportunities, *American Journal of Public Health*, 88, 735–8.

Yach, D. and Bencher, D. (1998). The globalization of public health, II: the convergence of self-interest and altruism. *American Journal of Public Health*, 88, 738–41.

22 Pedagogy of the oppressed: an extract

Paulo Freire (trans. Myra Bergman Ramos)*

Cultural invasion

In this phenomenon, the invaders penetrate the cultural context of another group, in disrespect of the latter's potentialities; they impose their own view of the world upon those they invade and inhibit the creativity of the invaded by curbing their expression.

Whether urbane or harsh, cultural invasion is thus always an act of violence against the persons of the invaded culture, who lose their originality or face the threat of losing it. In cultural invasion (as in all the modalities of antidialogical action) the invaders are the authors of, and actors in, the process; those they invade are the objects. The invaders mold; those they invade are molded. The invaders choose; those they invade follow that choice – or are expected to follow it. The invaders act; those they invade have only the illusion of acting, through the action of the invaders.

All domination involves invasion – at times physical and overt, at times camouflaged, with the invader assuming the role of a helping friend. In the last analysis, invasion is a form of economic and cultural domination. Invasion may be practiced by a metropolitan society upon a dependent society, or it may be implicit in the domination of one class over another within the same society.

Cultural conquest leads to the cultural inauthenticity of those who are invaded; they begin to respond to the values, the standards, and the goals of the invaders. In their passion to dominate, to mold others to their patterns and their way of life, the invaders desire to know how those they have invaded apprehend reality – but only so they can dominate the latter more effectively.[1] In cultural invasion it is essential that those who are invaded come to see their reality with the outlook of the invaders rather than their own; for the more they mimic the invaders, the more stable the position of the latter becomes.

For cultural invasion to succeed, it is essential that those invaded become convinced of their intrinsic inferiority. Since everything has its opposite, if those who are invaded consider themselves inferior, they must necessarily recognize the superiority of the invaders. The values of

---

* From Paulo Freire (1972). *Pedagogy of the Oppressed*, Ch. 4, 150–86. London: Sheed & Ward.

the latter thereby become the pattern for the former. The more invasion is accentuated and those invaded are alienated from the spirit of their own culture and from themselves, the more the latter want to be like the invaders: to walk like them, dress like them, talk like them.

The social *I* of the invaded person, like every social *I*, is formed in the socio-cultural relations of the social structure, and therefore reflects the duality of the invaded culture. This duality (which was described earlier) explains why invaded and dominated individuals, at a certain moment of their existential experience, almost 'adhere' to the oppressor *Thou*. The oppressed *I* must break with this near adhesion to the oppressor *Thou*, drawing away from the latter in order to see him more objectively, at which point he critically recognizes himself to be in contradiction with the oppressor. In so doing, he 'considers' as a dehumanizing reality the structure in which he is being oppressed. This qualitative change in the perception of the world can only be achieved in the praxis.

Cultural invasion is on the one hand an *instrument* of domination, and on the other, the *result* of domination. Thus, cultural action of a dominating character (like other forms of antidialogical action), in addition to being deliberate and planned, is in another sense simply a product of oppressive reality.

For example, a rigid and oppressive social structure necessarily influences the institutions of child rearing and education within that structure. These institutions pattern their action after the style of the structure, and transmit the myths of the latter. Homes and schools (from nurseries to universities) exist not in the abstract, but in time and space. Within the structures of domination they function largely as agencies which prepare the invaders of the future.

The parent–child relationship in the home usually reflects the objective cultural conditions of the surrounding social structure. If the conditions which penetrate the home are authoritarian, rigid, and dominating, the home will increase the climate of oppression.[2] As these authoritarian relations between parents and children intensify, children in their infancy increasingly internalize the paternal authority.

Presenting (with his customary clarity) the problem of necrophilia and biophilia, Fromm analyzes the objective conditions which generate each condition, whether in the home (parent–child relations in a climate of indifference and oppression or of love and freedom), or in a socio-cultural context. If children reared in an atmosphere of lovelessness and oppression, children whose potency has been frustrated, do not manage during their youth to take the path of authentic rebellion, they will either drift into total indifference, alienated from reality by the authorities and the myths the latter have used to 'shape' them; or they may engage in forms of destructive action.

The atmosphere of the home is prolonged in the school, where the students soon discover that (as in the home) in order to achieve some satisfaction they must adapt to the precepts which have been set from above. One of these precepts is not to think.

Internalizing paternal authority through the rigid relationship structure emphasized by the school, these young people tend when they become professionals (because of the very fear of freedom instilled by these relationships) to repeat the rigid patterns in which they were miseducated. This phenomenon, in addition to their class position, perhaps explains why so many professionals adhere to antidialogical action.[3] Whatever the specialty that brings them into contact with the people, they are almost unshakably convinced that it is their mission to 'give' the latter their knowledge and techniques. They see themselves as 'promoters' of the people. Their programs of action (which might have been prescribed by any good theorist of oppressive action) include their own objectives, their own convictions, and their own preoccupations. They do not listen to the people, but instead plan to teach them how to 'cast off the laziness which creates underdevelopment'. To these professionals, it seems absurd to consider the necessity of respecting the 'view of the world' held by the people. The professionals are the ones with a 'world view'. They regard as equally absurd the affirmation that one must necessarily consult the people when organizing the program content of educational action. They feel that the ignorance of the people is so complete that they are unfit for anything except to receive the teachings of the professionals.

When, however, at a certain point of their existential experience, those who have been invaded begin in one way or another to reject this invasion (to which they might earlier have adapted), the professionals, in order to justify their failure, say that the members of the invaded group are 'inferior' because they are 'ingrates', 'shiftless', 'diseased', or of 'mixed blood'.

Well-intentioned professionals (those who use 'invasion' not as deliberate ideology but as the expression of their own upbringing) eventually discover that certain of their educational failures must be ascribed, not to the intrinsic inferiority of the 'simple men of the people', but to the violence of their own act of invasion. Those who make this discovery face a difficult alternative: they feel the need to renounce invasion, but patterns of domination are so entrenched within them that this renunciation would become a threat to their own identities. To renounce invasion would mean ending their dual status as dominated and dominators. It would mean abandoning all the myths which nourish invasion, and starting to incarnate dialogical action. For this very reason, it would mean to cease being *over* or *inside* (as foreigners) in order to be *with* (as comrades). And so the fear of freedom takes hold of these men. During this traumatic process, they naturally tend to rationalize their fear with a series of evasions.

The fear of freedom is greater still in professionals who have not yet discovered for themselves the invasive nature of their action, and who are told that their action is dehumanizing. Not infrequently, especially at the point of decoding concrete situations, training course participants ask the coordinator in an irritated manner: 'Where do you think you're steering us, anyway?' The coordinator isn't trying to 'steer' them anywhere; it is just that in facing a concrete situation as a problem, the participants begin to realize that if their analysis of the situation goes any deeper they will either have to divest themselves of their myths, or reaffirm them. Divesting themselves of and renouncing their myths represents, at that moment, an act of self-violence. On the other hand, to reaffirm those myths is to reveal themselves. The only way out (which functions as a defense mechanism) is to project onto the coordinator their own usual practices: *steering, conquering,* and *invading* . . . [4]

Cultural invasion, which serves the ends of conquest and the preservation of oppression, always involves a parochial view of reality, a static perception of the world, and the imposition of one world view upon another. It implies the 'superiority' of the invader and the 'inferiority' of those who are invaded, as well as the imposition of values by the former, who possess the latter and are afraid of losing them.

Cultural invasion further signifies that the ultimate seat of decision regarding the action of those who are invaded lies not with them but with the invaders. And when the power of decision is located outside rather than within the one who should decide, the latter has only the illusion of deciding. This is why there can be no socio-economic development in a dual, 'reflex', invaded society. For development to occur it is necessary: (a) that there be a movement of search and creativity having its seat of decision in the searcher; (b) that this movement occur not only in space, but in the existential time of the conscious searcher . . .

Cultural synthesis

Cultural action is always a systematic and deliberate form of action which operates upon the social structure, either with the objective of preserving that structure or of transforming it. As a form of deliberate and systematic action, all cultural action has its theory which determines its ends and thereby defines its methods. Cultural action either serves domination (consciously or unconsciously) or it serves the liberation of men. As these dialectically opposed types of cultural action operate in and upon the social structure, they create dialectical relations of *permanence* and *change*.

The social structure, in order to *be*, must *become*; in other words, *becoming* is the way the social structure expresses '*duration*', in the Bergsonian sense of the term.[5]

Dialogical cultural action does not have as its aim the disappearance of the permanence–change dialectic (an impossible aim, since disappearance of the dialectic would require the disappearance of the social structure itself and thus of men); it aims, rather, at surmounting the antagonistic contradictions of the social structure, thereby achieving the liberation of men.

Antidialogical cultural action, on the other hand, aims at mythicising such contradictions, thereby hoping to avoid (or hinder insofar as possible) the radical transformation of reality. Antidialogical action explicitly or implicitly aims to preserve, within the social structure, situations which favor its own agents. While the latter would never accept a transformation of the structure sufficiently radical to over come its antagonistic contradictions, they may accept reforms which do not affect their power of decision over the oppressed. Hence, this modality of action involves the *conquest* of the people, their *division*, their *manipulation*, and *cultural invasion*. It is necessarily and fundamentally an *induced* action. Dialogical action, however, is characterized by the supersedence of any induced aspect. The incapacity of antidialogical cultural action to supersede its induced character results from its objective: domination; the capacity of dialogical cultural action to do this lies in its objective: liberation.

In cultural invasion, the actors draw the thematic content of their action from their own values and ideology, their starting point is their own world, from which they enter the world of those they invade. In cultural synthesis, the actors who come from 'another world' to the world of the people do so not as invaders. They do not come to *teach* or to *transmit* or to *give* anything, but rather to learn, with the people, about the people's world.

In cultural invasion the actors (who need not even go personally to the invaded culture; increasingly, their action is carried out by technological instruments) superimpose themselves on the people, who are assigned the role of spectators, of objects. In cultural synthesis, the actors become integrated with the people, who are co-authors of the action that both perform upon the world.

In cultural invasion, both the spectators and the reality to be preserved are objects of the actors' action. In cultural synthesis, there are no spectators; the object of the actors' action is the reality to be transformed for the liberation of men.

Cultural synthesis is thus a mode of action for confronting culture itself, as the preserver of the very structures by which it was formed. Cultural action, as historical action, is an instrument for superseding the dominant alienated and alienating culture. In this sense, every authentic revolution is a cultural revolution.

The investigation of the people's generative themes or meaningful thematics constitutes the starting point for the process of action as cultural synthesis. Indeed, it is not really possible to divide this process into two separate steps: first, *thematic investigation*, and then *action as cultural synthesis*. Such a dichotomy would imply an initial phase in which the people, as passive objects, would be studied, analyzed, and investigated by the investigators – a procedure congruent with antidialogical action. Such division would lead to the naive conclusion that action as synthesis follows from action as invasion.

In dialogical theory, this division cannot occur. The Subjects of thematic investigation are not only the professional investigators but also the men of the people whose thematic universe is being sought. Investigation – the first moment of action as cultural synthesis – establishes a climate of creativity which will tend to develop in the subsequent stages of action. Such a climate does not exist in cultural invasion, which through alienation kills the creative enthusiasm of those who are invaded, leaving them hopeless and fearful of risking experimentation, without which there is no true creativity.

Those who are invaded, whatever their level, rarely go beyond the models which the invaders prescribe for them. In cultural synthesis there are no invaders; hence, there are no imposed models. In their stead, there are actors who critically analyze reality (never separating this analysis from action) and intervene as Subjects in the historical process.

Instead of following predetermined plans, leaders and people, mutually identified, together create the guidelines of their action. In this synthesis, leaders and people are somehow reborn in new knowledge and new action. Knowledge of the alienated culture leads to transforming action resulting in a culture which is being freed from alienation. The more sophisticated knowledge of the leaders is remade in the empirical knowledge of the people, while the latter is refined by the former.

In cultural synthesis – and only in cultural synthesis – it is possible to resolve the contradiction between the world view of the leaders and that of the people, to the enrichment of both. Cultural synthesis does not deny the differences between the two views; indeed, it is based on these differences. It does deny the invasion of one by the other, but affirms the undeniable support each gives to the other. . .

Notes

1. To this end, the invaders are making increasing use of the social sciences and technology, and to some extent the physical sciences as well, to improve and refine their action. It is indispensable for the invaders to know the past and present of those invaded in order to discern the alternatives of the latter's future and thereby attempt to guide the evolution of that future along lines that will favor their own interests.
2. Young people increasingly view parent and teacher authoritarianism as inimical to their own freedom. For this very reason they increasingly oppose forms of action which minimize their expressiveness and hinder their self-affirmation This very positive phenomenon is not accidental. It is actually a symptom of the historical climate which . . . characterizes our epoch as an anthropological one. For this

reason one cannot (unless he has a personal interest in doing so) see the youth rebellion as a mere example of the traditional differences between generations. Something deeper is involved here. Young people in their rebellion are denouncing and condemning the unjust model of a society of domination. This rebellion with its special dimension, however, is very recent; society continues to be authoritarian in character.

3. It perhaps also explains the antidialogical behavior of persons who, although convinced of their revolutionary commitment, continue to mistrust the people and fear communion with them. Unconsciously, such persons retain the oppressor within themselves; and because they 'house' the master, they fear freedom.

4. See my 'Extansão ou Comunicação?', in *Introducción a la Acción Cultural* (Santiago, 1969).

5. What makes a structure a *social* structure (and thus historical–cultural) is neither permanence nor change, taken absolutely, but the dialectical relations between the two. In the last analysis, what endures in the social structure is neither permanence nor change; it is the permanence–change dialectic itself.

23 Addressing the contradictions: health promotion and community health action in the United Kingdom*

Wendy Farrant

Introduction

In the United Kingdom, as elsewhere, the 1980s saw a rapid growth and development of the community health movement (Community Projects Foundation, 1988; Blennerhassett *et al.*, 1989). The emergence of the UK community health movement in the late 1970s can be linked to a number of influences, including the women's movement, health action by black and minority ethnic groups; increasing public dissatisfaction with conventional approaches to health care; community workers becoming involved with local health issues; and health workers seeking more democratic ways of working that address the social, economic and political determinants of health. The movement encompasses a diverse and increasing number of groups, projects and initiatives that are applying a community development approach to health. Central to these initiatives is a concern with redressing inequalities in health, by facilitating collective responses to community-defined health needs and enabling powerless and disadvantaged groups to have an effective voice in policy decisions that affect their lives and health. During the 1980s the movement gained added strength and cohesion through the setting up of the National Community Health Resource (NCHR), a national vol- untary organization with responsibility for supporting, developing and promoting the community health movement. Accounts of the develop- ment, composition and activities of the UK community health move- ment and descriptions of individual community development health initiatives, are contained in various publications produced by the NCHR [which changed its name to Community Health UK in 1993], for example see Kenner (1986).

Up until the mid-1980s, there was little meeting point between the community health movement and the National Health Service (NHS). The initial wave of local community development health projects in the

---

* From *Critical Public Health*, (1994), 5, 5–19. © Baywood Publishing Co. Inc. 1991.

late 1970s and early 1980s were largely initiated, funded and located outside the NHS, mainly in the voluntary sector (Rosenthal, 1983). Although some NHS workers, particularly health education officers, were pioneering community development approaches, health and prevention policy and practice within the NHS continued to be dominated by an individualistic perspective. A study carried out during the first half of the 1980s highlighted the marginalization of community development approaches to health education at both central and local levels within the NHS, and the perceived political constraints that militated against the national Health Education Council and local Health Education Departments taking this approach on board (Farrant and Russell, 1986).

The latter half of the 1980s, in contrast, was marked by increasing lip service within the NHS to community development in health, stimulated in part by the World Health Organization's 'Health for All by the Year 2000' (HFA 2000) and Health Promotion initiatives. A development project in an inner city health district during this period highlighted the possibilities, as well as the constraints and dilemmas, of utilizing HFA 2000 principles as a framework for promoting a community development approach to health promotion policy (Farrant and Taft, 1989). It also underlined the profound contradictions of 'community participation for health for all' coming into vogue at a time of major national policy shifts toward inequality and non-accountability.

This chapter focuses on the contradictory implications for the community health movement of recent developments in health promotion policy within the United Kingdom, and aims to illuminate the contradictions by locating them within a historical and international context. The NHS interest in community development in health is examined in relation to broader health and welfare policy of the 1980s, the history of community development in health in former British colonial territories, and the background to the WHO health promotion initiative. The possibilities and limitations of utilizsing the rhetoric, to support community health action, are explored with reference to moves by the UK community health movement to 'reclaim' Health for All . . .

Community participation or community manipulation?

For those involved in community health action outside the NHS, the later 1980s saw the opening up of opportunities, contradictions and dilemmas. Within mainstream health promotion, there were signs of community development moving from the periphery to centre stage and being seen as less of a threat than a panacea. Terms such as 'community participation' and 'community empowerment' became commonplace in the literature.

The principles of community development received endorsement from the WHO in its HFA 2000 strategy. As noted by the WHO Regional Office for Europe: 'It is a basic tenet of the health for all philosophy . . . health developments in communities are made not only for but with and by the people' (WHO, 1985). References to HFA 2000 became increasingly prominent in UK policy statements. There was little evidence, however, of this official endorsement being translated into increased support for community development health initiatives and devolution of power in decision-making. Health promotion and 'the new public health' were becoming arenas for intersectoral competition as much as collaboration, and in the power struggles between different professional groups and statutory sectors for resources and control the community health movement was hardly getting a look-in (NCHR, 1988). Health promotion priorities were adopting the language of community development without taking on board the fundamental principal of community control over the definition of health needs and solutions.

Meanwhile, as government policies served to intensify inequalities in health, the burden of caring was being thrown ever more on the shoulders of unpaid women in the family and the voluntary sector. Under such circumstances, the notion of health by the people begins to look like a convenient cover-up for the erosion of health *for* the people.

Community development and ideology

Beattie (1986), in arguing for the crucial importance of a critical analysis of the relationships of power and control embedded in different approaches to community development, observed: 'Too often in the health promotion field, the community development approach has been seized upon uncritically and simplistically, as offering radical promise in and of itself . . . It is essential to see that community work is bound up with the whole historical development of the social welfare sector in the modern state.'

Accounts of the historical emergence of community development suggest that far from being inherently radical, it has often been employed to safeguard and further the interests of the ruling class (Cockburn, 1977). The label 'community development' has been applied to many different, often coexisting activities and approaches, ranging from the programme initiated by the British Colonial Office in response to demands for self government for the colonies and by the UK and US governments in response to urban unrest in the 1960s, to oppositional forms of community-based action, and comprehensive development strategies introduced by countries such as China in pursuit of major social transformation. If the potential of community development for challenging rather than reinforcing power relations is to be realized, then it is essential to identify where the impetus for community development is coming from and to differentiate between the ideologies underlying various approaches.

Community development health work in the UK largely originated outside the NHS, in response to the rapid growth of public interest in health from the late 1970s onward. The belated interest of the NHS in community development needs to be seen in relation to the crisis of the welfare state, and broader debates around such issues as community care, volunteerism, decentralization and consumerism. It is also illuminating to examine the much longer history of state interest in community development in health in the Third World, and the background to the WHO health for all initiative.

The NHS policy content

The increasing reference to concepts of community development/ participation/involvement/empowerment in the health promotion literature in the late 1980s was backed up by the rhetoric about responsiveness to community needs in Department of Health policy documents such as *Care in Action* (DHSS, 1981), the Griffiths Report on NHS management (1983) and the Cumberledge report on community nursing (DHSS, 1986).

Davies analysed a series of policy interventions within the NHS introduced during the first two administrations of the Thatcher government, which can be seen as amounting to successful establishment of the conditions for a new mix of services, public and private, statutory, voluntary and commercial, in the arena of heath care delivery. She argues that 'self-help, new forms of volunteering, and community empowerment are some of the terms in which a more limited statutory involvement is being cast' (Davies, 1987). This trend toward welfare pluralism has been subjected to more critical scrutiny in the field of social services than in the health sector. Although the opening of the door for expansion of the commercial sector might be regarded as perhaps the most serious implication of the ideology of welfare pluralism, a major focus of the debate has been the relationship between the state and the voluntary sector. While the potential of voluntary and community initiatives for challenging the non-accountability of state bureaucracies and official definitions of need is recognized by both the advocates and critics of welfare pluralism, Beresford and Croft (1984) point out that it is essential to distinguish between allocation of resourccs to the voluntary sector versus promotion of unpaid voluntary and informal care, and between voluntary initiatives that seek to change statutory provision versus those that provide a substitute for it. It is the notion of unpaid voluntary and informal care as a substitute for statutory provision that is so strongly supported by Tory government policy: the negative implications for women as the main providers of unpaid care in the family and the community have been well documented (Finch and Groves, 1983).

Debates around policies of decentralization highlighted the ways in which concepts such as 'decentralization', 'patch planning', 'accountability', 'community participation', 'public involvement', 'partnership with the voluntary sector' and so on, can have very different meanings and very different implications in practice, depending on where they are coming from and the political ideology of their advocates (Hambleton and Hoggett, 1984). The model of decentralisation that can be seen as dominating the growing popularity of 'pack' and locality planning within health authorities is a managerialist–consumerist approach that has little to do with notions of democratization and shifting of the balance of power between providers and users of service (Dun, 1987) . . .

Health for who by the year 2000?

The limitations of conventional approaches to health development were documented in WHO-commissioned studies published in the mid-1970s. The search for alternative solutions (Djukanovic and Mach, 1975), drew heavily on the socialist development strategies of China, Cuba and Tanzania. The major conditions for success identified by WHO analysts were: a commitment to reallocation of resources toward meeting the basic health needs of the impoverished majority; integration of the health sector within a comprehensive programme of social and economic development; and community participation in health planning and implementation. These principles formed the basis of the 1978 Alma-Ata declaration on Primary Health Care (PHC) and the subsequent global HFA 2000 strategy . . .

Health promotion: a new panacea?

Whereas the initial impetus for HFA 2000 came from demands for new approaches to health development in the Third World, the WHO health promotion initiative can be linked to the health crisis and social movements in advanced capitalist societies. To quote from the introduction to the report of the First International Conference on Health Promotion (1987):

> This first conference was intended primarily to bring together people from industrialised countries . . . In the industrialised countries inequalities in health are increasing between social groups while health costs continue to rise. The gap between the potential for health of people in industrialised countries and their current health status has indicated a need for new strategies and pro-

grammes . . . Moreover, the public interest in health, self-care and mutual aid has led to the questioning of professional approaches and definitions in health problems . . . Health promotion is an effort to crystallise a wide range of activities that have contributed towards a changing model of public health.

Some insight was provided by Stacey (1988) at a workshop in which she shared her experiences as a social scientist on the WHO European Committee for Research for Health for All (RFHFA). She described the background of the RFHFA strategy as a continual struggle between individualistically orientated biomedical approaches and more socially orientated perspectives.

Such tensions are reflected in the products of WHO consultations on health promotion. The WHO concept of health promotion is explicitly informed by a sociological perspective that sees health and lifestyle as inextricably linked to the social and economic environment, and acknowledges the social nature of the movement for health (Kickbusch, 1986). In many places, however, the publications of the WHO Regional Office for Europe continue to reflect the influence of the biomedical model. A clear example is the 'Targets for HFA' documents, in which the socially orientated perspective of the 'lifestyle' section is juxtaposed with the biomedical perspective of the section on disease prevention.

Although the underlying principles of the WHO concept of health promotion can be seen as profoundly radical in their implications, the model of social change that is implicit in policy statements is inevitably constrained by the political and ideological position of WHO discussed above (Ineson, 1986). Whereas the central HFA focus on redressing inequalities would imply an emphasis on empowering oppressed and disadvantaged groups, 'the community' and 'the public' are frequently referred to as a homogeneous whole, with little encouragement to systematically analyse power relations within and between communities. Insofar as mention is made of the need to secure the participation of the disenfranchised, it is rarely acknowledged that participation involves conflict and confrontation as well as consensus and co-operation and, to be effective, would require a fundamental shift in the distribution of power. While support of spontaneous community action around health is encouraged, community activists tend to be treated as just one set of actors in an equal partnership between the powerful and powerless. The profound significance of the community health movement in challenging social relations that are antithetical to health is at best underplayed.

As with the implementation of HFA in the Third World, the contradictions inherent in the strategy documents of the WHO Regional Office for Europe leave them open to misappropriation by professional and other vested interests. There are clear parallels, for example, between the pro-

motion of selective PHC in the Third World and the selective interpretation of HFA targets by some health authorities within the UK to support
a conventional medical model (Farrant, 1987).

Reclaiming Health for All

In contrast to the gap between the rhetoric and reality of official health
promotion, the HFA principles of redressing inequalities, community
participation and intersectorial collaboration are central to the aims,
values and ways of working of community development health projects
and initiatives.

The growth of the UK community health movement has been paralleled by similar developments in other industrialized countries. As indicated above, the WHO health promotion initiative can be seen as, in
part at least, a response to this movement. As noted in the report of the
workshop on 'Strengthening Communities' at the First International
Conference on Health Promotion (1987):

> Though this has been an international conference of local, national
> and international delegates, the deliberations were primarily a
> response to the rising and changing expectations of populations
> around the world, who are demanding assistance in achieving their
> self-set goals . . . People are seeking a broader social response to
> improving their personal, social and health environments.

If the potential of this social movement is not be be stultified, then a priority for all concerned about Health for All must be to safeguard against
its appropriation.

The Ottawa Charter for Health Promotion (WHO, 1986) emphasizes
that 'Health promotion works through concrete and effective *community
action* in setting priorities, making decisions, planning strategies, and
implementing them to achieve better health. At the heart of this process
is the *empowerment of communities*, their *ownership* and *control* of their
own destinies'. Endorsement of this principle implies at the very least:

- *Acknowledging* inequalities in power, ownership and control, and
  vested interests in maintaining inequalities;
- *Challenging* professional control of health promotion; and
- *Validating* and *supporting* community health initiatives that are seeking
  to transform the distribution of power, ownership and control.

As the implications of professional misappropriation of HFA 2000 have
become more apparent, the response of the UK community health
movement to 'Health for All' has shifted from detached cynicism to

active attempts to 'reclaim' it. An important trigger was the First UK
Healthy Cities Conference in Liverpool in 1988, at which community
activists produced a statement commenting on the contradiction
between the rhetoric of community participation and the planning and
structure of the conference, which precluded the participation of local
community groups and particularly women and the black community
(Thornley, 1988). A week later, at the other end of the world, community activists representing the Central Australian Aboriginal Congress
similarly seized possession of the podium at the Second International
Conference on Health Promotion, to challenge the Australian Health
Minister's expressed commitment to reducing the health gap between
white and aboriginal peoples and to seek support for a community
health initiative by and for aboriginal women (Farrant and Taft, 1988).

The implications of HFA 2000 for the UK community health movement were the subject of the Summer 1988 issue of *Community Health
Action*, the newsletter of the (then) NCHR. A leading article noted that:

> an important point – which seems to have been misused by some
> who are keen to leap on to the Health for All bandwagon – is that
> the fundamental principles of Health for All are also principles of
> community development. More importantly, there is already a
> wealth of experience and expertise in this area, which needs to be
> recognised and acknowledged. Health for All might currently be
> 'flavour of the month', but those who have been battling for years
> to get community development work adequately resourced might
> take a more cynical view of what really lies behind the enthusiasm.
> (National Community Health Resource 1988).

Conclusion

This article has focused on the contradictory implications for the community health movement of developments in health promotion policy
during the late 1980s, whilst the scarcity of resources to back up the
rhetoric about strengthening community action remained a major contradiction, the trend toward increased NHS support for community
development health projects inevitably gave rise to a new set of
dilemmas.

At the national level, some of the contradictions were played out in
the relationship between the community health movement, the Health
Education Authority and government. As HFA 2000 began to capture the
imagination of the community health movement and progressive local
government and health authorities, and staff within the Health
Education Authority began to utilize it as a framework for a systematic
strategy of support for community development, there were signs of the

government's response to HFA 2000 shifting from apathy to opposition. An indication was a widely publicized ministerial review of the Health Education Authority's 1989/90 operational strategy, when pressure was placed on the Authority to channel its activities even more narrowly into high-profile government-initiated mass media campaigns, and questions were asked about 'the proposed concentration on a community development approach' (West and Jones, 1989). This reaction was not new, but was an endemic feature of the relationship between government and the central body for health education.

The research community did not escape the backlash. A study of dampness and health, carried out by the Edinburgh Research Unit for Health and Behavioural Research at the initiation of, and in collaboration with, a local tenants' group, came under critical scrutiny at the Unit's review by its main funding body, the Scottish Office (West and Jones, 1989). The Scottish Office made clear that it would not welcome a continuation of such research. In terms of both the content and process of the research, the study in question was an exemplary model of 'Research for Health for All'.

Despite the contradictions, the HFA 2000 principles of redressing inequalities, community participation and intersectoral collaboration provide a useful framework for:

- Monitoring the gap between the rhetoric and reality of official health promotion policy and practice;
- Stimulating debate about the structural barriers to translating HFA principles into practice;
- Challenging the monopolization of health promotion by health professionals;
- Legitimizing and promoting approaches that are rooted in community health action.

The indications were that the last decade before the year 2000 would be marked by further retrenchment of material support for community health action, accompanied by the continued propagation of consumerist notions of community participation that undermine the fundamental principles of community development. The challenge for the community health movement will be to utilize the rhetoric, at the same time as exposing the contradictions and safeguarding against its own colonization. For activists both within and outside the statutory sector, there is a need to critically re-examine the meaning of *In and Against the State* (London Edinburgh Weekend Return Group, 1979) in the current cold political climate.

References

Beattie, A. (1986). Community development for health: from practice to theory? *Radical Health Promotion*, 4, 13.

Beresford, P. and Croft, S. (1984). Welfare pluralism: the new face of fabianism, *Critical Social Policy*, 9, 19–39.

Blennerhassett, S., Farrant, W. and Jones, J. (1989). Support for community health projects in the UK: a role for the National Health Service, *Health Promotion*, 4(3), 199–206.

Cockburn, C. (1977). *The Local State*. London: Pluto Press.

Community Projects Foundation (1988). *Action for Health: Initiatives in Local Communities*. London: Health Education Authority.

Davies, C. (1987). Viewpoint: things to come: the NHS in the next decade, *Sociology of Health and Illness*, 9(3), 302–17.

Department of Health and Social Security (DHSS) (1981). *Care in Action*. London: HMSO.

Department of Health and Social Security (1986). *Neighbourhood Nursing – A focus for care*. London: HMSO.

Dun, R. (1987). *Going Local? A Study of West Lambeth District Health Authority*. London: West Lambeth Health Authority.

Djukanovic, V. and Mach, E. P. (1975) *Alternative Approaches to Meeting Basic Needs in Developing Countries*. Geneva: World Health Organization.

Farrant, W. (1987) Health for WHO by the year 2000? – choices for district health promotion strategies. *Radical Community Medicine*, 28, 19–26.

Farrant, W. and Taft, A. (1988). WHO Healthy Public Policy conference, *Community Health Action*, 9, 16–17.

Farrant, W. and Taft, A. (1989). Building healthy public policy in an unhealthy political climate – a case study from Paddington and North Kensington. In Evers, A., Farrant, W. and Trojan, A. (eds), *Healthy Public Policy at Local Level*. Boulder, Col.: Westview Press, 135–43.

Farrant, W. and Russell, J. (1986). *The Politics of Health Information: 'Beating heart disease' as a case study in the production of Health Education Council Publications, Bedford Way Papers, 28*. London: Kogan Page.

Finch, J. and Groves, D. (1983). *A Labour of Love: Work and caring*. London: Routledge & Kegan Paul.

Griffiths, E. R. (1983). *NHS Management Inquiry*. London: HMSO.

Hambleton, R. and Hoggett, P. (eds) (1984). *The Politics of Decentralisation: Theory and practice of a radical local government initiative*. Bristol: School of Advanced Urban Studies.

Ineson, A. (1986). O s for obscurantism – a review of Health Promotion Glossary 1, *Radical Health Promotion*, 3, 49–51.

Kenner, C. (1986). *Whose Needs Count? Community action for health*. London: Bedford Way Press.

Kickbusch, I. (1986). Lifestyles and health, *Social Science Medicine*, 22, 117-24.

London Edinburgh Weekend Return Group (1979) *In and Against the State*. London: Publications Distributions Co-op.

National Community Health Resource (1988) Health for All by year 2000?, *Community Health Action*, 9, 4–6.

Report of the First International Conference on Health Promotion (1987). *Health Promotion*, 1(4), 407.

Rosenthal, H. (1983). Neighbourhood health projects – some new approaches to health and community work in parts of the United Kingdom, *Community Development Journal*, 18(2), 120–30.

Stacey, M. (1988). Background to the Research for Health for All initiative, unpublished paper presented at Workshop and Information Exchange on Research for HFA, convened by the British Sociological Association Medical Sociology Group, Aston University, Birmingham (March).

Thornley, P. (1988). Community participation – rhetoric or reality?, *Community Health Action*, 9, 7–10.

West, J. and Jones, L. (1989). Bound, gagged and blindfolded, *Health Matters*, 2, 12–13.

World Health Organization Regional Office for Europe (1985). *Targets for Health for All*. Copenhagen: WHO.

World Health Organization (1986). *Ottawa Charter for Health Promotion*. Copenhagen: WHO.

24 Dialogical evaluation and health projects: a discourse of change*

Alan Beattie

Mainstream approaches to evaluation: the limits of linear thinking

Evaluating health programmes and projects is a huge and growing area of investment in the NHS, indeed an 'evaluative culture' has come to dominate the working lives of staff in statutory agencies across all sectors of public provision of services (Henkel, 1991). But evaluation is itself a fiercely contested terrain: there are many distinct and competing views as to what form an evaluation should take and how it should be conducted (Fox, 1991; Øvretveit, 1998).

For hard-pressed practitioners working at local level – say, on health improvement programmes, community health projects, area-based health initiatives, or innovations in primary health care – the discourse of the mainstream evaluative culture that they come into contact with is often seriously ill-suited to the challenges they face in their kinds of context. The approaches to evaluation that are best-known in the official health service world – often taken for granted as the only ones that exist – are of three kinds. All three emphasise quantitative investigation, but each comes from a different professional or academic discipline, each has a distinctive focus of interest, and offers a characteristic blueprint for research design, and a typical set of tools for evaluative inquiry and data-collection (see Table 24.1).

Not only does the official evaluative culture strongly favour evaluation through the collection of numerical data; there is a further hierarchy of merit even within this domain, whereby experimental study designs – in particular randomized controlled trials – are established as a 'gold standard' against which all evaluative inquiry is compared, as seen in the National Service Framework for mental health (NHS/OHN, 1999). The specific merits and shortcomings of each of the three mainstream approaches are summarized in Table 24.2.

The relevance of the mainstream approaches in certain contexts need not be denied. But their limitations arise from the 'linear logic' behind all these approaches. This derives from the biostatistical analysis of experi-

---

* Commissioned for this volume.

239

Table 24.1 Key features of three mainstream approaches to evaluating health projects

Approach	Distinctive focus of interest	Characteristic study design	Typical tools
1 Experimental (epidemiological) evaluation	Analysis of causal relations between input variables and outcome variables, and strength of such relationships	Trials Before and after Randomization Control of variables Randomized controlled trial	Input survey Outcomes trail
2 Economic evaluation	measurement of resources and how they are allocated/distributed, and with what effect	Cost-effectiveness appraisal (CEA) Cost–benefit appraisal (CBA) Cost–utility appraisal (CUA)	'Willingness-to-pay' criteria and scales Standard wager
3 Managerial evaluation	Identification of standards of performance, and measurement and monitoring of compliance with these	Design of performance indicators Audit/monitoring frameworks and cycles	Standard-setting

Source: Drawing partly on Øvretveit 1998)

Table 24.2 Merits and shortcomings of three mainstream approaches to evaluating health projects

Approach	Merits	Shortcomings
1 Experimental (epidemiological) evaluation	Precise and explicit in defining/comparing the 'variables' of the system studied; Focusing on the outcomes of projects; Effects are attributable to specific inputs Reduces bias (by randomization)	Difficult to set up, not always generalisable Time-scale often too short to track all 'effects' Not all relevant variables known or quantifiable Randomisation unacceptable in some situations Sampling bias often present but difficult to see
2 Economic evaluation	Takes account of resource limitations Opportunity costs, & competing criteria Can make value decisions transparent	Deals with costs better than utility/benefits/values Value criteria often poorly grounded, and debatable Fails to resolve competition/conflict between values
3 Managerial evaluation	Offers way to monitor key indicators of performance and to review progress and compare across projects or times	PIs are often simplistic, arbitrary: = 'blunt tools' Useful if used to raise questions, not answer them Difficulties with time-scale and with quantifiability

ments (formulated for research in medicine and the life sciences) or from budgetary calculations (devised for economic appraisals, and financial audits and accounts). It is a logic that is concerned to link outputs and outcomes (dependent variables) to initial inputs (independent variables) through exact and calculable lines of cause–effect connection. But this ambition can be seriously jeopardised by the many difficulties – practical and conceptual – that arise when trying to apply hard, linear analysis to the initiatives typical of contemporary innovations in clinical practice (Jelinek, 1992) and community health (Newell, 1992). Such initiatives are most often complex rather than simple, entailing multiple and recursive loops of influence rather than separate and independent lines of causation; and even the input or output variables of interest are sometimes elusive or unknown – hard to identify with confidence, let alone to measure and/or control for experimental purposes (Oakley, 1990).

The limits of the experimental/epidemiological approach are highlighted in a recent systematic appraisal of the literature on the evaluation of health-promoting schools. This review was carried out as part of the NHS Health Technology Assessment Programme, and used the most rigorous, explicit and methodical search procedures. It started with the randomized control trial as its 'gold standard' for evaluative inquiry, and therefore excluded all studies that did not use controlled comparison or before-and-after designs, or did not report explicit health outcomes. However, after reviewing the few research papers that met their search criteria, this report noted several issues of theory and methodology that such studies raise and that need further debate (see boxed text).

Issues of the theory and methods of RCTs raised by a review of the evaluation of health-promoting schools

Studies of this approach remain methodologically challenging, and too little attention has been given to the way in which the intervention and the evaluation impact on each other. There is a need for more widespread understanding of the aims of health promoting schools as well as further debate on the optimum way of evaluating such interventions ... The process of randomization [necessary to conduct a randomized control trial] is difficult to reconcile with readiness to change, which is likely to be important in achieving the active participation of schools ... [therefore research agencies should ...]

- encourage and enable further debate on the value of including studies using observational and qualitative methodologies in reviews of effectiveness of health promotion interventions ...
- ensure that process evaluation – which describes the way in

> which programmes have been implemented – is undertaken and
> reported in all studies of health promotion in schools ....
> - ensure, in publications of studies of school health promotion
>   interventions, that the following are reported:
>   the theoretical basis or assumptions underpinning the interven-
>   tions;
>   the content of the interventions;
>   the process of delivery.

(Summarized from Lister-Sharp *et al.*1999, pp. 24; 113; 115–16)

In economic evaluation (Ludbrook, 1990; Watson, 1997), the shortcomings of linear thinking are reinforced by the abstract and axiomatic
manoeuvres entailed in setting up a CEA (cost effective analysis), CBA
(cost benefit analysis) or CUA (cost utitlity analysis). In a review of the
field, an influential health economist concedes (Mooney, 1992, p. 157)
that: 'perhaps economists have generally been guilty of overselling economic appraisal'.

In managerial evaluation, the general shortcomings associated with
linear thinking are compounded by the specific additional difficulty that
this area of work remains dominated by a largely uncritical use of the
'3Es model' – a value for money (VfM) framework first brought into
public life by the Audit Commission in its conduct of performance
review in town halls (Local Government and Finance Acts 1982; Audit
Commission, 1985) – and extended into the National Health Service
(NHS) in 1989.This model is shown in Table 24.3.

The Audit Commission itself acknowledged in 1990 that 'economy'
had been the dominant and traditional focus of performance review;
that 'efficiency' had come more to attention in the 1980s; and that
'effectiveness' was still 'at the leading edge of performance review', as yet
given less attention than the first two Es (Audit Commission, 1990).
Nevertheless, the 3Es model has been used widely in the NHS since then,
in both hospital and community health settings (Henkel, 1991; Perkins,
1996; Renshaw, 1996) and is often presented as a straightforward and
unproblematic application of basic 'economics of health care' (Mooney,

Table 24.3 The 3 Es of 'value for money' in performance review and managerial
evaluation

VfM criterion	Definition
E1 Economy	How much *input* of resources used to provide services within specified budget headings
E2 Efficiency	How much *output* (specified quantity and quality of services) provided for the lowest possible input of resources
E3 Effectiveness	How far a project/service is achieving previously specified *outcomes* or goals

Table 24.4 Three critiques of the 3 Es/'Value for Money' approach in managerial evaluation

Critique	Argument
1 'Technical'	The 3Es are conceptually impoverished and narrow in scope (Metcalfe and Richards, 1987)
	The 3Es fail to do justice to the organizational complexities of the NHS (Klein, 1982)
	The 3Es are too blunt/crude to deal with rapidly-changing science-based practice (Pollitt, 1984, 1986)
2 'Moral'	The 3Es seriously neglect questions of ethics and value conflicts
	The value criteria need to be widened, to incorporate further Es, e.g. E4 = 'Ethics' (Balogh, 1988, 1989; Balogh *et al.*, 1989; Beattie, 1989); or ' equity' (Goddard, 1989); *or* 'excellence + enterprise' (Gunn, 1989)
3 'Political'	The 3Es framework over-emphasises monetary criteria and seriously neglects questions about who owns public services and whose views should therefore count in deciding their value (Kline and Mallaber, 1986; Mallaber and Kline, 1987)

1992), for example in the construction of minimum data sets suitable for use as performance indicators (Reid, 1986).

The standard argument in favour of the use of VfM and the 3Es in evaluating health systems is an economic one (Donaldson and Gerard, 1993): when resources are scarce, and insufficient to meet all of the needs (or demands) that exist, then VfM criteria can provide a discipline for making choices among different options for expenditure. But arguments against application of the VfM/3Es framework in the health sector have been widespread, and are of three kinds, as shown in Table 24.4.

Alternative evaluation paradigms: a change of discourse?

Since the 1980s or earlier, a wide variety of efforts have been made to evaluate new initiatives in health in many different contexts, and these efforts have helped to shape and define alternative ways of dealing with questions of worth that try to go beyond the limitations of the 'linear thinking' of the three mainstream evaluation strategies. Some of these approaches try to do this by holding on to a linear logic, but enriching it. In an effort to combine the different strands of mainstream evaluation so as to complement each other and compensate for their individual shortcomings, Øvretveit (1998) has suggested linking quality assurance tools to wider experimental methods of project evaluation and he describes a further strategy of inquiry (which he calls 'developmental evaluation'), in which the emphasis is on feeding back a range of evaluation and monitoring data to inform directly and guide 'formatively' the processes of project implementation. An approach devised by Pawson and Tilley (1997) – which they label 'realistic evaluation' – extends still further the scope of traditional 'linear' evaluative investigations (see boxed text below).

A summary of 'realistic evaluation'

'Realistic evaluation' focuses on the basic formula:
  context + mechanism = outcome

Key features are that:

1 A 'realist' methodology must adopt a rigorous, scientific, objective methodology, but it will not fall into the trap of using the 'over-simple, mechanical, experimental format' that historically has bedevilled evaluation of public sector projects; and
2 To be realistic, evaluation must attempt to 'inform the thinking of policy-makers, practitioners, program participants and public', within the specific *circumstances* of each specific project: it must be orientated firmly on action and decisions about action.

The task of the evaluation is then to try to find out which context–mechanism–outcome configurations are efficacious'. On this approach, there is not one single standard formula or design for an evaluation study, but key *processes* are likely to include the following:

1 Methods of data collection are likely always to combine qualitative as well as quantitative, retrospective as well as prospective, and responsive (interactive) as well as remote (hands-off) methods;
2 Data collection must be put alongside the building and testing of theory, drawn from wider bodies of relevant social research, especially, for example, to throw light on the role that all the many and different groups of practitioners and subjects play in the operation of the programme;
3 Data collection must be guided by these theoretical accounts, in particular by the questions that they prompt, eg as to how well particular aspects of the programme appear to be working, and why: 'what works for whom in what circumstances';
4 The evaluation process should 'marshal' the fragmentary expertise and insights of multiple stakeholders, and thereby initiate and support learning processes for all – can, in fact, encourage the building of a 'learning organization' around the project under scrutiny.

Source: Drawing on Pawson and Tilley (1997)

These two examples – Øvretveit's 'developmental evaluation', and Pawson and Tilley's 'realistic evaluation' can serve as a first illustration of some features that are basic to the alternative paradigms that are emerging:

1 They do not necessarily give primacy to quantification and biostatistical analysis; they may emphasize ethnographic methods, including observations, interviews, document analysis, narrative reportage;
2 They examine and analyse the theoretical foundations and working procedures of projects as well as their outcomes or impact; and
3 They invest considerable effort in the 'action-orientation'; giving priority within an evaluation study to ensuring that evaluative findings are taken on to the agendas of relevant decision makers.

As a tool for further analysis and development of this shift in thinking about evaluation, I would like now to call on 'critical discourse analysis' (CDA), which affords a way of looking at texts at a number of levels 'beyond the text itself' (here, we are looking at documents that record evaluative studies of health projects). A framework for CDA devised by Fairclough (1992, 1995) offers a way of analysing and categorizing the wider discourse practices and sociocultural practices that must always be drawn on in the production of a specific text. It suggests three levels of question we should ask about the 'functions' – 'textual' and beyond – of any text (see boxed text).

Three functions of discourse, 'text and beyond': a preliminary framework for critical discourse analysis

1 **The textual function**
   How is the text ordered? How do parts of the text link together?
2 **The interpersonal function**
   Which particular social identities and relationships are 'privileged' by a specific text/discourse practice?
3 **The ideational function**
   Which particular pictures of the world are shown/concealed by a specific text/discourse practice?

Source: Drawing on Fairclough (1992, 1995)

This scheme highlights the most distinctive and crucial feature of evaluation approaches that seek to go beyond the mainstream 'linear' thinking. Mainstream approaches (as set out in Fig 24.1) are concerned to track linear structures and linkages within the projects that are the subject of evaluative inquiry. But alternative approaches to evaluation (in varying degree) move forward to encompass the *interpersonal* and the *ideational* 'functions' – sometimes alongside a concern for linear order (as in 'developmental evaluation' and 'realistic evaluation', described above), but sometimes going further and giving precedence to the *'interpersonal* and *ideational* functions' by starting with these. This latter shift is seen in what I have called 'dialogical evaluation' (see Beattie, 1984, 1995), and in the remainder of this chapter I want to offer an analysis in terms of the two 'functions beyond the text' set out in the boxed text above. I will argue that dialogical evaluation is by now beginning to constitute a coherent, structured way of thinking, and amounts (by comparison with mainstream evaluation) to a decisive 'change in discourse'.

Engaging multiple stakeholders: the 'interpersonal function' in evaluation

One the most important prompts to the rise of new paradigm evaluation has been frustration with the common practice in mainstream evaluation of starting with technical questions, concerning how to order, sequence and design the evaluative study. One key feature of the alternative paradigm has been to start with questions about participants, power and ownership, about 'stakeholders': Who has a stake in the project that is to be evaluated? Whose interests are likely to be affected by the project? Who has authority in resource allocation and decision making related to the project? How close to the project are such stakeholders? In what ways does the evaluation process for a project engage different stakeholders? The 'interpersonal function' can be opened up on several fronts by this 'stakeholder perspective' in evaluation:

Pluralistic evaluation

In some ways, the most fundamental and difficult challenge in the conduct of evaluation is to appreciate that multiple stakeholders exist, and that there is almost always a range of different views among different stakeholders, and that these form the basis for disagreement and power play within the life of most health projects. 'Pluralistic evaluation' is an approach that has shown how to give a full account of these multiple views, to portray them, to provide what ethnographers call a 'thick description' of these sources of diversity and conflict – as demonstrated by Smith and Cantley (1983, 1984, 1985) in an evaluation of a day care unit for the elderly mentally infirm.

Collaborative evaluation

A second stance in 'stakeholder' evaluation (which Smith and Cantley did not move on to) is to attempt to ensure that the findings about multiple views are taken up and acted upon in the agendas of decision making for the project that is being evaluated. After all, if the findings about multiple views are not fed back into such deliberations, a crucial opportunity to enhance democratic procedure is missed. This stance brings evaluation closely into line with the 'action research' tradition. Making a reality of the link to action can be a lengthy, time-consuming and exhausting phase in the cycle of 'interpersonal negotiation', and it may need to be repeated frequently. But some evaluation studies that have attempted such work have shown remarkable success, as seen in Springett's (1998) report on evaluating the Liverpool Healthy City project.

Participatory evaluation

A further step that can be taken in exploring the interpersonal function is to take the view that project participants (staff, clients) may be the people best placed to figure out what data may be most relevant, and how best to collect it, make sense of it, and act upon it. On this view, priority is given to building evaluative capacity within a project, by training participants and encouraging them to work as 'co-researchers'. This is often found to have a marked impact on the self-confidence and sense of ownership of project participants (Feuerstein, 1982), and like other forms of 'participatory action research' (of which this is an instance) it can become highly prized as a means by which local people can enfranchise and empower themselves. It is now used extensively in evaluating health projects in less-developed countries (Feuerstein, 1986, 1988), and is becoming familiar in local community health projects in the UK (Jones, 1998).

Reflexive evaluation

A final turn in the cycle of interpersonal negotiation occurs when the researcher/evaluator (whether they have the status of insider or outsider) explores and reports on the extent to which their own presence may have an impact on participants' experience of the process of evaluation. For example, regular exchange of views between 'insider' and 'outsider' may have a crucial influence on both (Bond and Hart, 1998). Or an outside evaluator whose presence is temporary and tangential to the project – may be faced with challenging questions about his/her acceptability to participants who are themselves long-term residents in the neighbourhood (Hunt, 1987). Or the choice of ways of gathering data and interpreting them that are shaped by feminist views on reciprocity in the researcher–informant relationship may lead to resistance or hostility in some quarters (Kirkup, 1986). This loop of evaluative inquiry

HIGH GRID

Privileges fixed, closed categories

	Pluralistic evaluation Portray/describe multiple stakeholders disagreements, power-play	Collaborative evaluation Play-back findings into decision-making agendas; seek official action/response	
LOW GROUP **Privileges** **individual** **responsibility**	Reflexive evaluation Give an account of evaluator presence/role/ impact; Acknowledge own learning process	Participatory evaluation build on-site evaluative capacity: Train participants as co-researchers; Encourage group self- determination	**HIGH GROUP** **Privileges** **collective** **responsibility**

Privileges negotiable, open categories

LOW GRID

Figure 24.1   Ways of engaging stakeholders in evaluation: as forms of cultural bias

Source: Beattie (1991c, 1993)

connects to wider issues and developments related to 'reflexivity' in research and practice.

Through these four steps, evaluation studies can trace and reveal *'which particular social identities and relationships are being privileged'*. It is tempting to view this in terms of the grid/group analysis devised in social anthropology for identifying different forms of cultural bias (Beattie, 1991c, 1993), as shown in Figure 24.1.

Addressing contested concepts: the ideational function in evaluation

The rise of new paradigm evaluation has also been fuelled by a second concern. Frequently during the conduct of an evaluation study, crucial new insights emerge, or new ideas are brought to light that substantially change the way in which some or all of the stakeholders conceive of the project and its aims and processes. In mainstream evaluation approaches the study design is usually fixed and predetermined, so shifts in under-standing what a project might appropriately try to do cannot be accom-modated by the research. But new paradigm evaluation regards the conceptual positions and movements within a project as a crucial part of the picture. It asks a set of questions along the lines of: What key ideas informed the setting up of this project? What issues have been raised during the life of the project? Around what concepts does disagreement and power-play most often arise? What agendas for debate have been taken up? Are there some issues that are raised but then discarded or ignored? By addressing the contested concepts in play within a project, evaluation can decipher the 'ideational function', and again it can do so on several fronts or in several stages.

Illuminative evaluation

A readiness to watch, listen, wait and pick up key insights when they arise, often at unexpected moments, is crucial. Like the 'pluralistic' stance, this is a basic standpoint, sometimes difficult to grasp, yet essential to opening up this second cycle of work. 'Illuminative evaluation' shows how to do this: to seize ideas, issues and debates as they surface or subside; to dig out a new, previously hidden insight, and to focus it and use it to throw light on other aspects of the project that is being evaluated. It was pioneered in evaluations of educational innovations (Parlett and Hamilton, 1972; Hamilton *et al.*, 1977), before its application in health promotion (Levane *et al.*, 1981; Prout, 1992); it has affinities with the 'grounded theory' approach in wider social research.

Critical evaluation

This approaches the theoretical issues raised by a project from a different direction. Rather than seek out and focus ideas that emerge from within the project under scrutiny, it draws on wider (and usually well-established) frameworks of theoretical debate – say, in sociology, or social policy – and uses these to ask searching questions of the project, its underpinnings, its aims, its ways of working, its internal debates, its pattern of development, its future plans etc. Often a sharp new perspective on a project and its distinctive strengths and weaknesses may be brought to bear by this modality of evaluation: say, for example, highlighting issues around equal opportunities policies; or around ways of working to reduce health inequalities (Everitt and Hardiker, 1996, 1997).

Creative evaluation

Another rich vein of growth in new paradigm evaluation has arisen from the development of methods and tools that can help project participants who are less confident or less comfortable with conventional textual and verbal formats as vehicles for expressing their thoughts and feelings about the project, to explore other media through which they might be better able to articulate their views. Some recent evaluations of urban public health projects have used creative writing and story-telling to elicit personal accounts (Wilkinson, 1999) – like the use of such approaches in wider strategies for the management of change (Amtoft, 1994; Weil, 1994). Other evaluators have found it helpful to employ exercises and activities which explore the metaphors that are often embedded in people's everyday talk about services, about health, about evaluation itself – as a way of prising open taken-for-granted assumptions and bringing fresh ideas to projects – e.g. by exposing for discussion and debate the 'machine/production line' metaphor that runs through mainstream health service evaluation – and generating relevant and useful new metaphors (see House, 1986; Smith, 1981).

Dialectical evaluation

This step in the cycle of 'addressing concepts' in project evaluation is less well documented than other phases, but it seems likely to be a major growth point for the future – in an era characterized by postmodern flux, and the collapse of master narratives and commanding grand theories. As in other spheres, in project evaluation the dialectical position entails drawing out opposed theories, mapping key ideas and their opposites, but then trying to move beyond simple dualities, divisions and polarizations – by seeking new 'syntheses', shared common ground – moving into what some call 'thirdspace'. Through this process, none of the parties to an encounter 'across a bar' of different beliefs remains the same; rather, all change by learning from each other (Bhabha, 1994; Soja, 1996). Glimpses of this are given in evaluation studies by Beattie, 1991a, 1991b, 1995; Fox, 1991; and Scott, 1992.

In these four steps, evaluation studies can trace and reveal *'which particular pictures of the world are being privileged'*. This phase of work can be

HOW KNOWLEDGE IS CLASSIFIED

Public: clear and fixed boundaries

	Illuminative evaluation Excavate emerging insights; Use these to focus/ refocus the study	Critical evaluation Juxtapose project against backdrop of wider social theory; Expose strengths and weaknesses	
HOW KNOWLEDGE IS SELECTED Within the project	Creative evaluation Generate personal accounts through story and metaphor; Use these to open up private views	Dialectical evaluation Bring together polarised views, Encourage/facilitate structured debate; Seek shared common ground	HOW KNOWLEDGE IS SELECTED Beyond the project

Private: blurred and negotiable boundaries

HOW KNOWLEDGE IS CLASSIFIED

Figure 24.2   Ways of addressing contested concepts in evaluation: as knowledge codes

Source: Beattie (1991c, 1993)

depicted in terms of the 'classification-and-framing' scheme devised in sociolinguistics to map competing codes of knowledge (Beattie, 1991c, 1993), as shown in Figure 24.2.

Dialogical evaluation as a discourse of change

The approach to evaluation outlined here is one that is far more appropriate to the circumstances of precarious projects and hard-pressed practitioners (usually) than are mainstream approaches. It puts a premium on the cultural (interpersonal and ideational) rather than on the technical/formal dimensions of the project under scrutiny. Because of this emphasis it can grapple directly with the wicked, messy and at times chaotic situations characteristic of practice innovations in health settings – and not see such complexities as a distraction and a disappointment. It can capture the interplay of 'multiple voices' and 'contested concepts' that is probably unavoidable, and that some regard as highly desirable as part of wider moves to strengthen 'civil society' and 'deliberative democracy'. In choosing the label 'dialogical' for this double-cycle framework for evaluation, I am consciously invoking the parallels with some other current discourses with which it has important common ground and useful points of contact. The dialogical approach to evaluation recommended here echoes numerous areas of development in 'complex systems thinking' (Harries *et al.*, 1998; Plamping *et al.*, 1998; Pratt *et al.*, 1999) and I would like to finish by making just one connection (of many that could be made). An approach to bringing about change that has generated a great deal of interest in recent years and has a well-developed theory and evidence base is the 'learning organization' (LO) strategy, which Pedler, *et al.* (1997, p. 3) define as 'an organization that facilitates the learning of all its members and consciously transforms itself and its context'.

One of the sources of the LO strategy is whole systems thinking, which argues that, for successful management of strategic change, it is vital to invest in the *structuring and sharing of information across the organization*. This is described by Argyris and Schon (1978, p. 313) as the way to 'extend the capacity for multiple viewing of organizational phenomena ... to tolerate and deal with conflict ... to learn to model good organizational dialectic'. Thus 'dialogue' has come to be seen as an essential tool for building a learning organization (see boxed text)

A précis of 'Dialogue as a Tool for Building a Learning Organization'

Dialogue is a key reflective learning process, a form of conversation that can bring to the surface, and alter, the tacit infrastructures of thought, the taken for granted assumptions, the polarization of opinions, the rules for acceptable and unacceptable conversation, and the methods for managing differences. It is how a group learns to watch or experience its own tacit processes in action. Too often discussion is more orientated towards the 'advocacy' styles of raw debate – discussing to win, challenging each other, one-upmanship, beating one another down, 'having ideas against each other' in adversarial or accusatorial mode – and not enough to 'inquiry', attending to the sources of group thought and trying to deliberate on and illuminate them. Disciplined dialogue differs from unproductive discussion or debate because the participants are not merely engaged in 'advocacy wars'. They develop a repertoire of techniques (encompassing collaborative reflection and inquiry skills) for seeing how the components of their situation fit together, and they develop a more penetrating understanding of the forces at play among the team members themselves. In discussion you may make a choice; but in disciplined dialogue you discover the nature of choice. Dialogue is a sustained collective inquiry into everyday experience and what we take for granted. The goal of dialogue is to open new ground by establishing a 'container' or 'field' for inquiry: a setting where people can become aware of the context around their experience and of the processes of thought and feeling that created that experience ... The serious lack of balance between 'advocacy' and 'inquiry' causes common misunderstandings, miscommunications, and poor decisions. The building of shared meanings requires a better balance between the two.

Source: Summarised from Senge (1994, pp. 352–4; 359–63; 385–91)

Evaluative inquiries that work their way around the twin cycles of 'interpersonal and ideational negotiation' in dialogical evaluation (described above) can be a uniquely powerful resource for setting up the 'structured dialogue' required to build a learning organization. In summation, dialogical evaluation offers a 'change of discourse' by comparison with mainstream approaches; and it brings to bear a 'discourse of change' that links dialogue to action, as set out in the boxed text below.

Dialogical evaluation as a discourse of change: ten precepts

1 Map the diverse questions asked by different stakeholders, about aims, processes, outcomes;
2 Generate data at multiple levels, to answer the questions posed by different stakeholders;
3 Facilitate the learning of all stakeholders;

4 Investigate the shifting coalitions and power-plays that occur within the project and its context;

5 Tolerate and deal with conflict;

6 Identify and use new explanatory or analytical insights as they emerge during evaluation;

7 Report fully and examine critically the contested concepts explicit or implicit in the project;

8 Prompt and inform debate about aims/processes/outcomes and relate it to theoretical issues;

9 Extend the capacity of all stakeholders for 'multiple viewing of organizational phenomena'; and

10 Ensure that the conduct of the evaluation itself models 'good organizational dialectic'.

Sources: Drawing partly on Beattie (1984, 1995); Springett *et al.* (1995); WHO (1999)

References

Amtoft, M. (1994). Storytelling as a support tool for project management, *International Journal of Project Management*, 12(4) 230–33.

Argyris, C., Schon, D. (1978). *Organizational Learning: A theory of action perspective*. New York: Addison-Wesley.

Audit Commission (1985). *Good Management in Local Government*. London: Local Government Training Board.

Audit Commission (1990). *Performance Review Action Guide*. Milton Keynes: Learning Materials Design.

Balogh, R. and Beattie, A. (1988). Performance review, *Nursing Times*, 94(18), 4 May.

Balogh, R. and Beattie, A. (1989). *Monitoring Performance and Quality in Training Institutions*. London: English National Board.

Balogh, R. Beattie, A. and Beckerleg, S. (1989). *Figuring Out Performance: A guide to assessing performance and quality in nursing and midwifery training institutions*. Sheffield: English National Board.

Beattie, A. (1984). Evaluating community health initiatives. In Somerville, G. (ed.) *Community Development in Health: Addressing the confusions*. London: King's Fund.

Beattie, A. (1989). From quantity to quality: the 4 Es of evaluation, *Community Health Action*, 12, 7–9.

Beattie, A. (1991a). *Success and Failure in Community Development for Health in the NHS: 8 case studies*. Milton Keynes: Open University Health Education Unit Occasional Papers, 1(1).

Beattie, A. (1991b). *The Evaluation of Community Development Initiatives in Health Promotion: A review of current strategies*. Milton Keynes: Open University Health Education Unit Occasional Papers, 1(3).

Beattie, A. (1991c). Knowledge and control in health promotion: a test-case for social theory and social policy. In Gabe, J., Calnan, M., Bury, M. (eds), *Sociology of the Health Service*. London: Routledge.

Beattie, A. (1993). The changing boundaries of health. In Beattie, A., Gott, M., Jones, L. and Sidell, M. (eds), *Health and Wellbeing: A book of readings*. London: Macmillan.

Beattie, A. (1995). Evaluation in community development for health: an opportunity for dialogue?, *Health Education Journal*, 54, 465–72.

Bhabha, H. (1994). 'How newness enters the world: postmodern space, postcolonial times and the trials of cultural translation'. In Bhaba, H., *The Location of Culture*. London: Routledge.

Bond, M. and Hart, E. (1998). Exploring the roles and contributions of outside evaluators in an action research project, *Socal Sciences in Health*, 4(3) 176–86.

Donaldson, C. and Gerard, K. (1993). *Economics of Health Care Financing: The invisible hand*. London: Macmillan.

Everitt, A., Hardiker, P. (1996). *Evaluating for Good Practice*. London: Macmillan.

Everitt, A., Hardiker, P. (1997). Towards a critical approach to evaluation. In Sidell, M. *et al*. (eds), *Debates and Dilemmas in Promoting Health*. London: Macmillan.

Fairclough, N. (1992). *Discourse and Social Change*. Cambridge: Polity Press.

Fairclough, N. (1995). *Media Discourse*. London: Arnold.

Feuerstein, M. T. (1982). Participatory evaluation: by, with and for the people, Idea: Reading Bulletin 14, Agricultural Extension and Rural Development Centre, University of Reading, March 18–23.

Feuerstein, M. T. (1986). *Partners in Evaluation: Evaluating development and community programmes with participants*. London: Macmillan.

Feuerstein, M. T. (1988). Finding the methods to fit the people: training for participatory evaluation, *Comminity Development Journal* 23(1).

Fox, N. J. (1991). Postmodernism, rationality and the evaluation of health care, *Sociology Review*, 39(4), 709–44.

Goddard, A. (1989). Are three Es enough? Assessing value for money in the public sector. OR Insight 2, September 16-19.

Gunn, L. (1989). A public management approach to the NHS, *Health Services Management Research*, 2(1), 10–19.

Hamilton, D., Jenkins, D., King, C., MacDonald, B., Parlett, M. (1977). *Beyond the Numbers Game: A reader in educational evaluation*. London: Macmillan.

Harries, J., Gordon, P., Plamping, D. and Fischer, M. (1998). *Elephant Problems and Fixes that Fail*. London, King's Fund.

Henkel, M. (1991). *Government, Evaluation and Change*. London: Jessica Kingsley.

House, E. (1986). How we think about evaluation. In House, E. R. (ed.), *New Directions in Educational Evaluation*. London: Falmer.

Hunt, S. (1987). Evaluating a community development project: issues of acceptability, *British Journal of Social Work* 17, 661–7.

Jelinek, M. (1992). The clinician and the randomised controlled trial. In Daly, J., McDonald, I. and Willis, E. (eds), *Researching Healthcare: designs, dilemmas, discipline*. London: Routledge.

Jones, J. (1998). *Private Troubles and Public Issues: A community development approach to health*. Edinburgh: Community Learning Scotland.

Kirkup, G. (1986). The feminist evaluator. In House, E. R. (ed.), *New Directions in Educational Evaluation*. London: Falmer.

Klein, R. (1982). Performance management and the NHS: a case study in conceptual perplexity and organizational complexity, *Public Administration*, 60 (Winter), 385–407.

Kline, R., and Mallaber, J. (1986). *Whose Value? Whose Money? – How to assess the real value of council services*. Birmingham: Local Government Information Unit.

Levane, L., Beattie, A., Plamping, D. and Thorne, S. (1981). *The Children's Health Club: An evaluation*. London, King's Fund.

Lister-Sharp, D., Chapman, S., Stewart-Brown, S. and Sowden, A. (1999). Health promoting schools and health promotion in schools: two systematic reviews, *Health Technology Assessment*, 3(22).

Local Government and Finance Act (1982). London: HMSO.

Ludbrook, A. (1990). Using economic appraisal in health services research, *Health Bulletin*, 48(2).

Mallaber, J. and Kline, R. (1987). Counting what can't be counted, *Social Services Insight* (March 13), 12–19.

Metcalfe, L., and Richards, S. (1986). The efficiency strategy in central government: an impoverished concept of management, *Public Money* (9 June), 29–32.

Mooney, G. (1992). *Economics, Medicine and Health Care* (2nd edn). London: Harvester Wheatsheaf.

Newell, D. J. (1992). Randomised controlled trials in health care research. In Daly, J., McDonald, I. and Willis, E. (eds), *Researching Healthcare: designs, dilemmas, discipline*. London: Routledge.

NHS/OHN (National Health Service/Our Healthier Nation) (1999). *National Service Framework for Mental Health*. London: Department of Health.

Oakley, A. (1990). Who's afraid of the randomized controlled trial? In Roberts, H. (ed.) *Women's Health Counts*. London: Routledge.

Øvretveit, J. (1998). *Evaluating Health Interventions*. Buckingham: Open University Press.

Parlett, M. and Hamilton, D. (1972). *Illuminative Evaluation: A new approach to the study of innovatory programs*, Edinburgh: University of Edinburgh Centre for Research in Educational Sciences, Occasional Paper 9.

Pawson, R. and Tilley, N. (1997). *Realistic Evaluation*. London: Sage.

Pedler, M., Burgoyne, J. and Boydell, T. (eds) (1997). *The Learning Company* (2nd edn). Maidenhead: McGraw-Hill.

Perkins, D. A. (1996). Effectiveness and efficiency in health care. In Glynn, J. J., Perkins, D. A., Stewart, S. (eds), *Achieving Value for Money*. London: W. B. Saunders.

Plamping, D., Gordon, P. and Pratt, J. (1998). *Action Zones and Large Numbers*. London: King's Fund.

Pollitt, C. (1984). Blunt tools: performance measurement in policies for health care, OMEGA: International Journal of Management Science, 12, 131–40.

Pollitt, C. (1986). Beyond the managerial model: the case for broadening performance assessment in government and the public services, *Financial Accountability and Management*, 2(3) 155–70

Pratt, J., Gordon, P. and Plamping, D. (1999). *Working Whole Systems*. London: King's Fund.

Prout, A. (1992). Illumination, collaboration, facilitation, negotiation: evaluating the MESMAC Project. In Aggleton, P. Young, A., Moody, D., Kapila, M. and Pye, M. (eds), *Does it Work? Perspectives on the evaluation of HIV/AIDS health promotion*. London: Health Education Authority.

Reid, E. (1986). Performance indicators, *Nursing Times*, 82(37) (Sept 10), 44–8.

Renshaw, J. (1996). Measuring efficiency in health care: the role of the Audit Commission. In Glynn, J. J., Perkins, D. A. and Stewart, S. (eds), *Achieving Value for Money*. London: W. B. Saunders.

Scott, S. (1992). Evaluation may change your life but it won't solve all your problems. In Aggleton, P., Young, A., Moody, D., Kapila, M. and Pye, M. (eds), *Does it Work? Perspectives on the evaluation of HIV/AIDS health promotion*. London: Health Education Authority.

Senge, P., Kleiner, A., Roberts, C., Ross, R. and Smith, B. (1990). *The Fifth Discipline: The art and practice of the learning organization*. New York: Doubleday.

Senge, P., Kleiner, A., Roberts, C., Ross, R. and Smith, B. (1994). *The Fifth Discipline Fieldbook: Strategies and tools for building a learning organization*. London: Brealey.

Senge P., Kleiner, A., Roberts, C., Ross, R. and Smith, B. (1999). *The Dance of Change: The challenges of sustaining momentum in learning organizations*. London: Brealey.

Smith, G. and Cantley, C. (1983). *Pluralistic Evaluation: A study in day care for the elderly mentally infirm*. Hull: Hull University, Dept of Social Administration, Occasional Paper.

Smith, G. and Cantley, C. (1984). Pluralistic evaluation. In Lishman, J. (ed.), *Evaluation*. Aberdeen: Aberdeen University Research Highlights No. 8.

Smith, G., Cantley, C. (1985). Directions in Evaluative Research. In Smith, G. and Cantley, C., *Assessing Health Care*. Milton Keynes: Open University Press.

Smith, N. L. (1981). Metaphors for evaluation. In Smith, N. L., *Metaphors for Evaluation: Sources of New Methods*. London: Sage.

Soja, E. W. (1996). *Thirdspace: Journeys to Los Angeles and other real-and-imagined places*. Oxford: Blackwell.

Springett, J., Costongs, C., Dugdill, J. (1995). Towards a framework for evaluation in health promotion: the importance of process. *Journal of Contemporary Health*, 2, 61–5.

Springett, J. (1998). Quality measures and evaluation of Healthy City policy initiatives: the Liverpool experience. In Davies, J. K., Macdonald, G. (eds), *Quality, Evidence and Effectiveness in Health Promotion*. London: Routledge.

Stenhouse, L. (1982). The conduct, analysis and reporting of case study in educational research and evaluation. In McCormick, R. (ed.), *Calling Education to Account*. London: Heinemann.

Watson, K. (1997). Economic evaluation of health care. In Jenkinson, C. (ed.), *Assessment and Evaluation of Health and Medical Care: A methods text*. Buckingham: Open University Press.

Weil, S. (1994). Bringing about cultural change in colleges and universities: The power and potential of story. In Weil, S. (ed.) *Introducing Change from the Top in Universities and Colleges*. London:, Kogan Page.

WHO (World Health Organization) (1999). *Health Promotion Evaluation: Recommendations to Policymakers*. Copenhagen: WHO.

Wilkinson, M. (1999). *Creative Writing: Its role in evaluation*. London: King's Fund.

25 User movements, community development and health promotion*

Marian Barnes

Contested Communities

Community has been a focus for sociological research and analysis for many years (see, for example, Young and Willmott 1962; Williamson, 1982; Bulmer, 1987; Etzioni, 1995). It has also been the subject of a range of policy initiatives, such as community care, community regeneration and community safety, which have all made assumptions about the nature of the links between people who live in geographical proximity or who share characteristics or interests with each other. Often such policies have sought to encourage or enforce forms of behaviour based in normative assumptions about how people should relate to others. This is perhaps most evident in the policy of community care. This is based not only in a belief that older people, disabled people and those experiencing psychological distress should receive support 'in the community', rather than segregated from the rest of society in long-stay institutions, but also in the assumption that care by family and friends is both the best and the preferred option in such circumstances (Barnes, 1997). There has not always been a close link between the analysis of community deriving from research, and the assumptions that have driven policy. In particular, the emphasis within official community care policy on family care not only conflated 'community' with 'family' as the source of support for individuals. but also largely failed to address the potential of communities to exclude those they regard as 'different'.

'Community' can be based in identity and interest as well as locality. Shared ethnicity, gender and sexuality can provide a basis for friendship, support and political action for people who may not identify themselves primarily in relation to the locality in which they live. Similarly, the 1980s and 1990s saw a substantial development of collective action among those who identify themselves as users of health and social care services – as disabled people, as survivors of psychological distress and/or of mental health services, or as carers. Disabled people, users and survivors are working together to support each other and to achieve change

---

* From Adams, L. and Munro, J., (eds) (2002) *Promoting Health: politics and practice*, London: Sage.

within welfare services and in society more broadly. They draw on their collective experiences to propose action to overcome the barriers they face, and to provide support which enables community participation.

For those who have experienced stigma and exclusion, such 'communities of identity' can be more significant than a community defined by locality. Collective action of this type can also contribute to the diversity of identities which may be included within the population of any particular locality. Action which might be considered as 'community development' among people previously separated from 'ordinary life' in long-stay hospitals and residential units has been important not only in supporting disabled people and others to take part in community, but also in changing communities to enable that participation (Barnes, 1997).

User movements

Collective action among disabled people and mental health service users has been theorized by reference to 'new social movements' (Barnes and Bowl, 2001; Campbell and Oliver, 1996; Shakespeare, 1993). Melucci (1985) has suggested that a shared identity 'constructed and negotiated through a repeated process of "activation" of social relationships connecting the actors' distinguishes 'new' from 'old' social movements. Identities are created and re-created not simply by 'being', but through action within such movements. New social movements are not solely or primarily concerned with redistribution, structural revolution or reform, as in the case of class-based movements, but with cultural and expressive objectives based in identity formation or consciousness raising (Cohen, 1985). Touraine (2000, p. 92) has described it in these terms: 'A social movement is never reducible to the defence of the interests of the dominated. Its ambition is always to abolish a relationship of domination, to bring about the triumph of a principle of equality, or to create a new society which breaks with the old forms of production, management and hierarchy.' The overarching objective can be expressed as one of transformation rather than restructuring and the means by which this is to be achieved is through a transformation of the values and meanings predominating in what has been variously termed the 'postindustrial' or 'postmodern' world.

We can see this in both the strategies and objectives of user groups. They seek change in the nature of health and social care services, and in the social policies which shape both the provision of welfare services and broader public policy. But their *underlying* objectives are concerned with transforming the way in which mental illness and disability are understood, and the way in which disabled people and people experiencing severe psychological distress are perceived. The methods they use to achieve this include user-led research and training, cultural expression and public awareness campaigns, as well as more direct involvement in policy making.

There might be some reluctance among activists to define this as 'health promotion'. Within the disability movement there has been a powerful analysis of the inadequacy of the medical model and an assertion of the difference between illness and disability. Mental health service users and survivors have also challenged clinical perspectives on distress and madness. The motivation for action comes more from the experience of exclusion than of poor health. Where groups have organized around particular 'mental health problems', most notably in the case of the Hearing Voices movement (Romme and Escher, 1993), the aim has been to reclaim and redefine the meaning of such experiences. rather than to achieve a reduction in 'symptoms'.

Another dilemma in locating such action within the health promotion arena has been the response of some clinicians to user organization, particularly in the area of mental health. Constructions by clinicians of the purpose of 'user involvement' as *therapy* rather than *empowerment* have led to conflict (Barnes and Wistow, 1994), and expectations that users will conform to bureaucratic 'rules of the game' in the context of consultation or participation exercises have, in some cases, contributed to stress (Barnes and Bowl, 2001).

Nevertheless, both the process and outcome of such action can contribute to promoting health and well-being. It can achieve this directly as a result of the development of skills and the enhancement of self-esteem, and indirectly through producing more health promoting services, and by contributing to the development of a more inclusive society. Models of health promotion which locate this within practices which have the aims of reducing inequalities and social exclusion, rather than of individual health improvement, are more consistent with the transformative objectives of user movements.

Achieving change

Some examples will illustrate how user groups are pursuing their objectives, and the issues they face in doing so.

One of the longest-established mental health user groups in the UK is the Nottingham Advocacy Group (NAG). NAG grew out of patients' meetings on hospital wards. It was strongly influenced by the Dutch user movement and has grown to become an umbrella organization for user groups within different service settings, advocacy projects and user representation within a wide range of decision making fora in the city. Activists in NAG have played an important role in supporting, the development of similar user-led initiatives elsewhere and in the formation of the UK Advocacy Network (UKAN) in 1991.

Interviews with NAG activists carried out for research in the early 1990s illustrated the importance of active involvement in such groups for the participants themselves, as well as the impact they achieved:

> In some ways it turned out to be a positive step for me. It changed my life around from something that was killing me, virtually, to something that I finally got some kind of reward in.

> ... it's given me a life and without it I wouldn't have dreamed of doing half the things I do now. It's given me confidence, assurance ... I get up now and speak at a conference quite happily. A few years ago I would have no more done that than fly! So really we are here for ourselves as well as other people. (Quoted in Barnes and Shardlow, 1996)

But the importance of this goes beyond individual personal development. Activists also spoke of the way in which their involvement in decision making demonstrated that mental health service users, who are often regarded as being incapable of decision making on their own behalf, can play an important role in shaping policies and services. This has an impact on wider perceptions of what it means to be someone with a mental health problem.

NAG has faced problems. While it is influential within the local mental health system, it has continually faced the problem of resourcing its work, and of persuading officials in all parts of the system that it has a role to play. There have also been differences of philosophy within the group: not all service users hold the same views about 'mental illness' nor about the priorities to be given to different strategies to support service users. One development initially under the NAG umbrella and later established as a separate initiative, was 'Ecoworks'. Brian Davey, who played a key role in this, locates Ecoworks within the community development tradition (Davey, 1999). Its aim is to enable people who have used mental health services to become involved in small-scale work projects based on ecological principles. Rather than prioritizing changes in the mental health system, this initiative aims to address more directly social exclusion and the conditions which create this.

Elsewhere mental health service users, disabled people and others have become involved in user-led research which has the joint aims of exploring and disseminating, users' views and of demonstrating the value of research in which users are fully represented in determining the subject matter and in carrying it out (e.g. Barnes and Mercer, 1997; Faulkner and Layzell, 2000). Others have become trainers and some are employed on postgraduate and professional training, programmes, taking part in the education of professionals who will subsequently deliver services. Involvement in the process of knowledge production and dissemination is a potent demonstration of the challenge offered to traditional assumptions about professional knowledge and the power associated with it.

Older people constitute the largest group of people using community care and health services. Self-organization among older people is less developed than among other groups, but examples are emerging (e.g., Thornton and Tozer 1994; Cormie, 1999; Barnes and Shaw, 2000). Once again, studies of such experiences demonstrate the impact that collective action which values people's experiences can make on the individuals who take part: 'one of the best things that's ever happened to me is getting to go there so that I could voice my opinion on things and say to them what I think. I feel, you feel, you are getting somewhere by doing that and being able to do it, whereas before I couldn't.' (Barnes and Bennet, 1998). But, as with the experience of mental health service users, the reluctance of some professionals to hear what users have to say, and the struggle to obtain the resources necessary to sustain and develop such initiatives, are never far away.

There is also a tendency among officials to construct the voices of service users as 'self interested' and thus to question their legitimacy. Involvement in a user group *per se* is sometimes considered to mean that the users concerned are no longer 'representative' of the silent majority. The way in which people make their contributions can also be dismissed as 'over-emotional' or as expressing 'mere anecdotes' which do not have the same legitimacy as rational scientific argument. User organisation has provided an important source of alternative knowledge and expertise, and has produced real improvements for participants and the services they have sought to influence. But the balance of power is still firmly in favour of the professionals.

New policy directions

The late 1990s saw important shifts in the construction of social problems and of policy responses to them. The identification of social exclusion as *the* problem for which social policy solutions were required marked official recognition that deprivation and inequality in material circumstances are associated with deprivation and inequality in terms of physical environments, educational and health status. There are three key aspects to this that are of central relevance to this discussion:

- There is a chancing focus from a service delivery to an issue or locality-based approach to policy making;
- There is an increasing focus on people as members of communities; and
- Communities are identified as deliverers of policy and creators of solu-

tions as well as the context within which problems have to be understood. (For a longer discussion of this, see Barnes and Prior, 2000.)

These changes should provide a more fertile environment within which user, movements can play a role in challenging the social exclusion experienced by their members. In practical policy terms this will extend beyond the community care arena. It will take place within the context of Health Action Zones (HAZs) and Health Improvement Programmes as well as other locality-based initiatives to reduce social exclusion. For example, some HAZs have developed programmes focusing on mental health issues, on older people or on disabled people. The challenge will be to ensure that *locality*-based action to address the root causes of ill health can also include these groups, who have often found local communities to be unsupportive of the experiences of people regarded as 'different'.

References

Barnes, C. and Mercer, G. (eds) (1997). *Doing Disability Research*, Leeds: The Disability Press.

Barnes, M. (1997). *Care, Communities and Citizens*. Harlow: Addison-Wesley Longman.

Barnes, M. and Bennet, G. (1998). Frail bodies, courageous voices: older people influencing community care, *Health and Social Care in the Community*, 6(2), 102—11.

Barnes, M. and Bowl, R. (2001) *Taking Over the Asylum: empowerment and mental health*. Basingstoke: Palgrave Macmillan.

Barnes, M. and Prior, D. (2000) *Private Lives as Public Policy*. Birmingham: Venture Press.

Barnes, M. and Shardlow, P. (1996). Identity crisis? Mental Health User Groups and the 'problem' of identity. In Barnes, C. and Mercer, G. (eds), *Exploring the Divide: Illness and disability*. Leeds: The Disability Press.

Barnes, M. and Shaw, S. (2000). Older People, Citizenship and Collective Action, In Warnes, A., Warren, L. and Nolan, M. (eds), *Care Services in Later Life*. London: Jessica Kingsley.

Barnes, M. and Wistow, G. (1994). Learning to Hear Voices: listening, to users of mental health services, *Journal of Mental Health*, 3, 525–40.

Bulmer, M. (1987). *The Social Basis of Community Care*. London: Allen & Unwin.

Campbell, J. and Oliver, M. (1996). *Disability Politics: Understanding our Past, Changing our Future*, London: Routledge.

Cohen, I. L. (1985). Strategy or identity: new theoretical paradigms and contemporary social movements, *Social Research*, 52(4), 663–716.

Cormie, J. (1999). The Fife user panels project: empowering older people. In Barnes, M. and Warren, L. (eds.) *Paths to Empowerment*, Bristol: The Policy Press.

Davey, B. (1999). Solving economic, social and environmental problems together: an empowerment strategy for losers. In   Barnes, M. and Warren, L. (eds), *Paths to Empowerment*, Bristol: The Policy Press.

Eizioni, A. (1995). *The Spirit of Community*. London: Fontana.

Faulkner, A. and Layzell, S. (2000). *Strategies for Living: A report of user led research into people's strategies for living with mental distress*. London: Mental Health Foundation.

Melucci, A. (1985). The symbolic challenge of contemporary movements, *Social Research*, 52(4), 789–816.

Romme, M. and Escher, S. (1993). *Accepting Voices*. London: MIND.

Shakespeare, T. (1993). Disabled people's self-organisation: a new social movement?, *Disability, Handicap and Society*, 8(3), 249–64.

Thornton, P. and Tozer, R. (1995). *Having a Say in Change: Older people and community care*, York: Joseph Rowntree Foundation.

Touraine, A. (2000). *Can We Live Together? Equality and difference*. Cambridge: Polity Press.

Williamson, B. (1982). *Class, Culture and Community*. London: Routledge & Kegan Paul.

Young, M. and Willmott, P. (1962). *Family and Kinship in East London*. Harmondsworth: Penguin.

26 Promoting health with black and minority ethnic communities: developing strategies to address social inequalities and social exclusion*

Jenny Douglas

Introduction

This chapter aims to explore the role of health promotion in opposing the impact of racism and racial discrimination on the health of black and minority ethnic communities in the United Kingdom. First, it examines some of the constraints and dilemmas health promotion faces at the time of writing, particularly in relation to addressing inequality in these communities. Second, it considers information currently available on the health of black communities, concentrating on differential health experience and health status in relation to mortality and morbidity, and the way in which work on health issues has tended to be conceptualized within minority ethnic communities.

The chapter then discusses lessons emerging from health promotion strategies which aim to tackle inequality in black and minority ethnic communities, drawing on work that has been developed in Sandwell, West Midlands, and focusing on the Smethwick Heart Action Research Project. This project has set out to document the health experience of those communities, opening up the links between poverty, racism and health, and highlighting gaps in service provision. The project has also encouraged the participation of voluntary organizations and community groups in determining appropriate methods for health promotion. However, its initiatives, too, emerge as being subject to current constraints on health promotion.

* Originally published (adapted from) P. Bywaters and E. McLeod (eds) (1996) *Working for Equity in Health*, Chapter 12, pp. 179–96, London: Routledge.

The role of health promotion

Current theories and concepts of health promotion do not tend to focus on the contemporary realities of racial oppression. Where anti-oppressive practice has been developed, this has not arisen out of prevailing health promotion theories, but has tended to represent the attempt of individual practitioners to develop health promotion programmes and strategies that seek to address oppression (Douglas, 1995a). The predominant approach adopted within health promotion campaigns and strategies is a multi-cultural one which concentrates on the particular cultures of black and minority ethnic communities. It attempts to develop health promotion programmes and resources targeted at specific black and minority ethnic communities; but without acknowledging the association between material inequality and ill health in the communities concerned. It also fails to move beyond a focus on the biological causes of ill health and their treatment by medical intervention (Douglas, 1995b). In these respects it echoes some of the dominant assumptions informing medical research and health initiatives more generally within black and minority ethnic communities. These are discussed next.

The health of black and minority ethnic communities

An emphasis on the relative incidence of ill health

There is now a diverse and growing literature on the health of black and minority ethnic communities (Smaje, 1995; Modood *et al.*, 1997; Nazroo, 1997; Davey Smith *et al.*, 2000; Karlsen and Nazroo, 2002a). A review by Smaje (1995) demonstrated its emphasis on a biomedical model, with a focus on illness and disease affecting the aforementioned communities. He argued that epidemiological work on mortality and morbidity has tended to concentrate on two approaches in examining the health of particular ethnic groups. The first approach is to outline the frequency of disease within each ethnic group by looking at the prevalence or incidence of particular diseases or conditions, while the second approach is concerned with differences between ethnic groups. This is measured by relative risk or standardized mortality ratios which indicate the degree of difference between such groups. Bhopal (1988) has argued that the medical literature on the health of black and minority ethnic communities has been dominated inappropriately by studies of relative risk. There has been an over-emphasis on diseases with high relative risk among black and minority ethnic populations as compared to white populations, considered as the norm. Such an approach reinforces an emphasis on diseases such as tuberculosis and thalassaemia, where the diseases in question are ones where occurrence may reflect geographical or genetic aetiology. This is rather than concentrating on illness and conditions which affect larger populations of black and minority ethnic people, such as coronary heart disease, where there may be explanations that relate to racially disadvantaged economic and social conditions.

In relation to morbidity, there has been little literature on the subjective experiences black and minority ethnic communities have in relation to illness or disability. Where there is information this has not, until recently, been available at a national level, but has been based on small local studies of chronic illness or self-reported morbidity (Pilgrim et al., 1993; Thompson et al., 1994a, 1994b). Moreover, early health and lifestyle surveys were based on predominantly white populations (Blaxter, 1990), and there was little national data available on the health and lifestyles of black and minority ethnic communities. To counteract this tendency, the Health Education Authority commissioned MORI's (Market and Opinion Research International) Health Research Unit to carry out a programme of health and lifestyle research on its behalf (Rudat, 1994). This survey demonstrated that there were significant differences between white and other ethnic groups in relation to health status and perceptions of health. At least twice as many African Caribbean, Indian, Pakistani and Bangladeshi respondents defined their health status as poor when compared with white respondents. In 1994, the Fourth National Survey of Ethnic Minorities was undertaken by the Policy Studies Institute and Social and Community Planning Research (Modood et al., 1997). It was the first fully representative national survey to include detailed information on the health of minority ethnic groups, and started to explore differences in health status between black and minority ethnic communities. A second health and lifestyle survey was commissioned by the Health Education Authority (2000) which focused on the demography, language and religion of black and minority ethnic communities in Britain, and further reported on ethnic inequalities in health. The ninth Health Survey for England was undertaken in 1999 on behalf of the Department of Health, and focused for the first time on the health of minority ethnic groups. It included minority ethnic children as well as adults (Erens et al., 2001). Thus, since the mid-1990s we have seen a burgeoning literature on the health experiences of minority ethnic communities which has facilitated a more detailed examination of inequalities in health and has initiated a more sophisticated exploration of the intersections of health, inequality, ethnicity, social class and gender. What has become clear is that although the construction of 'ethnicity' is often used in health research in a relatively unproblematic way, such ethnic categories are not fixed and are subject to a changing social, political and cultural context such that their use in epidemiological research needs more careful consideration to reflect more accurately the complex nature of individual realities (Davey Smith et al., 2000; Fenton and Charsley, 2000).

The health agenda within black and minority ethnic communities

The health agenda coming from black communities has also tended to focus on the incidence of freedom from disease and on securing appropriate medical intervention. These have been important issues in their own right. For black communities, community initiatives or campaigns around health issues have arisen out of the link between racial discrimination and the lack of appropriate service provision, as in the case of sickle cell anaemia, thalassaemias, coronary heart disease, diabetes, hypertension and circumcision (Douglas, 1991) or misdiagnosis based on racial and cultural stereotypes, as in the case of mental illness (Wilson, 1993). However, there has been little attention paid to the association between poverty, racism and ill health. Moreover, the women's health movement has not focused on the needs of black and minority ethnic groups, and on the possible association between sexism, relative poverty, racism and ill health (Douglas, 1992, 1998b). Also, little attention has been focused on learning why some minority ethnic groups experience lower levels of certain diagnoses than the white majority population (Blakemore and Boneham, 1993)

The association between socio-economic conditions and the health of black and minority ethnic communities

A number of studies have indicated that black and minority ethnic communities experience relative disadvantage in relation to poverty and discrimination. During the 1980s, with the exception of Chinese communities and East African Indians, unemployment rates for minority ethnic communities were much higher than for the white population (Brown, 1984; Amin and Oppenheim, 1992; Jones, 1993). Rates of long-term unemployment were greater for most minority ethnic groups, and the differential between minority ethnic communities and white communities widened during the 1980s and was even wider amongst young people (Amin and Oppenheim, 1992; Jones, 1993). Black people were also employed disproportionately in low paid occupations and in poor working conditions such as night work and shift work (Brown, 1984). A greater proportion of black people were employed as home workers, compared to white people. Housing tenure shows ethnic patterns (Jones, 1993). Caribbean and Bangladeshi people were more likely to be living in rented council accommodation compared to the white population. Although people from Indian and Pakistani communities tended to be owner-occupiers, there was evidence that such ownership still reflected occupancy of less expensive housing stock (Rudat, 1994).

The Fourth National Survey of Ethnic Minorities in Britain (Modood *et al.*, 1997) analysed the position of black and minority ethnic communities in British society and examined the different experiences of specific ethnic groups. They demonstrated that, while Pakistani and Bangladeshi groups were consistently disadvantaged when compared to white groups and other minority ethnic groups, people of Caribbean and Indian origin (excluding African Asians) experienced less severe disadvantage than those from Pakistan and Bangladesh and that Chinese people and African Asians seemed to occupy a similar position to white populations. Furthermore they found that the relative health of each group followed the general socio-economic patters, with Chinese, African Asian and Indian people experiencing similar health status to that of white communities, and Bangladeshi, Pakistani and Caribbean people experiencing poorer health.

An association between low socio-economic status and poor health in the white population has been demonstrated, as discussed earlier; the poor health is shown to be associated with poverty, unemployment, poor housing and poor working conditions. We have also discussed an association between minority ethnic status and disadvantage. Therefore, material disadvantage caused by racism is a plausible explanation for poor health among black and minority ethnic groups. However, there has been little research on the impact of racial disadvantage on material disadvantage and the subsequent impact, on the health experience of these groups. Some research has also suggested that poor health and ethnic differences in disease prevalence can be explained by other factors, such as the geographical distribution of black and minority ethnic populations, who reside primarily in inner cities (MacIntyre, 1986; Williams et al.,1994).

In 1996, the ESRC (Economic and Social Research Council), under the Health Variations Programme, funded a number of research projects to explore the association between socio-economic status and health. One of the research projects (Karlsen and Nazroo (2000, 2002a, 2002b) set out to explore the associations between racism, social class and health among minority ethnic people in England and Wales. Through an examination of different manifestations of racism – be they socio-economic disadvantage, inter-personal violence or institutional discrimination, Karlsen and Nazroo demonstrated that all forms of racism had independent detrimental effects on health (Karlsen and Nazroo, 2002b).

There is growing evidence about the effect of material disadvantage and racial discrimination on black and minority ethnic communities' health in the United Kingdom. What follows from this is that at the least this issue should be a focus for further research, and should be taken into account as a possibly significant factor in health promotion projects.

Introduction to Smethwick Heart Action Research Project (SHARP)

The Smethwick Heart Action Research Project was located within the framework of Healthy Sandwell 2000 and was a collaborative project between a number of agencies – the health authority, the family health services authority, the Health Education Authority – but located within Sandwell Health Promotion Unit. SHARP grew from the community-based approach of Sandwell Health Promotion Unit, supported by and building upon networks and resources which had already been established. As a piece of action research in line with Torkington's discussion of similar work in Liverpool (1991), the project was designed to provide data which could reflect issues of relevance for local communities and hence influence local policies aimed at improving the health of the population in general, and black and minority ethnic communities in particular.

The project was funded by the Health Education Authority for three years from April 1991, with its aims being to identify risk factors for black and minority ethnic communities in Smethwick in relation to coronary heart disease and stroke. Although the focus was pre-determined as being on the incidence of disease, the project sought to examine social, economic and political factors that might affect the health of these communities in Smethwick, and to identify the priorities that members of black communities worked to in terms of improving health.

Key findings

Detailed discussion of the research methodology and further findings is provided elsewhere (Thompson *et al.*, 1994a, 1994b; Douglas 1998a, 1998c). Overall, on the basis of self-report evidence in this study, Bangladeshi and Pakistani communities appear to experience greater relative poverty, with higher rates of unemployment and more worries about money. However, the data outlines a complex picture of the differences between ethnic groups in terms of perception of health, social disadvantage, experiences of racial discrimination, money worries and debt, and communication. The first three issues are focused on here.

Perception of health
The findings demonstrated clear differences between black and minority ethnic groups and white groups in relation to perceptions of health status. When asked, 'How healthy do you feel?', at least 17/60 in each of the black and minority ethnic groups, compared with only 5/60 in the white group, answered 'not healthy' or 'not healthy at all'. The numbers were greatest for Pakistani (23/60) and Bangladeshi (22/60) respondents (Thompson *et al.*, 1994a).

Social disadvantage

With the exception of Indian respondents, respondents from other minority groups were, for example, consistently less likely to be car owners than were white respondents. When asked about housing problems – for example, damp, condensation or mould, major repairs outstanding or problems maintaining adequate heating – 63 per cent of people from the Bangladeshi group, 40 per cent of people from the Pakistani group, 28 per cent of African Caribbeans and whites, and 15 per cent of Indians stated that they had housing problems.

Racial discrimination

Nine per cent of the black and minority ethnic sample reported racial discrimination and attacks as being a problem in the locality. This result can be compared to Pilgrim *et al.*'s Bristol survey (1993), where 11 per cent of people had experienced racial insults in the streets. Fifteen per cent of the black and minority ethnic sample also felt that racism had affected their access to health services.

These findings illustrate the difficulty, but also the importance, of beginning to disentangle such issues and their possible bearing on health, by obtaining information from different minority ethnic groups and not simply by contrasting the position of members of one minority ethnic group with the white population.

The survey also sought to explore possible gender differences in health experience. However, for example, in relation to experience of signs of stress indications of women being at some disadvantage here have emerged. Although such differences require some qualification, there is evidence of the interaction of gender and ethnic identity. Respondents were interviewed about feeling angry or irritable; feeling tired, and finding it hard to relax. Of women in the survey, 43 per cent compared to 25 per cent of men said that they often felt angry or irritable with those around them. However, this was more frequently experienced by African Caribbean and white women than other groups. In the African Caribbean and white groups, just over half the women interviewed said that they often felt angry or irritable. At least a third of women in each group agreed that they felt very tired, with little energy. Overall, 47 per cent of women, compared with 33 per cent of men, experienced this, and 41 per cent of women overall and 31 per cent of men found it hard to relax and unwind.

Following on from such responses, the people interviewed highlighted a range of initiatives which they felt would improve their health. Across both white and minority ethnic groups, these related not only to initiatives they could pursue as private individuals, such as to take more exercise, eat more healthily and to take steps to be happier in close relationships. They also concerned initiatives which drew on social policy measures such as provision of employment, good working conditions, a good standard of housing, a good education, to be reunited with family members abroad who were separated by immigration legislation, and to live in a safe, clean environment. Thus the survey covered the way in which initiatives identified by black and minority ethnic communities as having the potential to improve their health moved away from a 'medical model' focus. The respondents identified environmental, economic, political and cultural factors as affecting their health, and their comments were much more aligned to the Health For All model of health (World Health Organization, 1978).

In the context of one-to-one interviews, the SHARP project therefore picked up a much broader definition of health than that featured in earlier research or community consultations (Douglas, 1991). The reason for this may be that, previously, community consultations had often focused on black health issues that had already become politicized – sickle cell disorders and thalassaemia, mental health and circumcision (Douglas, 1991). In responding to health concerns, health promotion workers must, however, be able to address both this narrower health agenda, and the wider health agenda revealed by our survey. Because, unless the lack of health service provision is addressed, community support and trust will not be harnessed in order to tackle the much bigger issues of poverty, poor housing, and material and racial disadvantage.

Further outcomes of the project

The project therefore broke new ground in establishing that health promotion workers and respondents from black and minority ethnic communities shared concerns about the impact of unequal social conditions on health, and about the importance of addressing these issues. This has also provided a focus for subsequent practice. A series of health promotion initiatives has arisen out of the needs identified by black and minority ethnic communities during the survey. These have involved black and minority ethnic communities in their planning, implementation and evaluation and have endeavoured to tackle aspects of disadvantage and discrimination injurious to health. Four are presented in detail here.

Interpreting services
In relation to communication, the survey showed that a third of the Bangladeshi group was literate only in Bengali, approximately a quarter of the Pakistani group was literate only in Urdu, and almost a quarter of the Indian group were literate only in Punjabi. Thus the research demonstrated that in Smethwick almost a quarter to a third of Asian communities were literate only in their first language, suggesting the need for appropriate translation and interpreting services. These research findings on language and experiences of discrimination were then fed directly

into the health services commissioning machinery. This led to a further investigation of interpreting services and a review of the overall provision of multi-lingual information.

SHARP training project

This project aimed to develop skills and confidence among black and minority ethnic people/community workers in organizing health promotion activities. One of the reasons for this initiative was that, during community consultations, black and minority ethnic people described how they felt that health promotion activities did not target black and minority ethnic communities, and that there should be more health promotion activities organized within temples, Gurdwaras and community centres used by black and minority ethnic groups.

A training course was developed on 'Organizing groups and activities in the Community'. This course was accredited by the Black Country Access Federation. Eight people attended the course, which provided:

- Personal development in a supportive environment;
- Demystification of 'health promotion' – enabling local people/community workers to develop skills in health promotion;
- Networking between local community workers; and
- Development of health provision and awareness of health issues in organizations/community groups.

Promoting Asian foods as healthy

When asked about their health, one of the reasons people from black and minority ethnic communities cited for feeling less healthy than white populations was their diet. Asian respondents described themselves as 'not eating the right foods', and Asian foods as being 'rich in fat', i.e. they appeared to view their food as unhealthy. Among respondents and workers, there was also the impression that white health professionals lacked an awareness of Asian and African Caribbean foods, and therefore perpetuated racist stereotypes about unhealthy Asian and Caribbean food customs/practices.

The Community Action Steering Group for this project felt that it was important to:

- Challenge myths about Asian foods with local Asian women and health professionals; and
- Promote healthy eating with Asian foods.

The health promotion project therefore organized one day seminars on Food and Diet in a Multi-racial Society, aimed at health visitors, community workers and local authority workers: to look at broader aspects of healthy eating in a multi-racial society, as well as at the difficulties of affording food in low-income families. This second focal point was a crucial matter of concern as in the SHARP survey: 24 per cent of respondents overall had said that affording food was sometimes, often, or very difficult. Bangladeshi (41 per cent) and white groups (31 per cent) stressed that affording food was difficult; 25 per cent of African Caribbean and 10 per cent of Indian and Pakistani groups said affording food was difficult.

Cookery demonstrations were also organized at a local community centre run by Asian Community liaison officers from the Family Health Services Authority (FHSA), who had been involved with the SHARP project. The aim of the workshops was to raise awareness of healthy eating with Asian foods, and to demonstrate methods of reducing the fat content of meals. The demonstrations also included the use of cheaper English vegetables, for example, leeks and potatoes, in place of more expensive traditional Asian vegetables, but using Asian methods.

Sustaining health promotion initiatives

One of the shortcomings of SHARP was that it was a short-term funded project and hence it was important to try to ensure that its activities and initiatives were sustainable, by building on networks that had been created. In achieving sustainability, it is important to work with existing structures, representatives and workers within existing localities. It is important to involve established organizations, including youth and community services, voluntary agencies, places of worship, community centres, local shops and health centres in any health promotion initiatives. So, for example, the SHARP survey had indicated low rates of physical/leisure activity among the Muslim population and 'Asian' women. Bangladeshi and Pakistani groups participated least in leisure exercise, as there were few facilities which catered for the needs and wishes of these communities. Facilities clearly needed to become more generally user-friendly: providing privacy for women, and with women instructors and information available in Asian languages. Two key issues that emerged as the availability of appropriate facilities was explored were the lack of local authority leisure services' provision of sessions for women only in Smethwick; and stereotypical views among white professionals and organizations about Asian women, such as the idea that religious beliefs prohibited them from participation in physical activities.

Consequently, two options were explored and developed in conjunction with the leisure department: providing Bhangra aerobics sessions at a community centre, and providing swimming sessions for Asian women in Smethwick. The local authority Leisure Services Department employed an Asian woman Sports Development Officer who worked with the SHARP team to develop the initiatives described above – which were then continued by the Leisure Services Department after initial piloting and evaluation through the SHARP project.

Democratic, participatory forms of evaluation also need to be built into all health promotion programmes and initiatives, which involve local people and communities not only in identifying their own ideal objectives but also in reviewing the outcomes. Each health promotion initiative developed as part of the Smethwick Heart Action Research Project had a community action steering group with members drawn from local community groups and voluntary organizations, which consulted with local people and organizations before the development of health promotion programmes – identifying the possible options and in implementing the health promotion programmes – as well as in evaluating their success (Malik *et al.*, 1994)

Conclusion

The Smethwick Heart Action Research Project has demonstrated that health promotion can start to identify key issues and concerns for local people trying to maintain and improve health against a backcloth of social disadvantage, and notably for black and minority ethnic communities, against racism and racial discrimination. The findings from SHARP show that black and minority ethnic communities are in fact aware of the social, economic and environmental factors influencing their health. What is more difficult is to develop health promotion programmes which address such concerns, once having identified them. This project, within the limitations of its funding, tried to achieve small changes in policies within health and local authorities, and to empower local communities to develop health promotion programmes which focused not only on lifestyle approaches to heart health but which also acknowledged the impact of material factors. SHARP also demonstrates that it is possible to make progress on the self-direction of health promotion initiatives by members of the local community, which address these issues.

However, in other respects, the experience of SHARP makes sobering reading. At the time of the project very little research had been done regarding the health needs of black and minority ethnic communities. However, since that time, more sophisticated methods have been developed to assess the health needs of black and minority communities which reflect the intersections of ethnicity, 'race', culture, class, gender and disadvantage. At the time of the SHARP project, the remit of health promotion practice was constrained by the national Health of the Nation strategy, which did not offer an incentive to move beyond a narrow focus on individual behaviour change as affecting the incidence of disease.

More recently, the *Our Healthier Nation* strategy and the associated programmes aimed at tackling health inequalities have, on the surface, placed the health of black and minority ethnic communities higher on the agenda. However, health promotion programmes aimed at minority ethnic communities, continue to a large extent to be funded on a short-term basis and to focus on medicalized concerns such as coronary heart disease and diabetes, With the abolition of NHS regional offices and health authorities in April 2002, many health promotion departments in England have moved to Primary Care Trusts rather than to Strategic Health Authorities. This may further reinforce a focus on health improvement programmes concentrated on specific diseases (Douglas, *et al.*, 2002).

It is important for health promotion to develop methodologies and practices that recognize the social, economic and environmental factors affecting health. In doing so, as SHARP's experience demonstrates, there is a need for health promotion to develop strategies to work with other organizations which are better placed to effect changes in policy to improve health. Local respondents to SHARP's survey clarified, for example, that substantial improvements in employment conditions and immigration policy are germane to their health: both are matters which are beyond the remit of short-term health promotion projects.

Acknowledgements

The author was project manager for SHARP; Helen Thompson was research co-ordinator; Ameen Malik project officer; Dawn Henry and Minara Khatun were research assistants, and Lorna McKee was the research consultant. The project was funded as a demonstration project by the Health Education Authority, Look After Your Heart programme, as part of the community grant scheme. The views expressed in this article are those of the author and do not represent the views of any other person, or the views of the authorities concerned.

References

Amin, K. and Oppenheim, C. (1992). *Poverty in Black and White.* London: Child Poverty Action Group/Runnymede Trust.

Bhopal, R. (1988). *Setting Priorities for Health Care for Ethnic Minority Groups.* Newcastle upon Tyne: Department of Epidemiology and Public Health, University of Newcastle upon Tyne.

Blakemore, K. and Boneham, M. (1993). *Age, Race and Ethnicity – A comparative approach.* Buckingham: Open University Press.

Blaxter, M. (1990). *Health and Lifestyles.* London: Routledge.

Brown, C. (1984). *Black and White Britain: The Third PSI Survey.* Aldershot: Gower.

Davey Smith, G., Charsley, K., Lambert, H., Paul, S., Fenton, S. and Ahmad, W. (2000) Ethnicity, health and the meaning of socio-economic position in. Graham, H. (ed.) *Understanding Health Inequalities.* Buckingham: Open University Press.

Davey Smith, G., Chaturvedi, N., Harding, S., Nazroo, J. and Williams, R. (2000). Ethnic inequalities in health: a review of UK epidemiological evidence, *Critical Public Health,* 10(4) 375–408.

Douglas, J. (1991). Influences on the community development and health movement

– a personal view. In Health Education Unit, The Open University (ed.), *Roots and Branches: Papers from the Open University Health Education Council Winter School on Community Development and Health*. Milton Keynes: Health Education Unit, The Open University.

Douglas, J. (1992). Black women's health matters: putting Black women on the research agenda. In Roberts, H. (ed.), *Women's Health Matters*. London: Routledge.

Douglas, J. (1995a). Developing anti-racist health promotion strategies. In Bunton, R., Nettleton, S. and Burrows, R. (eds), *The Sociology of Health Promotion*. London: Routledge.

Douglas, J. (1995b). Developing appropriate research methodologies for health and social care research with black and minority ethnic communities. Conference report, West Bromwich: SHARP/Sandwell Health Promotion Unit.

Douglas, J. (1998a). Health needs assessment: health promotion – the Sandwell experience. In Rawaf, S. and Bahl, V. (eds) *Assessing the Health Needs of People from Black and Minority Ethnic Communities*. London, Royal College of Physicians.

Douglas, J. (1998b). Meeting the health needs of women from black and minority ethnic communities. In Doyal, L. (ed.) *Women and Health Services*. Buckingham, Open University Press.

Douglas, J. (1998c). Developing appropriate research methodologies with black and minority ethnic communities, Part 1: Reflections on the research process, *Health Education Journal*, 57(4) (December), 329–38.

Douglas, J., Heller, T. and Russell, J. (2002). The potential for promoting health with local communities: working with primary care organisations. In Jones, L., Sidell, M. and Douglas, J. (eds), *The Challenge of Promoting Health: Exploration and Action*. Basingstoke: Palgrave Macmillan/Open University.

Erens, B., Primatesta, P., and Prior, G. (2001). Health Survey for England – The health of minority ethnic groups 1999. London: The Stationery Office.

Fenton, S. and Charsley, K. (2000). 'Epidemiology and Sociology as incommensurate games: accounts from the study of health and ethnicity', *Health* 4(4) 403–425.

Health Education Authority (2000) *Black and Minority Ethnic Groups in England: The second health and lifestyles survey*. London: Health Education Authority.

Jones, T. (1993). Britain's Ethnic Minorities. London: Policy Studies Institute.

Karlsen, S. and Nazroo, J. (2000). Identity and structure: rethinking ethnic inequalities in health. In Graham, H. (ed.) *Understanding Health Inequalities*. Buckingham: Open University Press.

Karlsen, S. and Nazroo, J. (2002a). Agency and structure: the impact of ethnic identity and racism on the health of ethnic minority people, *Sociology of Health and Illness*, 24(1) 1–20.

Karlsen, S. and Nazroo, J. (2002b). Relation between racial discrimination, social class and health among ethnic minority groups. *American Journal of Public Health*, 92(4) 624–31.

Macintyre, S. (1986). The patterning of health by social position in contemporary Britain: directions for sociological research, *Social Science and Medicine*, 23(4), 393–415.

Malik, A., Thompson, H., Douglas, J. and McKee, L. (1994). *Smethwick Heart Action Research Project – Developing heart health initiatives with black and minority ethnic communities*. West Bromwich: SHARP/Sandwell Health Promotion Unit.

Modood, T. I., Berthoud, R., Lakey, J., Nazroo, J., Smith, P., Virdee, S. and Beishon, S. (1997). *Ethnic Minorities in Britain: Diversity and disadvantage*. London: Policy Studies Institute.

Nazroo, J. Y. (1997). *The Health of Britain's Ethnic Minorities*. London: Policy Studies Institute.

Pilgrim, S., Fenton, S., Hughes, T., Hine, C. and Tibbs, N. (1993). *The Bristol Black and Ethnic Minorities Health Survey*. Bristol: University of Bristol.

Rudat, K. (1994). *Health and Lifestyles. Black and minority ethnic groups in England.* London: Health Education Authority.

Smaje, C. (1995). *Health, Race and Ethnicity – Making sense of the evidence.* London: King's Fund Institute/SHARE.

Thompson, H., Malik, A., Douglas, J. and McKee, L. (1994a). *Smethwick Heart Action Research Project. Results of a health survey with the African-Caribbean, Bangladeshi, Indian, Pakistani and white communities in Smethwick.* West Bromwich: SHARP/Sandwell Health Promotion Unit.

Thompson, H., Malik, A., Douglas, J. and McKee, L. (1994b). *Smethwick Heart Action Research Project, Final Report.* West Bromwich: SHARP/Sandwell Health Promotion Unit.

Torkington, P. (1991). *Black Health – A political issue.* London: Catholic Association for Racial Justice.

Williams, D., Lavizzo-Mourney, R. and Warren, R. (1994). The concept of race and health status in America, *Public Health Reports,* 109(1), 26–41.

Wilson, M. (1993). *Mental Health and Britain's Communities.* London: King's Fund Centre/NHSME Mental Health Task Force/Prince of Wales Advisory Group on Disability.

World Health Organization (1978). *Alma-Ata 1978. Primary health care.* Copenhagen: WHO.

27 Econology: integrating health and sustainable development. Guiding principles for decision-making*

Ronald Labonté

Introduction

The concept of sustainable development ('development that meets the needs of the present without compromising the ability of future generations to meet their own needs', World Commission on Environment and Development, 1987) is becoming central to political and economic discourse in most countries, and in international fora. . . .

Health has been embedded in the concept of sustainable development since its inception. Until recently, however, the health sector, and more specifically the public health sector, has not been actively engaged in decision making or policy setting discussions on sustainable development. Three unique patterns of relationships emerge when health is placed alongside the two major dimensions of sustainable development, the environment and economy.

The health–environment relationship is described by research on the human health impact of environmental hazards. Traditional public health has focused on protecting individuals from environmental hazards; this comprises one set of health–environment relations. The obvious shift herein is from toxins (biological hazards) to toxics (chemical hazards). However, data on the human health effects of toxics is rarely unequivocal and largely absent. Environmental protection policy must begin to use biological markers (health effects in other species and experimental animal research) as proxy human measures where human data are equivocal or absent, and must begin to study subtle effects (e.g. immunotoxic, developmental) as well as gross effects (e.g. cancer, reproductive failures). At a paradigmatic-shift level, public health must also shift its emphasis from protecting humans from environmental hazards, to protecting the environment from human hazards. The most threatening, and least quantifiable or certain, threats to human health are those relating to global ecosystem change, notably the enhanced greenhouse effect.

* From *Health Promotion International*, 6(2) (1991), 147–56. Oxford University Press. © Oxford University Press 1991.

The health–economy relationship pertains to the well documented relationship between poverty and disease. Less well known is research linking improved health status to social support systems, psychosocial emotional states and relatively flat income or power hierarchies. When human health in its broadest sense becomes the endpoint for sustainable development decision-making, 'trickle-down' theories of wealth creation and continuous economic growth become far less important than the equitable distribution of wealth related resources within a community or nation. Indeed, the most powerful amendment public health can make to the concept of sustainable development is the fundamental relationship between social justice, environmental protection and economic development.

The final relationship, that of economy–environment, represents both a value shift from what Daly and Cobb (1989) describe as 'chrematistics' ('the manipulation of property and wealth so as to maximise short-term exchange value to the owner') to 'oikonomia' ('the management of the household so as to increase its value to all members of the household over the long run'); and a correction in market economics so that 'externalities' such as the costs of pollution control and resource renewal are internalized in commodity prices, thus sending consumers a true price of consumption while generating the revenues necessary to invest in environmental protection.

Respectively, these three relationships can be captured by the imperatives to consume less, share more equitably and account more accurately.

It is possible now to articulate a set of principles for sustainable development that give full expression to human health and its social and environmental underpinnings. . .

The principles offered below are intended to provide ethical and health-biased guidelines for addressing the most fundamental question: When conflicts arise within the environment–health–economy triad, what values will guide the process of conflict resolution? These principles are not given in any order of importance, nor are they separate from each other. One might increase intra-national equity while worsening transnational inequities and increasing pollution, or vice versa. Neither situation is sustainable, nor healthy. The principles are a packaged set.

Principle 1: the necessity of principle-based decision-making

Principles are fundamental to the process of sustainable development decision-making. Scientific data can only inform, but neither predict nor dictate, sustainable development decision-making.

Comment
Greater support for scientific research into the health implications of sustainable development is required. Nevertheless, decisions on global-

scale environmental effects (greenhouse gas emissions, stratospheric ozone depletion, loss of carbon sink capacity and increased appropriation of net primary product) cannot await scientific certainty . . . To anticipate is to make best guesses about what might happen, and to act upon those guesses.

Principle 2: inclusiveness of information

Scientifically generated data should encompass as broad a pattern of complex relations as possible: environment–health (risk assessments); economy–health (equity assessments); environment–economy (full-cost accounting). It should not be restricted to only one set of relationships.

Comment
With respect to environment–economy relationships, an ecosystems approach is required, and not one that separately assesses environmental impacts on air, water, flora, fauna, etc . . . [Very] small toxic emissions or system-wide perturbations may be sufficient to create profound and health damaging changes, and the need to integrate 'total carrying capacity' for ecosystems and humans into risk assessments. Whenever disputes over data interpretation arise, particularly concerning environment–health effects, the most health-conservative findings or models should be used, that is, any benefit of scientific doubt should be given to human health.

Principle 3: shrinking global inequities

Sustainable development, globally, requires that a proposed activity increase global equity, that is, it lessen the wealth (income) gap between nations.

Comment
The Third World debt is the global economy's current greatest threat to sustainable development. It was largely incurred for the benefit of few. It must be forgiven or postponed, and not simply through debt–equity swaps such as rainforest preservation which, by themselves, are inadequate to meet the population growth and resource depletion crises faced by most poor nations. This is a radical suggestion, though not without precedent. (It also begs an interesting question: what is more important, the health of the species and sustainability of the planetary ecosystem, or colourful pieces of paper with the faces of dead politicians and rulers?) At the very least, the implications of monetary policy on environmental sustainability must be made explicit.

There are several ways in which this principle can be implemented. In the case of transnational projects, international agreements could require the retention and reinvestment within the poor country of more earned income than is repatriated. In the case of strictly national projects within a rich country, this might be achieved through a combination of national taxation policies and untied foreign aid, or specific trading and sharing policies for poor countries related to the project's goods or production technology . . . One suggestion would have each nation pay a carbon tax based on consumption, with revenues collected by an international body and used, in part, to fund clean technology transfer to poorer countries . . .

The environmental and occupational conditions under which the products are manufactured should equal those required for First World production. Increased foreign aid to Second and Third World countries could be dedicated to supporting these countries in achieving this equity in sustainable development . . .

Emphasis should be placed not on international trade, but on intranational, bioregional market development. This approach would foster, rather than remove, trade barriers. Daly and Cobb argue that free trade, by allowing capital to move wherever labour is cheapest, lowers living standards for most of the world's workers, creating a global 'rush towards poverty'. This stimulates unsustainable economic activities in rich countries in order to compete with the cheap labour productivity of poor countries . . .

Principle 4: shrinking national inequities

Sustainable development, nationally, requires that a proposed activity increase national equity, that is, it lessen the wealth (income) gap between have and have-not citizens.

Comment
This principle might be achieved through taxation policies (e.g. negative income tax), and equity oriented development permits . . . [It] might also be also be achieved through various forms of employment equity policies (regarding the hiring of women, ethnic minorities, disabled workers, and so on) and legislation supporting more equitable forms of remuneration.   Taxation and other fiscal policy instruments will need to be used to offset the income inequities that will arise as full-cost accounting of environmental resource use is achieved.

Principle 5: empowering equally

Sustainable development, both globally and nationally, requires that a proposed activity increase equity in power.

Comment

Power is not quite the same as wealth, although the two are certainly related. Empowerment requires an increase in access to decision-making by less powerful individuals, groups and communities. This might be achieved through provision of resources (economic, technical, organizational) to such groups to assist them in participating in the decision-making on the proposed activity. It takes as fundamental the participation by all interested parties and requires regular environmental audits and reporting by the private and public sectors, including reports of international activities.

Principle 6: producing fairly, healthily

Sustainable development requires that each proposed activity increase worker control and workplace democracy relative to past practices.

Comment

Increasing workplace democracy may include, but is not restricted to, unionization of the labour force; specific agreements regarding health and safety measures that comply with, or exceed, legislated minimums; worker–ownership agreements; voting worker representation on management boards and committees; and the existence of workplace policies reflecting Emery's six basic criteria for healthful work (cited in Levi, 1983).

- The job should be reasonably demanding in terms other than sheer endurance, and should provide variety.
- The worker should be able to learn on the job, and to go on learning.
- The job should include some area of decision-making that the worker can call his or her own.
- There should be some degree of social support and recognition in the workplace.
- The worker should be able to relate what he or she does or produces to social life (that is, feel that his or her labour contributes to improved social welfare).
- The worker should feel that the job leads to some sort of desirable future, at a personal and collective level.

Principle 7: sustaining communities

Sustainable development requires that each proposed activity create, sustain or re-create 'community'. This means that the activity, at a minimum, must address how it will:

- Increase opportunities for social interaction and development of social networks;

- Diversify the community's economic base;
- Increase proximity between production, consumption and disposal;
- Support a more active, democratic participation of community citizens in political and economic decision-making, including that pertaining to the proposed project.

Comment

This principle together with principles 3 to 6, comprise a social contract between capital (business, economy) and community. This principle also requires novel methodologies to capture community perceptions and future scenarios that draw heavily on participatory learning theories, ethnographic research and sociology.

The notion of increasing proximity between what is produced, consumed and disposed is sometimes dismissed as urging a return to pre-industrial, agrarian forms of economic and social organization. This is not so. Rather, the need to increase proximity recognizes the absolute necessity of decreasing fossil fuel use and greenhouse gas emissions. This requires a dramatic decline in the scale of transport, and in the energy inputs for food production . . . Relatively self-sufficient communities form the base of relatively self-sufficient nation-states.

Principle 8: replenishing and replacing

Sustainable development locates a proposed activity along a hierarchy that asks if the product the activity produces, or the process by which it is fashioned:

- Replenishes the planet, putting in more resources (i.e. 'carbon sink') than it extracts?
- Replaces what is taken, achieving a steady-state economy-environment systems relation?
- Reduces energy and renewable/non-renewable resource consumption, and reduces the production/consumption of toxics?
- Reuses (or allows for the reuse of) constituent materials ('resources')?
- Recycles (or allows for the recycling of) constituent materials?

This is a hierarchy of sustainable development. Human sustainability is commensurate with any given activity's ability to address higher tiered concerns. Any proposed activity that does not, at a minimum, replace what it takes (the notion of 'living off the interest') is not, by definition, environmentally sustainable.

Comment

Implementation of this principle includes a 'best available' precept, in which the best available technologies, legislation, regulations and standards, conditions, enforcement practices and policies internationally are incorporated into proposed activity decision-making.

Principle 9: internalising all the costs

Sustainable development requires that each proposed activity employ full-cost accounting, and internalize all of its externalities to the fullest extent that these externalities can be estimated.

Comment
Externalities are effects that create costs outside of the market-mediated relationship between producer and consumer, e.g. replacement of natural resources, clean-up of pollution. The costs of these externalities are to be borne by the proposer(s) of the activity. Since full-cost accounting is a novel activity and subject to debate over value estimates, preference should be given to those estimates most conservative in terms of human health and environmental integrity. Full-cost accounting must take place in public, and be accompanied by an 'open-book' policy by government and industry.

Principle 10: sustaining diversities

Sustainable development requires that each proposed activity respects, by not actively or passively decreasing, ecosystem (including genetic stock) and human system (cultural) diversity.

Comment
Environmental impact assessments may provide the scientific data regarding ecosystem diversity; human system diversity requires that such assessments and decision-making fora incorporate and utilize other forms of cultural knowledge. Social impact assessments offer some potential to do so, although such assessments tend to be positivist and to accept *a priori* certain impact categories which reflect certain cultural biases (Rickson and Chu, 1990). How problems are defined and economic activities selected, and the relationship between information and political decision making, may be more important issues than impact assessments *per se*.

Principle 11: nurturing the intangibles

Sustainable development requires that each proposed activity include statements about how it will nurture the intangible quality of life for the citizens affected by it.

Comment
There are many things besides a healthy planet and a healthy body that create the self-actualizing experience of human well-being. These things might include aesthetic experiences, feelings of history or continuity in one's family or community, cultural identification, respect for and feelings of oneness with nature, and other spiritual phenomena . . .

As intangibles are identified they become tangible, but never in quite the same way as events that can be represented by data . . . These intangibles, will vary across cultures and communities.

Principle 12: planning across the generations

Sustainable development requires that each proposed activity state how it will ensure equity in future generations, that is, how it will maintain the natural capital and the sustainability of human cultures. It demands that economic activity extend the notion of full-cost accounting across time, as well as across the resource base. . .

Conclusion: the role of health promotion professionals

. . . Health professionals should not wait to be invited into sustainable development discussions. They must invite themselves. As they do so, they should consider that, just as principles are only as good as the actions they generate and the decisions they inform, increased public health participation in sustainable development fora will only be as good as the degree to which health professionals are clear about their unique contributions. These contributions can be summed as:

- The limitations of scientific data, and the ethics of decision-making when epidemiological data are equivocal;
- A broad construction of health, particularly the role of political/economic equity in creating individual and population health;
- The limitations of 'lifestyle' (individual) based strategies;
- The concept of empowerment, its relationship to personal and community health, and its implication for sustainable development decision-making processes.

Health promotion has emerged in recent years as an attempt to synthesize the relative interplay of biomedical, behavioural and socio-environmental systems in creating health or disease. It represents to the health sector what sustainable development represents to the environment–economy sectors: an effort to articulate value-based strategies that sustain humans. The Ottawa Charter for Health Promotion (WHO, 1986) identifies several strategies that health promotion must address: reorient health services, develop personal skills, build healthy public policy, create supportive environments, and strengthen community action. These can be, and have been, applied to sustainable development; they have also raised political challenges that any sustainable development decision-making process must face.

Reorientating health services speaks to the need to develop more effective and efficient community-based systems of health care. Large health care institutions, predicated on a narrow bio-medical model of disease, often lose the human quality of caring in their relationships with ill people. There is also declining marginal utility in disease treatment, and the amount of public revenue that currently goes into health care services may now be unsustainable . . .

Developing personal skills can be narrowly construed as promoting healthy lifestyles. However, it is being more broadly interpreted by many health promotion practitioners as encouraging skills in community organizing, policy advocacy, political decision-making and other forms of participatory democracy that constitute the larger personal responsibility of citizenship, (Hancock, 1989; Labonté, 1989). It intersects nicely with the rhetoric of broader community participation in sustainable development decision-making . . .

Developing healthy public policies means incorporating human health criteria into all policy sectors. It is a new public health truism that individual and community well-being are determined more by social, environmental and economic systems than by health care provision. Policies in such sectors as transportation, energy, economy, food and agriculture, waste management and urban design can either increase or decrease human health, just as they are either sustainable or not. Health promotion and sustainable development policies intersect in many areas. A low meat, low cholesterol, high fibre diet now recommended as a means of preventing cardio-vascular disease and, perhaps, cancer, requires far less land per capita than do current diets in Western industrialized countries. Health concerns are also driving increases in more sustainable, organic forms of agriculture that use fewer toxic petrochemical inputs . . . And so on.

The danger in the concept of healthy public policy is that it might imperialize existing forms of environmental decision-making, and risk further confusion rather than more concerted professional actions . . .

It is likely of greater strategic value for Public Health advocates to expand the parameters of existing environment–economy decision-making fora (such as environmental assessment procedures) to encompass a rigorously broad, social model of health, than to create cumbersome parallel structures.

Creating supportive environments essentially means ensuring that human social organizations enhance well-being . . . Choices are never simply 'personal'. One significant lesson from health promotion has been the importance of public policies in stimulating personal change.

Legislated workplace smoking bans are associated with markedly greater smoking cessation and maintenance rates; the carrot without the stick is simply a dangling vegetable.

Creating supportive environments also presumes the existence of a positive experience of community . . . The final strategy, 'strengthening community action', derives from the richer international literature on community development and community organizing, and is fundamentally about the re-creation of community . . . These ideas have become driving forces behind the several hundred healthy city/healthy community projects worldwide . . .

Community development successes in health promotion . . . speak to a point salient to sustainable development decision-making. Not only must actions accompany words; local actions are required. . . [Where] citizens can see, speak with and feel less intimidated by their municipal politicians and business leaders. They can also see directly the results of their participation in decision-making political processes.

There is, however, an important caveat to this finding: that of localizing global problems, and mystifying macro-level systems of power and decision-making . . . [M]ost economic decision-making is national and transnational in nature.Local decision-making at present can only be within narrow parameters at best, and is unlikely to include substantial control over economic resources. As Lester Brown (1989) of the Worldwatch Institute commented in his 1989 State of the World report, 'Small may be beautiful, but it may also be insignificant'. . .

Unless local actions are integrated with advocacy and political action strategies directed towards higher level government policies, our drive for decentralized decision-making and community development may unwittingly 'privatize', by rendering local, what are much larger issues. We risk mystifying the actual exercise of political power, just as green products mystify the sustainable limits of consumption. Local actions and green products are starting points only, and represent the community organizing rule 'to begin where the people are'. But where people are is not necessarily where they should be. The environmental motto to 'Think globally, act locally' may well need amending to 'Start locally, act globally'.

Empowerment, the ability to exercise choice, increasingly informs the individual and community work of health promotion professionals. It does not lack for problems of definition or co-optation, but it speaks to an emergent knowledge that the very act of organizing to alter conditions of relative powerlessness enhances individual health. 'Empower' is usually used transitively, as in we (health professionals) need to empower others (poor, marginalized individuals or groups). Empower is also a reflexive verb; the most enduring power (choice) is that which is taken, not that which is given. Health promotion professionals possess a power not yet seized, one that builds upon a discipline specific credibility while capitalizing on the relative lack of boundaries defining health promotion . . .

[T]o a considerable extent, health promotion is inherently multi-disciplinary, or a-disciplinary. It incorporates theory and practice from disciplines as diverse as social marketing, education, sociology, psychology, social work, anthropology, ecology, statistics, administration/management, to name only a few. The same might be said for the 'new' public health which, by focusing on the determinants of health, frees itself from the discipline boundaries of medicine and traditional infectious disease control. Few other professionals participating in sustainable development debates share this vague yet liberating generalism.

The most potent role of health promotion professionals in sustainable development decision-making, then, may be that of a cross-discipline interpreter. Using the metaphor of health, which shares its etymology with 'hello' and 'whole', the interpreter does not colonize the other disciplines or sectors with public health imperatives so much as seeks and seeds the commonalities, while raising to the conscious level the conflicts.

References

Brown, L. *et al.* (1989). *State of the World.* New York: Norton.

Daly, H. and Cobb, J. (1989). *For the Common Good.* Boston: Beacon Press.

Hancock, T. (1989). *Sustaining Health: Achieving Health For All in a Secure Environment.* (Conference background paper), Conference on Health–Environment–Economy. York University, Toronto (April 1989).

Labonté, R. (1989). Community empowerment: the need for a political analysis, *Canadian Journal of Public Health*, 80, 87–8.

Levi, L. (1983). Stress. In *Encyclopaedia of Occupational Health and Safety*, vol 2. Geneva: International Labour Organisation, 2106–111

Rickson, R. and Chu, C. (1990). Social impact assessments and the new public health, *Integrating Health and Environment Workshop Papers*. Nathan, Queensland: Griffith University.

World Commission on Environment and Development (1987). *Our Common Future.* New York: Oxford University Press.

World Health Organization (1986). *Ottawa Charter for Health Promotion.* Ottawa WHO.

28 Using sponsorship to create healthy environments for sport, racing and arts venues in Western Australia*

Billie Corti, C. D'Arcy J. Holman, Robert J. Donovan,
Shirley K. Frizzell and Addy M. Carroll

Introduction

Healthway

Healthway is an independent body established under the Tobacco Control Act 1990. Described more fully in Holman *et al.* (1993a), the main purpose of the Act is the active discouragement of tobacco smoking. Healthway's enabling legislation specifies a number of objectives. These include: funding activities related to the promotion of good health; offering an alternative source of funds for sport, racing and arts activities previously supported by tobacco sponsorship; and sponsoring sport, racing and arts activities that encourage healthy lifestyles and advance health promotion programmes.

As a funding organization, Healthway does not deliver its own health messages. In Western Australia, there is an active health promotion community with many local agencies involved in programme delivery. Healthway uses these established groups, known as 'support sponsors', to deliver health promotion messages at sponsored events. In 1990–1, some 132 sponsorships were awarded to sport (A$3.4 m), arts (A$ 1.7 m) and racing (A$0.06 m) organizations (Western Australian Health Promotion Foundation, 1992). Each sponsorship organization is allocated a support sponsor as part of its sponsorship contract. Overall, in 1990–1, support sponsors (including the National Heart Foundation, Cancer Foundation and the Health Department's Smoking and Health Programme) received A$1.3 m to promote health messages at sponsored events including the negotiation of related structural reforms . . .

* From *Health Promotion International*, 10(3) (1995), 185–97. Oxford University Press. © Oxford University Press 1995.

Sponsorship

Sponsorship is a relatively new tool to health promotion . . . Sponsorship dollars are exchanged for a range of sponsor 'benefits' designed to promote the sponsor's image and/or products. Examples of negotiated sponsor benefits include naming rights, signage, personal endorsement of a product by a performer or player, programme advertising and editorial, hospitality for sponsor guests and the distribution of promotional materials. For health sponsors, sponsored events provide promotional and educational opportunities for some of the hard-to-impact groups in the community (Egger *et al.*, 1993).

Sponsorship also provides the health sponsor with one additional and potentially powerful sponsor benefit – the introduction of structural reforms that support healthy behaviour at sponsored events. Examples of structural reform include the introduction of smoke-free policies; the provision of healthy food choices; and the introduction of appropriate sun protection for outdoor events (for example, 'legionnaire hats' rather than caps for baseball players). Unlike other sponsor benefits, it is possible that after sponsorship dollars have been depleted, structural reforms introduced during the sponsorship period will remain.

Healthway's approach to sponsorship reflects a broad interpretation of its charter and comprehensive health promotion practice. Taking the lead from the Victorian Health Promotion Foundation, Australia's first health promotion foundation, Healthway requires its sponsored organizations to introduce structural reform at sponsored events, particularly the creation of smoke-free environments.

Health Promotion Development and Evaluation Program

The Health Promotion Development and Evaluation Program (HPDEP) is an independent academic programme funded by Healthway. The role of the HPDEP is to evaluate Healthway's activities in terms of its legislative mandate . . .

This chapter describes how Healthway has used sponsorship to create healthy environments in sporting and cultural settings. Drawing from results of a HPDEP survey of Healthway-sponsored organizations, it describes the level of structural reform within sport, racing and arts organizations, and the potential reach of these reforms. There are many organizations contributing to structural reform in Australia, particularly in the tobacco control area. Some attempt is made to estimate the extent to which Healthway might have contributed to structural reform in Western Australia. It concludes with a discussion of how a funding body can use healthy public policy to influence intersectoral co-operation and to create healthier environments.

Methods

Sample selection

The sample consisted of sport, racing and arts organizations which had received Healthway sponsorship between May 1991 and June 1992. A questionnaire and an accompanying letter addressed to each organization's nominated 'contact person' (as specified in the grant application) was posted to 269 organizations. Organizations that failed to respond by a certain date (63 per cent of respondents) were contacted by telephone. Up to three follow-up telephone calls were made.

Survey instrument

The questionnaire, containing 118 separate questions, included eight items about structural reform. Organizations were asked:

(i) which of seven structural reforms they had in place within their groups and, where applicable, in the venues where these groups played, raced or performed: (a) before Healthway started (18 months prior to the survey); and (b) at the time of the survey (referred to hereinafter as 18 months later;
(ii) which structural reforms they had been asked by Healthway to implement; and
(iii) the extent of support for Healthway initiated structural reforms amongst: (a) key people in the organization; and (b) spectators or audiences of the organization's activities.

The seven structural reforms investigated were smoke-free areas; safe alcohol practices; sun protection measures; healthy food choices; access for disadvantaged groups; disability access; and safe exercise warm-up practices. The latter two reforms were not priority structural reform areas for Healthway and, although reported . . . in Corti *et al.*, 1993, are not discussed in this chapter.

Organizations also were asked for the number of individual members of the organization as well as how much Healthway sponsorship they had received, and over what period of time. The latter variables were used to calculate 'average annual sponsorship'.

Methods of analysis

The data were analysed using the Statistical Package for the Social Sciences. The statistical significance of a change in the proportion of organizations exhibiting a particular attribute was assessed by the McNemar Test. Organizations that claimed structural reform was not applicable to their organization (for example, committees constituted for the sole purpose of mounting a one-off event) and/or that had missing data were excluded from the analysis.

Results

Response rates

Of the 269 questionnaires forwarded to sport, racing and arts organizations, 260 were considered eligible to participate (i.e. excluding those returned-to-sender) and 209 organizations returned completed questionnaires. Response rates achieved were as follows: 81.4 per cent for arts, 80.7 per cent for sport and 70.6 per cent for racing organizations. Of organizations that failed to respond, 90 per cent had received sponsorship of A$15,000 or less from Healthway. The following analysis includes only those organisations that completed the questions relating to structural reform ($n = 171$).

Types of structural reforms in place

Figure 28.1 shows the types of structural reforms in place before Healthway started ($n = 158$, i.e. those for which structural reforms were applicable before Healthway started) and 18 months later ($n = 171$). The results show a substantial increase in the level of reform in all areas.

Eighteen months after Healthway's inception, smoke-free area policies

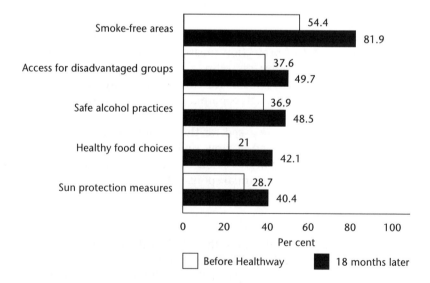

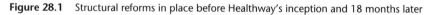

Figure 28.1   Structural reforms in place before Healthway's inception and 18 months later

were the most prevalent type of structural reform (81.9 per cent). More than one and a half (1.65) times as many organizations reported this policy compared with any other (Figure 28.1). Nearly one-half of the organizations surveyed reported having current policies related to access for disadvantaged groups (49.7 per cent) and safe alcohol practices (48.5 per cent).

Changes in the prevalence of structural reform since Healthway's inception

To examine any significant changes in the prevalence of structural reform that may have occurred since Healthway's inception, only organizations that provided data for both time periods (i.e. before Healthway started and 18 months later) were included in the following analysis ($n = 153$).

Since Healthway's inception, there has been a significant increase in the prevalence of structural reforms in all . . . [sponsored organizations]. While the prevalence of smoke-free areas increased the most (27 percentage points), there was also a 21.6 percentage-point increase in the prevalence of healthy food choice reforms.

Structural reform policies were more common among arts organizations. Nearly all arts organizations reported having a current smoke-free area policy (95.6 per cent) 18 months after Healthway's inception. Fewer arts than sports organizations reported having a sun protection policy, however, most arts events are conducted indoors. Arts organizations reported a significant increase in the prevalence of smoke-free policies, safe alcohol practices and access for disadvantage groups.

The majority of sport (69.9 per cent) and racing (60 per cent) organizations claimed to have smoke-free area policies 18 months after Healthway's inception, representing substantial increases since Healthway started. Sport organizations reported a significant increase in the prevalence of smoke-free areas, healthy food choices and sun protection measures.

Structural reforms requested by support sponsors or Healthway

The introduction of structural reform is one of the sponsor benefits negotiated by Healthway or its support sponsors, prior to execution of the contract of grant. Organizations surveyed were asked which, if any, structural reforms they had been requested to implement and which, if any, were not applicable to their organization (for example, because it was already in place). The results in this section relate to the prevalence of requests amongst organizations that stated a particular policy area was applicable to their organization.

In accordance with Healthway's legislative mandate, nearly three-quarters of organisations for which a smoke-free policy was applicable claimed that they had been asked to create smoke-free areas (72.8 per cent). Similarly, almost a half of organizations that claimed that healthy food choices were applicable to their organization, reported they had been asked to make healthy food choices available (46.8 per cent) at their sponsored event(s) . . .

Influence of the level of average annual sponsorship on the likelihood of Healthway requesting reforms

. . . On average, recipients of large sponsorships (i.e. in excess of A$100,000) received 66.5 times more sponsorship than organizations in the smallest sponsorship category (A$154,012 compared with A$2,316), they were requested to implement only 13 per cent more structural reforms (1.5 per organization compared with 1.33). There appeared to be a weak relationship between the amount of sponsorship received and the average number of requests for reform. However, little practical difference existed between groups receiving various levels of funding.

Healthway's contribution to the implementation of structural reform

Figure 28.2 shows the absolute percentage increase in the prevalence of structural reforms since Healthway's inception, comparing organizations requested to implement particular policies with other organizations

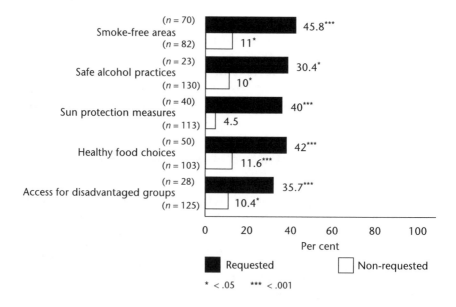

Figure 28.2 Absolute percentage increase in structural reform (before Healthway started versus 18 months later) for requested organizations and other non-requested organizations

funded by Healthway. Only organizations that provided data for time-points both before and after Healthway's inception were included in the analysis.

Amongst organizations requested to implement reforms, the level of increase was practically and statistically significant. For example, there was an increase of 45.8 percentage points in the prevalence of smoke-free areas and an increase of 30.4 percentage points in the prevalence of safe alcohol practices.

However Figure 28.2 illustrates that a movement towards the implementation of structural reform existed without Healthway's direct influence. That is, the prevalence of each type of structural reform also increased significantly in organizations not requested to implement changes. The average increases in percentage points were, however, far greater in organizations requested to implement changes compared with organizations not requested to implement reforms: 4.16 times greater for smoke-free areas (45.8 per cent compared with 11 per cent), 3.04 times greater for safe alcohol practices, 8.89 times greater for sun protection measures. 3.62 times greater for healthy food choices, and 3.43 times greater for access for disadvantaged groups. These data strongly suggest that Healthway has accelerated the rate of change.

Another way of considering the influence of Healthway on the implementation of structural reform was to examine the prevalence of structural reforms in place 18 months after Healthway's inception in organisations that did not have a reform in place before Healthway started (see Figure 28.3).

The creation of smoke-free areas represented the greatest gain in structural reform. Of organizations that had no such policy before Healthway's inception, 65.9 per cent reported having a policy 18 months later. Substantial gains were made also in the other areas. More than one-quarter of organizations that had no previous policies relating to safe alcohol practice (26.7 per cent), healthy food choices (28.8 per cent), or access for disadvantaged groups (27.2 per cent), claimed to have these reforms in place 18 months later.

The degree of institutionalization of pre-existing reforms in sporting and cultural venues is also demonstrated in Figure 28.3. As may be seen, the vast majority of organizations that had structural reforms in place before Healthway's inception persisted with the healthy policies 18 months later.

The influence of sponsorship level on the prevalence of structural reform

Regardless of the average amount of annual sponsorship received, significant increases were observed in the prevalence of smoke-free areas and healthy food choice reforms. In organizations receiving A$50,000 or

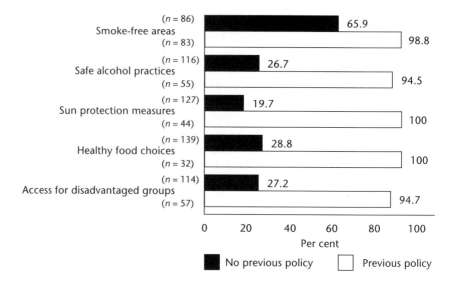

Figure 28.3   Prevalence of structural reforms 18 months after Healthway's inception: those that had no policy before Healthway versus those that did (excluding those reporting a policy 18 months later that was not applicable)

more, the percentage point increase in smoke-free area policies was 1.31 times higher than in organizations receiving A$5,000 or less (i.e. 35.7 per cent versus 27.3 per cent), while in the area of healthy food choices the ratio was 2.13 (28.5 per cent versus 13.4 per cent).

In other areas of structural reform, no clear pattern emerged based on the level of sponsorship received. Even organizations receiving A$5,000 or less reported significant increases in the prevalence of four out of the five reform areas.

Potential reach of structural reforms in organizations requested to implement changes

The potential reach of the structural reforms in organizations requested to implement changes (n = 136) was examined by calculating potential member reform-exposures (PMREs). The number of PMREs per organization was calculated by multiplying the number of reforms by the number of members of the organization. On average, each organization had 2.67 structural reforms in place 18 months after Healthway's inception, generating an average of 4,584 PMREs.

Regardless of the amount of sponsorship received from Healthway, there was very little difference in the average number of reforms reported. However, as might be expected, there was a considerable difference in the potential reach of these reforms among members.

Recipients of small sponsorship (≤A$5,000), on average, had the potential to generate 2,499 PMREs. This was 1.30 times more PMREs than in organizations receiving A$5,001–15,000 (1,927 PMREs). At the higher levels of sponsorship, the number of PMREs increased to an average of 28,828 for organizations receiving more than A$100,000 per annum. . .

Support for Healthway-initiated structural reform

It was a common view among organizations requested to implement reforms (*n* = 136), that all or most key people in the organization (for example, board members, players, actors) (83.1 per cent) and their spectators or audiences (73.5 per cent) supported Healthway initiated structural reforms . . . Nevertheless, while 45.6 per cent of organizations claimed that *all* of the key people in their organisation supported the changes, only half as many organizations perceived that *all* of their spectators or audience were supportive (22.3 per cent).

Discussion

Structural reform achievement

Although not all of the structural reform observed in this study can be attributed to Healthway, it has, nevertheless, been successful in using sponsorship to create healthier sporting and cultural venues. It has also achieved widespread support for its reform programme. While educational and promotional opportunities are an important component of the negotiated sponsor benefit package, tying the offer of sponsorship to a requirement to implement structural reform has the potential for longer-term impact if the reforms become institutionalized.

Considerable structural reform was achieved in all priority areas, but especially the creation of smoke-free areas. While arts organizations appear to be more receptive to reforms, the results also show that it is possible to make considerable progress towards healthier environments in racing and sporting organizations and venues. This is important because promoting health at sport and racing events provides opportunities to contact hard-to-impact audiences, such as blue-collar males (Egger *et al.*, 1993), and to associate health with positive role models and activities (Donovan *et al.*, 1993). A community survey conducted in 1992 found that sporting group members and spectators had above-average levels of smoking, low fruit and vegetable consumption, unsafe drinking and physical inactivity (spectators only) (Holman *et al.*, 1993b).

Although one might imagine that Healthway has more leverage to encourage recipients of larger sponsorships to implement more reforms, there was very little practical difference in the average number of reforms per organization amongst groups receiving different levels of funding. This may suggest that Healthway has not capitalised sufficiently on its larger sponsorships, but there are alternative explanations. Larger sponsorships provide greater overall population reach (see below), increased prospects for institutionalization of reform, and the mix of sponsorship benefits may be designed to take advantage of promotional opportunities associated with large spectator attendances and media coverage.

In addition, Healthway's staff and support sponsors have taken a 'small wins' approach to introducing healthy public policy. Weick (1984, p. 43) defines a small win as a 'concrete, complete, implemented outcome of moderate importance'. One small win may seem unimportant, but a series of small wins 'reveals a pattern that may attract allies, deter opponents, and lower resistance to subsequent proposals'. While committed to the creation of supportive environments. Healthway has remained cognisant of real, and potential, opposition to reform amongst its stakeholders. Rather than requiring radical immediate change, or the introduction of multiple reforms at the outset of a sponsorship project, it has moved groups along a continuum. No matter how large or small the sponsorship, or whether it is for a one-off event or a series of events, Healthway's strategy has been to introduce at least one type of reform at the outset and to work towards further reform as a project continues and/or is re-negotiated.

Potential reach of structural reforms

Promoting health through sporting and cultural events and venues has the potential to reach large numbers of people. Some 40 per cent of Western Australians claim to be members of one or more sport, racing or outdoor recreation club, while 1 per cent are members of an arts organization (Holman *et al.*, 1993b, 1993c).

On average, each Healthway-sponsored organization had the potential to generate 4,584 PMREs, and for every A$10,000 of sponsorship funds expended, 3,289 PMRE were generated. Although recipients of larger sponsorships produced many more per organization, when PMREs were quantified per A$10,000, smaller sponsorship recipients generated 4.44 times as many exposures.

While smaller organizations may represent good value for money in terms of exposure of members, omitted in the estimations of reform-exposures in this chapter is the potential reach among the event's spectators and audiences. Organizations receiving higher levels of sponsorship are more likely to be high-profile organizations and thus more likely to attract larger audiences. In addition, larger sponsored projects are more likely to attract media attention, providing promotional opportunities through television and print media coverage.

Healthway's contribution to reform

Not all of the structured reforms observed in this survey can be directly attributed to Healthway. Many Western Australian health agencies are active advocates of structural reforms related to tobacco control, nutrition and sun protection measures. However, with the exception of limited use by the Health Department of Western Australia prior to Healthway's establishment, no other health organization used sponsorship as a means of achieving health promotive reforms in recreational and cultural venues. Nor had any other organization promoted healthy public policy by tying the provision of funding directly to a reformist agenda.

While a sizeable proportion of the organizations surveyed had introduced structural reform prior to their association with Healthway, a substantial contribution was made by Healthway to the rate of policy development among 'structural reform laggards'. This is likely to have occurred through direct requests for reform, but also through indirect influence. As Healthway's objectives have become clear to potential recipients of sponsorship, it is possible that they have implemented structural reforms prior to submission of their sponsorship application in an attempt to strengthen their proposal's chance of success. . .

Policy and practice implications

There have been lessons gained from implementing the funding policy described in this chapter, and achieving community support for the introduction of structural reform. Key success factors have included a 'small wins' philosophy of change, developing co-operative working relationships with diverse organizations whose objectives are not related to health; developing an understanding and appreciation of the goals of sponsored organizations; winning over the trust and support of key individuals in the organizations; developing sound policy formation guidelines; working with individuals involved with the organization and its events at grass roots level (for example, caterers, coaches, front-of-house staff); learning how to promote health appropriately in different settings; and balancing a myriad of conflicting interests. Healthway has used pressure where appropriate, but has also made compromises, and remained committed to a participative model of social reform.

These results suggest that small sponsorship projects represent good value for money in terms of their potential member reform-exposure reach per A$10,000 expended and thus, an investment of A$100,000 in a series of A$5,000 sponsorships may yield more than four-fold the number of structural outputs than one large sponsorship to a single organization. While having important implications for sponsorship policy, this observation must be interpreted cautiously due to possible qualitative differences in the reforms that are purchased, quantitative differences in reach to spectators and audiences, and the extent to which reforms are enforced . . .

Although these results have been achieved by a system of health grants and sponsorships operating within the context of a relatively affluent developed country, we believe there is no reason to constrain the application of the basic principles outlined in this chapter within certain international borders or systems of health administration. Overseas aid organizations and many community-based granting schemes operate in developing countries, and opportunities exist to use these resource flows as a catalyst to facilitate healthy public policy development at the local provincial and state level.

Conclusion

The results indicate that it is possible to work inter-sectorally to achieve structural reform in sport, racing and arts organizations. Actively encouraging inter-sectoral co-operation by tying the provision of sponsorship with a requirement to introduce reform is an example of healthy public policy that will create healthier environments. Maximizing the institutionalization of reforms once sponsorship is removed, however, is likely to be achieved only if sponsored groups and the general public support the changes that are taking place. Working in genuine partnership with sponsored organizations, promoting positive community views of the intentions behind the creation of healthy environments, and communicating the results of supportive consumer research is therefore essential.

References

Corti, B., Holman, C. D. J. and Donovan, R. J. (1993). *Survey of the Impact of Healthway on Organisations It Funds 1992*. Health Promotion Development and Evaluation Program. Perth: University of Western Australia.

Donovan, R. J., Corti, B., Holman, C. D. J., West, D. and Petter, D. (1993). Evaluating sponsorship effectiveness, *Health Promotion Journal of Australia*, 3, 63–7.

Egger, G., Donovan, R. J. and Spark, R. (1993). *Health and the Media: Principles and practices for health promotion*. Sydney: McGraw-Hill.

Holman, C. D. J., Donovan, R. J. and Corti, B. (1993a). Evaluating projects funded by the Western Australian Health Promotion Foundation: a systematic approach, *Health Promotion Journal*, 8, 199–208.

Holman, C. D. J., Donovan, R. J. and Corti, B. (1993b). *Survey on Recreation and Health 1992. Vol. 1: Participation in Sports and Racing*. Health Promotion Development and Evaluation Program. Department of Public Health and Department of Management. Perth: University of Western Australia.

Holman. C. D. J., Donovan, R. J. and Corti, B. (1993c). *Survey on Recreation and Health 1992, Vol. 2: Participation in the Arts*. Health Promotion Development and Evaluation Program. Department of Public Health and Department of Management. Perth: University of Western Australia.

Weick, K. L. (1984). Small wins: revising the scale of social problems, *American Psychologist*, 39, 40–49.

Western Australian Health Promotion Foundation (1992). *Annual Report 1991–1992*. WEst Perth, Western Australia.

29 Can the health sector influence transport planning for better health?*

Adrian Davis

Introduction

This chapter considers whether the health sector can have a positive influence on transport policy at the local level in order to promote better health. The study examined collaboration between the health and transport sectors through the mechanism of the World Health Organization's (WHO) Health for All strategy. This seeks to address health concerns through policies beyond as well as within the health sector. In each of the study cities, Copenhagen (Denmark), Groningen (the Netherlands), and Sheffield (England) the research explored the work of the city Health for All projects in developing collaborative actions with their respective transport departments in order to achieve improvements in health. Using a comparative study approach, evidence was gathered by analysing national policies in the health and transport sectors in each country, and field work conducted in 1995–6 which consisted of interviews with key actors largely working at the city level within these sectors (Davies, 2001).

In the mid-1990s there was little reference in either the transport or health literature, including within Health for All, to the links between transport and health issues, beyond traditional areas of concern such as traffic injuries and pollution. Addressing health promotion issues such as walking and cycling as transport within Health for All projects was very much the exception during this period. This omission acted as a further stimulus to the research in order to assess whether there were any particular barriers which acted to discourage inter-sectoral action on transport and health.

Policy background: traditional links between transport and health

From the 1950s up to the mid 1990s, the road transport sector collaborated little with health professionals beyond the involvement of envi-

---

* Commissioned for this volume.

ronmental health officers in the monitoring of air and noise pollution, and the health services with regard to traffic casualties. Indeed, transport has been described as a hidden health issue (Jones, 1994), and there is little in either the transport or health policy literature to suggest that health concerns played a significant role in influencing transport policy in either England, Denmark or the Netherlands.

From the late 1980s there have been calls from within the public health movement in Europe for action on transport. This relates both to issues such as traffic injuries and pollution as well as to the environmental and social consequences of transport (Radical Community Medicine, 1989; Transport and Health Study Group, 1991). The calls were outcomes of renewed interest in public health in the 1980s. The Lalonde Report (Lalonde, 1974) and the work of McKeown (1976) were catalysts for the re-emergence of public health in the UK and elsewhere. They helped to raise awareness about the part that social and environmental factors play as determinants of ill health, so that health problems are seen as being influenced by factors beyond as well as under the control of the individual. In this, Lalonde and McKeown highlighted the need for consideration of environmental and social as well as biomedical factors as determinants of health.

The development of the Health for All strategy in 1985

The Health for All strategy was established by the WHO after the Declaration of Alma-Ata in 1978, and was followed by the development of the thirty-eight targets (World Health Organization, 1985). Health for All provided a framework through which national and local governments could develop initiatives to address the social and environmental determinants of health as well as the biomedical ones. National governments, including the Danish, Dutch and British, signed declarations of their commitment to Health for All in 1985. Some national governments provided initial financial support to the national networks which developed to service the growing number of towns and cities in Europe establishing Health for All projects from the late 1980s. The thirty-eight targets were designed to be a framework within which the various countries in the European Region could measure progress towards the attainment of Health for All. The targets covered a broad range of issues, and were divided into six themes. These were equity, health promotion, community participation, multi-sectoral co-operation, primary health care, and international co-operation.

Although transport issues were not identified explicitly in the Health for All targets and their summary notes[1] it is relatively easy to identify where transport issues can be located within a number of the targets beyond Target 11 (Accidents) and 21 (Air Quality). For example, transport, through the promotion of walking and cycling and less use of cars can contribute to Target 9 (Reducing Cardiovascular Disease), Target 18 (Policy on Environment and Health) and Target 24 (Human Ecology and Settlements).

In 1986, the WHO established the Healthy Cities project as a practical experiment to test out the implementation of Health for All at the local level. Copenhagen was designated a Healthy City in 1988. Designation of a city as a 'Healthy City' required the establishment of a project, the appointment of a project officer, an agreement to fulfil certain commitments such as to establish mechanisms to secure community participation in health promotion, and the development of a Healthy City Plan within a set timescale. By the mid 1990s the Healthy Cities project was in its second phase, involving forty two cities from twenty-three countries. In contrast, Health for All projects not designated 'Healthy Cities' were dependent on the level of political support within their municipality in terms of resources and ongoing political backing for any initiatives undertaken.

Evidence on sectoral barriers to inter-sectoral collaboration

Much of the health sector from which Health for All originates, and from which it needs support in order to be carried forward, is orientated around a narrow biomedical model of health. In England, as Hunter has noted, treatment of the sick is the central function of the National Health Service (NHS):[2] 'Despite the rhetoric and good intentions stretching back decades, the NHS is not a health service. Its whole ethos and bias is towards caring for the sick' (Hunter, 1995, p. 1589).

On a European level, Dekker has remarked that the focus of Health for All during the 1980s was on medical services and containment of the costs of those services. This marginalized Health for All not only in the Netherlands and England, but also in many other European countries. Health For All had therefore not achieved its aim of broadening health policy beyond the treatment of illness: 'For in those countries the health policy agenda contained items such as cost containment, planning of services, negotiation with care provider' organisations etc., in short, "traditional" items' (Dekker, 1994, p. 285).

In Denmark, by way of contrast, there had been less emphasis on the role of the free market and Health for All policy had not been so marginalized. Denmark's welfare policy is seen as an integral element of society, and concepts such as security and promoting good living conditions are highly valued (Swedish National Board of Health, 1993). During the late 1980s and early 1990s, the Danish Ministry of Health was supportive of health promotion and Health for All. It prepared its own health promotion programme in 1989, the first of its kind in Denmark, in response to the WHO Health for All strategy (City of Copenhagen, 1994).

The case studies

At the city level, inter-sectoral collaboration initiated by Health for All projects had some limited influence on transport departments. At best, health issues were taken up by transport departments as an additional justification for further action in pursuit of stated transport policy goals. This was the case in both Copenhagen and Sheffield. While health issues provided justification for action there was no evidence to show that health issues changed the general emphasis of transport planning policy.

Groningen

Groningen is the capital city of the province (region) of Groningen and was founded in the Middle Ages. The city is the sixth largest in the Netherlands, with a population of 170,000. It is in the north of the country, in an area with few large towns or cities nearby. Groningen municipality has six departments, including Health Services (GGD), Town Planning, Traffic, Transport and Economic Affairs.

In transport terms, the city had been recognized both within and beyond the Netherlands for its traffic restraint policies, a central feature of which was a traffic circulation plan introduced in 1978 which restricted private motor traffic access across the city centre while leaving this open to other modes of transport. The City Council had an overall goal of economic development and improving quality of life (Gronigen City Council, 1992). Groningen remains a compact city, so that many journeys can be made on foot, or by bicycle.

A Health for All project was established in the GGD in 1992, with a part-time co-ordinator. The Project had tried to initiate discussions with the transport department but this had not succeeded. One strategy had been to try to identify health orientated information about each department's work with which to open discussions. The lack of success was caused partly by lack of political support for Health for All among the City Council, and specifically a lack of such support among politicians responsible for transport:

> We want to work together with departments in the city but sometimes it is not possible for practical reasons and sometimes because politicians have missions and ideas other than the health ones. We have also tried to cooperate with other departments and met with lots of trouble [difficulties]. (Interview with Health for All co-ordinator, October 1995)

The interviewee from the Ministry of Health, who had overseen national policy work on Health for All for over a decade, put forward one reason for the lack of politician-led interest in collaboration with the Health for All Project. He stated that politicians tended to conceptualize health as ill health, so that health promotion and preventive measures became marginalized:

> Health is not really an important issue, that is the point. Because most people, if they talk of health, they talk in terms of diseases. Do you know our Alderman? He is the elected responsible board member, you can say, he or she when they ask about health it is always about hospitals and talk with general practitioners about care and health services. (Ministry of Health official, October 1995)

At officer level within the transport planning department there was little knowledge of the Health for All project. Collaborations beyond the department but within the Council were made largely with the Environment Department, where monitoring of air and noise pollution was undertaken:

> There is contact with people from the environmental health department. Not only the people who collect rubbish but more the people who will bring in the environmental aspects in the different policies. Especially air quality, and also with noise. That's the main health aspects of transportation. (Interview with transport planner, October, 1995)

Copenhagen

Copenhagen, the capital city of Denmark, lies within the region of Greater Copenhagen and on the eastern edge of Denmark's most easterly island. The city has a history of implementing traffic restraint policies since the 1960s and it has been policy for over a decade to reduce the overall level of motor traffic in the city (City of Copenhagen, 1991). It had already overseen a decline in motorized traffic in the city from the 1980s, and a significant reduction in traffic accidents.

In order to achieve the overall goal of Health for All, the Copenhagen Healthy City Project recognized that health promotion and disease prevention had to have a significantly more prominent role than previously in the work of the municipal authority (City of Copenhagen, 1994). For this reason, it was decided by the municipal government that the WHO Healthy Cities project provided an appropriate vehicle for the development of health promotion in Copenhagen with a distinct programme of projects to achieve this. Designation as a Healthy City came in June 1988.

The Healthy Cities project developed two initiatives which were to have some influence on transport planning. The first was a city-wide Health Profile, where more than 12,000 responses were received to a questionnaire which asked about how people perceived their own health. The profile results suggested that the public were concerned that their health and quality of life were being undermined by, among other things, 'too much traffic'. For example, in the district of Inner Nørebro, when asked 'What can the 'local authorities do?' over 50 per cent of respondents said that they wanted the local authorities to take action to reduce the problems caused by the traffic. This was the most frequent single proposal. Types of initiative proposed were those that would reduce the danger, noise, and air pollution from traffic: 'In particular, the people in Inner Nørebro want the local authorities to contribute to reducing inconveniences caused by the traffic . . . [they want] initiatives that reduce danger, noise and air pollution from the traffic' (Healthy City Project, 1992, p. 48).

The Health City Project then used the results from the Health Profile to highlight the public desire for action from the Council on traffic issues. The Healthy City project officer felt that the project was able to provide a valuable perspective, because health was not usually associated with transport planning.

> A lot of people urged us to do something about traffic because this is really a big issue . . . many people feel that there are a lot of decision makers in the field of traffic already so we were just an extra. So we were surrounded by decision makers who had many views on this aspect. But we started of course from a different angle which was the health angle. (Interview with Healthy City co-ordinator, July 1995)

The officer believed that the Health Profile was also important in influencing the transport planners, not least because the politicians were influenced by it. This was despite the fact that the profile was based on perceptions about quality of life and not ill health, as traditionally conceptualized by transport planning professionals as measurements of pollution and the counting of accidents:

> Of course, we discussed the figures in the health profile. How should we interpret it? Because when we look at the illness side we know that it is very difficult to see how much illness traffic creates. Anyway, we felt that the signal was very very clear to the politicians, even those who say that this is not health in the sense of illness, it's as much health in the sense of quality of life. But the signal is very very clear. (Interview with Healthy City co-ordinator, July 1995)

For the transport planners, residents' concerns provided the material for political discussions about what actions might be taken.

The second initiative of the Healthy City Project involving transport was the development of a Healthy City Plan. All WHO Healthy City projects are required to develop a Healthy City Plan, although how they undertake the preparation of the plan is for them and their respective municipal authorities to decide. According to the WHO, in Copenhagen the process by which the Plan was prepared illustrates the Health for All principle of intersectoral collaboration (World Health Organization, 1994). The Roads Department made a significant contribution to the plan during its drafting between 1992 and 1993. The Healthy City co-ordinator noted that, because of the political interest in traffic issues, proposals for traffic had to be included in the plan.

The Healthy City Plan was published in January 1994. The traffic chapter, which was informed by the 1991 Health Profile, set out new transport policy objectives as part of the Roads Department's contribution to the plan. This included specific targets to promote cycling by extending bicycle routes by 20 km over four years, improving public transport infrastructure, and undertaking further traffic management to route motor traffic away from sensitive areas (City of Copenhagen, 1994).

Sheffield

Sheffield is the fourth largest city in England, located in the south of Yorkshire and with a population of around 500,000. During the 1970s and 1980s Sheffield experienced a massive economic decline, losing a total of 60,000 jobs between 1978 and 1988. By 1995, 27,718 Sheffield residents were unemployed, an unemployment rate of 13 per cent (Sheffield Health, 1995). For such reasons, from the late 1980s, much emphasis was placed by Sheffield City Council, business interest groups and the city's two universities on the regeneration of the local economy.

Sheffield had operated a successful cheap fares policy on public transport between 1975 and 1986 before government legislation (bus deregulation) brought this to an end. The cheap fares policy was indicative of concerns for equity within Sheffield City Council. Transport policy, which was focused particularly on regaining public transport patronage 'lost' after 1986, was, however, secondary to regeneration of the city centre by enabling access by all modes of transport.

The impetus to establish Healthy Sheffield (in 1987) came originally from a combination of concerns raised through reports from Sheffield Health Authority and Sheffield City Council which highlighted issues of health inequalities and ill health in the city. These concerns were matched by local interest in the WHO Health for All initiative. The project was relatively well resourced with three staff, based within the

Environmental Health Department. The Department was responsible for, among other things, air pollution monitoring, and this determined that the main interest in transport from the Healthy Sheffield project was that of vehicle emissions. According to the Assistant Healthy Sheffield Co-ordinator, 'our head of department became very interested in the transport issue from the environmental air quality and the economic regeneration side. He was instrumental in holding a seminar last July at which issues of transport and health were brought up' (Interview with Assistant Healthy Sheffield Co-ordinator, February 1996).

From a transport planning perspective, officers within the Transport-ation Planning Unit noted that their interest in health had emerged through their concerns for environmental issues. Healthy Sheffield had had some influence on their perspectives about health work, although it had not instigated it. Rather, Healthy Sheffield was seen as a grouping which might be able to help the Transportation Planning Unit carry forward its own plans. In particular, the Transportation Planners were interested in getting help to develop health messages relating to trans-port in order to reduce car use, such as through disseminating facts about air pollution:

> I think we would say that we have arrived at our transport policies through our concerns for health, for the environment, just from our own professional point of view. And then found willing collabora-tors to develop it. Our first approach to environmental health was to say that there is a massive problem in changing peoples' atti-tudes, can you give us any help in establishing the facts about air pollution? (Interview with transportation planner, February 1996)

By mid-1996, some collaboration had been initiated between Healthy Sheffield and the Transportation Planning Unit. As a result, in November 1996, Healthy Sheffield and Rotherham Health for All issued a public consultation document 'Improving Health in Sheffield and Rotherham – the Transport Challenge'. However, there was no evidence of a change in transport policy, but rather an affirmation of the value of health argu-ments, focused strongly around pollution, in support of existing trans-port policies.

Conclusions

The findings from the study provide support for previous claims that health in itself does not have intrinsic value for policy makers at the city level. Indeed, the word 'health' can carry with it connotations of hospi-tals, medical services and the treatment of ill health. Consequently, this was a barrier to progressing Health for All targets relating to transport beyond those defined by a medical model of health. Therefore it is important for Health for All projects to ascertain what are the key policy drivers at the local level, and work through these so that health concerns inform other areas of public policy. Health then needs to be translated into values related to those policies (de Leeuw, 1998) to avoid being perceived as predominantly the responsibility of Health Service departments.

In this respect, in the two cities where there was least evidence of effective collaboration on transport and health there may have been untapped opportunities. In Groningen, where the Health for All project failed to gain political support within the Transport Planning department for collaboration, the fact that quality of life was an objective of the Council might have provided an opportunity if health objectives could have been aligned more with quality of life. Quality of life is contained within Target 2 (Health and Quality of Life) of the thirty-eight Health for All targets. Similarly, in Sheffield, equity issues, which featured so highly within the Council's perspective, might have been better used as a lever by the Healthy Sheffield project for earlier and more effective action on transport. Equity in Health is Target 1 of the thirty-eight Health for All targets.

The main policy drivers in transport planning varied in each city although in Groningen and Copenhagen these can be defined as largely environment-led, with a strong focus on traffic restraint and support for alternative modes of transport to the car. In Sheffield, the pressure for economic regeneration was powerful and so traffic restraint measures were not foremost in decision making. Where transport policies were environmentally led and there was political support for Health for All work (including resources), both at the national and local level, health concerns could provide support for further development of health-enhancing transport policies rather than initiatives which only sought to ameliorate the more widely recognized negative impacts of transport on health. These prerequisites were only found to be present in the Danish case study.

Moreover, the preconditions for inter-sectoral collaboration on health and transport occurred only where an official WHO Healthy City had been established, in Copenhagen. In addition, in Copenhagen the transport planning professionals were more open to Health for All initiatives as the transport sector had been successful in reducing traffic casualties while supporting modes of transport other than the car. None the less, Health for All collaboration was fruitful in the city only where the Healthy City Project was able to translate health into values such as quality of life concerns which had resonance with the transport planners and local politicians.

As a coda to this study, in 1999 the Member States of the European Region of the WHO at the 3rd Ministerial Conference on Environment and Health adopted the Charter on Transport, Environment and Health

(World Health Organisation, 1990). The importance of walking and cycling as means of achieving greater sustainability and attain health gains from transport was highlighted. The Charter has helped to raise the profile of health-promoting transport significantly across Europe, including within the Healthy Cities project. As the WHO has stated, 'Certain aspects of transport and land use policies protect the environment as well as promote public health. These synergisms need to be identified and emphasised' (World Health Organization, 2000).

Notes

1. 1991 edition.
2. In the Netherlands and Denmark, health services are provided largely by local municipal government.

References

City of Copenhagen (1991). *Municipal Plan for Copenhagen*. Copenhagen: Department of the Lord Mayor.

City of Copenhagen (1994). *Healthy City Plan and the City of Copenhagen 1994–1997*. Copenhagen: Copenhagen Health Services.

Davis, A. (2001). *Transport planning for health: explaining and evaluating barriers and opportunities to intersectoral collaboration*, unpublished Doctoral thesis, Open University.

Dekker, E. (1994). Health care reforms and public health, *European Journal of Public Health*, 4, 281–6.

de Leeuw, E. (1998). *Healthy Cities Second Phase Policy Evaluation: Final Report*. Maastricht University.

Groningen City Council (1992). *An Integrated Town Planning and Traffic Policy*, Department of Town Planning, Traffic, Transport and Economic Affairs.

Healthy City Project (1992). *Your District – Your Health*. Copenhagen: Copenhagen Health Services.

Hunter, D. (1995). The case for closer cooperation between local authorities and the NHS, *British Medical Journal*, 310, 1587–9.

Jones, L. (1994). *Transport and Health: The next move, Policy Statement. 2*. London: Association for Public Health.

Lalonde, M. (1974). *A New Perspective on the Health of Canadians*. Ottawa: Ministry of Supply and Services.

McKeown, T. (1976). *The Role of Medicine – Dream, Mirage, or Nemesis?*, London: Nuffield Provincial Hospitals Trust.

Radical Community Medicine (1989). *Autodestruction*, (Summer), 38.

Sheffield Health (1995). *Sheffield's Health into 1996: Director of Public Health 9th Annual Report*. Sheffield: Sheffield Health.

Swedish National Board of Health (1993). *Health Care and Social Services in Seven European Countries*. Stockholm: National Board of Health.

Transport and Health Study Group (1991). *Health on the Move: Policies for health promoting transport*. Birmingham: Public Health Alliance.

World Health Organization (1985). *Targets for Health for All: Targets in support of the European Regional Strategy*. Copenhagen: WHO.

World Health Organization (1994). *Action for Health in Cities*. Copenhagen: WHO Regional Office for Europe.

World Health Organization (1999). Charter on Transport, Environment and Health, Third Ministerial Conference on Environment and Health, London 16–18 June. Copenhagen: WHO Regional Office for Europe.

World Health Organization (2000). *A Review of Transport and Health*. Copenhagen: WHO Regional Office for Europe.

30 Crime is a public health problem*

John Middleton

Introduction

Crime and the fear of crime is a major cause of public ill health. In community surveys the biggest fear people always have is the fear of crime. They fear being attacked or burgled. From a health service perspective this might be disappointing – fear of heart disease, fear of cancer even, barely feature in the list.

There is a growing interest in health and criminal justice circles about the relationship between crime and public health. The Department of Health has commissioned the Public Health Alliance to report on the impact of crime on the public health and health services. The Home Office and Department of Health published a report in 1994 calling for greater collaboration between the health and probation services. The *Tackling Drugs Together* White Paper required health authorities to work with the police, probation, education and social services to reduce drug-related crime and public health problems (Home Office and Department of Health, 1994). In Sandwell, our report, *Safer Sandwell*, is an attempt to look at the impact of crime on the health of Sandwell's 300,000 people (Middleton, 1995).

Causes

The causes of crime and the causes of ill health are often the same. Poverty is the biggest among these. Between 1979 and 1992 the poorest 10 per cent of the United Kingdom population lost 17 per cent of their real income, while the richest 10 per cent became 62 per cent richer (Home Office 1995). During this period of divide between rich and poor, crime increased a staggering 75 per cent (from 3.5 million in 1979 to 5.5 million in 1993) (Townsend *et al.*, 1994). In Middleton (1995) very strong correlations were found between unemployment, no-car-ownership and overall social deprivation with high rates of crime. In the same period of this explosion in crime, the difference in life expectancy

---

* From Middleton, J. (1998) *Medicine, Conflict and Survival*, vol. 14, pp. 24–8, Frank Cass, London.

between very rich and very poor increased. From studies in the north of England (Townsend *et al.*, 1994) and Glasgow (McCarron *et al.*, 1994) there is now evidence of a decrease in life expectancy, particularly for young adult males. The same widening gap has been confirmed for the whole of the United Kingdom for the 1980s, with the publication of the Office of National Statistics *Occupational Mortality Decennial Supplement* (ONS, 1997). Unemployment and suicide are major factors in this. Poverty and inequalities in income are major causes of crime and inequalities in health.

Education

Education is often seen as the panacea for all ills. In health terms, the 'education' asked for is generally about 'health', but there is now growing objective evidence that education, in itself, is health promoting and crime preventing. The number of years spent in education is a powerful predictor of increasing life expectancy and other health outcomes. The US Highscope Perry project (Schweinhart *et al.*, 1993) randomly allocated three-year-olds from very deprived backgrounds to a programme of pre-school education, parental training as first educators and family support, or to a control group. After twenty-seven years of follow-up it was apparent that the programme group were more likely to have completed higher education and be homeowners in well paid jobs and less likely to have come in contact with health, social care, remedial education or criminal justice systems. Sandwell has a very high rate of pre-school placement from three years of age and a developing programme of parents as first educators on High Scope principles. We believe therefore that we have a good platform to improve education, health and safety in Sandwell, from our present lowly position in the national 'league tables'.

Problems of the young

Young people are disenfranchised from economic and political decision making; they are the major perpetrators, but also the major victims of crime and violence; they are less likely to use health services; life expectancy has been declining for 18–24-year-olds in Europe – not because of drugs and AIDS, but because of drinking and driving, accidental death and suicide. Teenagers, rightly, worry more about jobs than they do about AIDS. There is clearly a need for much greater participation by young people in local political decision making.

In Sandwell, we found that 43 per cent of 14-year-olds had tried or used illegal drugs regularly, in keeping with national figures. Marijuana,

LSD and amphetamine are most popular there. Ecstasy is more expensive and less prominent in the local drug fare. But the problems of illegal drugs are dwarfed by those created by alcohol. In the week that Leah Betts died from Ecstasy in 1995, forty-one UK 18–24-year-olds died on the roads, at least a third of these being attributed to drinking. We estimated that nearly 500 deaths in Sandwell alone are attributable to effects of alcohol (Office of National Statistics, personal communication).

Prevention

The health service has a major potential to reduce crime through its harm minimization approach to drug problems. Methadone substitution therapy can reduce the need for street drugs and so reduce crime and public ill health, We estimated that a minimum of 6,000 drug-related crimes in Sandwell would be preventable through harm minimization programmes.

If the causes of crime and ill health may be similar, some of the means of prevention are the same. Reducing poverty and inequality is the most important policy which health and safety professionals should lobby for to prevent ill health, crime and violence.

Community development

Community development is a major plank of local strategies for the promotion of health and community safety. Community development is a process of enabling communities to take control of decisions which affect them, and take action on the most important issues which they identify. Health professionals in the community may wish to work on smoking prevention or cancer or heart disease, but communities themselves may see accident prevention or safety of women, children's play, a factory emission or any number of other issues as more important. It is a duty of health professionals to respond to such locally expressed need, where possible – particularly if we want the chance to talk about smoking later, for example. Community development is a precarious business, with differing expectations from residents, community representatives, council officers and other workers. In Sandwell we have seen successful community partnerships built up in Tipton, in north Smethwick, and west Smethwick, and new partnerships developing in Hateley Heath, Cradley Heath and estates challenge renewal areas. While seeking to address the priorities of the residents, it Is important that partner agencies stay involved. Housing redevelopments, without educational training and economic, health and social care are likely to produce 'dormitories for the unemployed' – brand-new houses waiting to be vandalized.

Ethnic minorities

Community development has to address the needs of minority groups. In Sandwell, a particular concern is to secure the rights of the 42,000 black and ethnic minority community and the 4,000 long-term disabled, and to see they are represented in local decision-making. Fora of ethnic minorities, women, people with disabilities and young people are being built up to address their needs.

Ethnic minority issues in relation to crime are particularly important and controversial. Ethnic minorities, particularly black Caribbean young men, are portrayed as the perpetrators of crime. But Asian youths are significantly less likely to be involved in crime than white or Caribbean youths. Asians and Caribbeans are also significantly more likely to be victims of crime. Our report suggested all is not equal in the way the youth justice system deals with young black men. They are significantly more likely to receive custodial sentences for repeat offences. One in three black re-offenders are sent to prison, compared with one in five white youth re-offenders. The West Midlands police figures show that young black men were three times as likely as whites to be stopped and searched in 1994.

Role of the health service

The health service has a role to play in preventing crime and violence. Its place in the treatment of victims is obvious; its role in rehabilitating offenders is apparent, if often controversial.

In child protection, the health service is part of the policing and surveillance system which social services lead. Going back to 1988, *Working Together* (DHSS, 1988) exhorted social services and health authorities to put in place effective mechanisms for monitoring and managing child abuse, suspected child abuse, and children at risk. The health service is also a major employer, major landowner and therefore a security risk, with staff in danger of aggression and violence. The health services as a provider cares for victims of crime and is potentially a powerful source of information on assaults, domestic violence, alcohol-related violence and so on.

The role of the health service in preventing crime and violence is less apparent and less developed. Doctors still prescribe tranquillizers and ask for rehousing on medical grounds for people who need mediation over neighbour disputes. General practitioners, casualty staff and community health workers need to develop links with victim support, mediation schemes, women's refuges, domestic violence fora, Safer Cities groups, citizens' advice bureaux, crime reduction panels, community police and criminal justice agencies to identify problems of violent, and potentially violent, clients, and specify the needs and appropriate services for victims of crime. The health service is a major source of information on violent injury. Accident and emergency computer systems can be developed to provide a truer picture of common assaults, racial, domestic and alcohol-related violence. Community health staff need to network widely with other community workers and be advocates for improved services and facilities in the areas they serve. They should also be involved in the area-based initiatives that exist in many parts of the country now under various guises – estates renewal challenges, neighbourhood action areas, health action areas, locality health commissioning, local workers' fora and local residents' fora. Health workers can play a part in getting people the services they need to improve their health, their safety and their quality of life.

Crime and public health – a postscript

Since the original paper was published, a number of initiatives have been taken forward in Sandwell around personal safety, freedom from harassment and abuse, reviewing health needs of prisoners, developing the crime and disorder partnership and in building capacity for evidence-based policy on crime and public health related interventions.

'Personal safety' has become a catch-all for problems of harassment, violence and abuse in domestic and public settings. One of the Health for All principles has been freedom from violence and community safety, but this basic right to security – the right to walk down the street without fear has until recently rarely been considered a health issue.

McCabe and Raine's (1998) work for the Public Health Alliance described some of the interrelationships between crime and health services. More importantly, it showed clearly how the fear of crime has an adverse impact on people's mental health, their ability to function in the community and their ability to achieve a reasonable quality of life. Surveys of patients' experiences of crime were conducted in four GP surgeries in Sandwell and Bristol. The samples were by no means systematic, but the results were powerful and illustrative of the problems faced by patients and by the health system in responding (or not): Up to 6 per cent reported racial attacks; 12 per cent threatening or abusive behaviour; and 3–8 per cent domestic violence. Racial attacks and domestic violence were higher than the figures seen in British crime surveys of the time, but lower than in surveys looking for specific problems. Much higher figures for domestic violence have been reported, of 1 in 4 to 1 in 10 (Mullender, 1996; BMA, 1998).

McCabe and Raine (1998) highlighted the fact that GPs and other health professionals were unlikely or reluctant to identify domestic violence, preferring to treat only physical signs and symptoms. Other pro-

fessionals, health visitors, for example, might be willing to identify problems, but had only limited resources to respond effectively. This report
was a first attempt to look at issues common to the health and criminal
justice systems, and was undoubtedly influential in shaping the development of partnership approaches to problems of mutual concern to the
health and criminal justice services. (McCabe and Raine, 1998). Our
progress on domestic violence and the prison health needs assessment
were reported in the Sandwell public health report for 2000, *Heart and
Minds* (Middleton, 2001).

Domestic violence

The British crime survey of 1996 showed that a quarter of all violent
crimes were domestic, 44 per cent of all violent attacks on women were
domestic, with women with children, especially women aged 16–29
being most at risk.

Following Safer Sandwell, domestic violence was addressed as a priority. Mainstream health service funding was secured to support professional training, awareness raising and enhancing referral systems for
counselling and support. The health action zone gave further impetus to
this, seeing domestic violence as a mental health promotion issue.
Training in clinical areas extended into mental health and maternity
care. Peer education pilots on violence-free relationships have been
developed in schools. Multi-agency guidelines have been produced for
identification and appropriate referral. Much of this work has been led
by the voluntary sector, but now statutory agencies are accepting their
responsibility for tackling domestic violence as part of the work of the
crime and disorder partnership. A domestic violence strategy has been
developed and a post created under social inclusion and health to take
the work forward.

Racial harassment

Another aspect of personal safety which is receiving attention is racial
harassment. The relatively recent establishment of the racial attacks
monitoring unit has begun to provide some information on trends in
racial attacks. As with domestic violence, increased recognition of the
problem and a willingness to address it, has led to an increase in
recorded incidents, which we see as a necessary and welcome pointer to
success. A substantial programme of peer-led education has been developed, entitled, 'Hear no evil, see no evil', it is designed to reduce cultural
misconceptions and promote better relationships between different
ethnic groups. This has been rolled out across Sandwell and has been

commended by the Commission for Racial Equality as a model of good practice.

Sandwell health officialdom continues to be targeted by local extreme political parties for its alleged waste of public funds on ethnic minority health and social issues. The health authority, and now primary care trusts, continue to invest in community capacity building, seeing the promotion of strong community relations as an essential prerequisite for health improvement.

Health in prisons

The health of prisoners has long been the subject of criticism (Smith, 1984). The prison health service remains outside the NHS and there is concern about care standards, inappropriate placement of mentally ill people in prison, and unrecognized and untreated mental ill health and addictions.

Application of NHS standards to prison health care will have substantial resource consequences, but this should not be a justification for maintaining the status quo. The most recent prison health reforms (Joint Prison Service and NHS executive Working Group, 1999) have seen the creation of a joint NHS/Home Office policy board for prison health care development. Local health and prison services have set up partnerships with a first stage of assessing the health needs of prisoners and making local recommendations for service improvement. The West Midlands Institute for Public and Environmental Health has produced a helpful prison health needs assessment toolbox (West Midlands Institute for Public and Environmental Health, 2001). Unmet health needs in the prison population are manifold – drug users, 24 per cent are injecting drug users; cigarette consumption, 80 per cent; mental health problems, 90 per cent; HIV-positive males, 0.3 per cent; and 2 per cent attempt suicide per week.

Sandwell does not have a prison within its borders. However, in 2000, for the first time the number of Sandwell residents in prison was assessed, and 237 men and 7 women from Sandwell were identified in twelve units in the West Midlands. We have identified needs for better liaison between prison, probation and health services, particularly in relation to the pick up of released prisoners by the mental health services, but progress remains slow. Birmingham leads in the improvement of prison health care with Birmingham (Winson Green) Prison.

More fundamental change is undoubtedly needed with the full integration of prison health care under the NHS, and the NHS undoubtedly needs to acknowledge its responsibility and bring its considerable resources to bear to improve the health of prisoners.

Crime and disorder partnerships

Crime and disorder partnerships/crime and disorder steering groups 'responsible authority groups' have been required since the Crime and Disorder Act of 1998. Sandwell's experience has mirrored that of other partnerships. The initial preoccupations of the partnership were the somewhat mechanistic and prescribed requirements of the Crime and Disorder Act – getting anti-social behaviour orders in place, setting up the youth offending team and monitoring its progress, doing the crime audit. However, undertaking the crime audit became the key to identifying local priorities and developing relevant programmes for the partnership. The partnership was able to give greater prominence to drug and alcohol related crime, domestic violence and racial harassment, alongside mainstream policing concerns about burglary, robbery and car crime.

With the next round of crime audit and partnership strategy, we shall look to take our evidence base to a higher level. Sandwell has taken part in the development of evidence based public health policy in the West Midlands (Middleton *et al.*, 2001) We have used the York systematic reviews on the 'wider public health' as a start point to look at interventions which can promote health and reduce crime (NHS Centre for Reviews and Dissemination, 2000). We are taking this work forward as part of the emerging global Campbell collaboration for systematic reviews in criminal justice, education and social welfare (Davies and Boruch, 2001). A West Midlands 'Crime-GRIP' project has been set up, funded by the Government Office for the West Midlands, to look at how we get research into practice, promoting the use of interventions for which there is a strong evidence base. Strong evidence for effectiveness in promoting health and reducing crime exists for early years' education and family support; parenting skills education and low-level interventions to reduce mild to moderate behaviour problems in children; harm reduction and methadone maintenance in opiate drug dependence; and peer-led interactive personal social education programmes which include drugs education. Strong evidence for harm exists for the 'Scared straight' deterrence programme. Good quality evidence exists for the relatively weak effect of the popular American 'DARE' drugs education package, which is didactic and narrowly focused drugs education (Middleton *et al.*, 2001).

In Sandwell, we shall be seeking to complement this approach with better crime data being assembled through the police 'forensic local intelligence system', (FLINTS), which is a powerful tool for both geographical and temporal trend data.

There remains much to be done at both local and national level to enhance the effectiveness of partnerships in tackling ill health and crime. The need for criminal justice agencies to work together has only recently begun to be appreciated. Crime and the fear of crime remains a major threat to public health and quality of life.

References

BMA (British Medical Association) (1998). *Domestic Violence: A health care issue?* London: BMA.

Davies, P. and Boruch, R. (2001). The Campbell Collaboration, *British Medical Journal*, 294–5.

DHSS (Department of Health and Social Security) (1988). *Working Together*. London: DHSS.

Home Office and Department of Health (1994). *Tackling Drugs Together* (White Paper on drugs policy in the United Kingdom). London: HMSO.

Home Office (1995). *British Crime Survey 1994*. London: HMSO.

Joint Prison Service and National Health Service Executive Working Group (1999). *The Future Organisation and Delivery of Prison Health Care*. London: Department of Health and Home Office. HSC 1999/077.

McCabe, A. and Raine, J. (1998). *Framing the Debate: The impact of crime on public health*. Birmingham: Public Health Alliance.

McCarron, P. G., Davey-Smith, G., Womersley, J. (1994). Deprivation and mortality in Glasgow: changes from 1980–92. *British Medical Journal*, 309, 1481–2.

Middleton, J., (ed.) (1995). *Safer Sandwell: Seventh Annual Public Health Report for Sandwell*. West Bromwich: Sandwell Health Authority.

Middleton, J. (ed.) (2001). *Hearts and Minds: The 12th Annual Public Health Report for Sandwell 2000*. West Bromwich: Sandwell Health Authority.

Middleton, J., Reeves, E., Hyde, C., Howie, F. and Lilford, R. (2001). The Campbell Collaboration, 323, *British Medical Journal*, 323:1252.

Mullender, A. (1996). *Rethinking Domestic Violence: The social work and probation response*. London: Routledge.

NHS Centre for Reviews and Dissemination (2000). *Evidence from the Systematic Reviews of Research Relevant to Implementing the 'Wider Public Health' Agenda*. York: University of York.

ONS (Office of National Statistics) (1997). *Occupational Mortality: the Decennial Supplement for 1981–91*. London: ONS.

Schweinhart, L. J., Barnes, H. V., Weikart, D. P. (1993). *A Summary of Significant Benefits: The Highscope Perry pre-school study through age 27*. Ypsilanti, Mich.: High Scope Press.

Smith, R. (1984). *Prison Health Care*. London: British Medical Association.

Townsend, P., Phillimore, P., Beattie, A. (1994). Widening inequality of health in the north of England 1981–91, *British Medical Journal*, 308, 1125–8.

West Midlands Institute for Public and Environmental Health (2001). *Prison Health Needs Assessment Toolbox*. Birmingham: University of Birmingham WMIPEH (West Midlands Institute for Public and Environmental Health).

Looking forward – dilemmas in health promotion: introduction

In this section we consider an agenda for the twenty-first century. What are the issues that will grow in importance, and how best can we move forward with some confidence without losing sight of key debates and dilemmas? Section Four begins with two contributions relating to the growing focus on risk in health promotion.

The extent to which the government should use legislation to limit 'lifestyle' risks is the dilemma addressed by the first chapter in this section. Dan Beauchamp, in Chapter 31, arguing against the anti-paternalism that tends to characterize Western democracies, makes out a case for a limited public balance between individual liberty and the good of the community which is a delicate issue, and in declaring 'two cheers for paternalism' he carefully sketches out one way forward, using alcohol as the main example.

Developing the theme of surveillance and risk at a more abstract level, Sarah Nettleton in Chapter 32 explores the intimate relations between surveillance techniques and risk talk. In the process she presents a challenging critique of the ideological role of health promotion.

Turning to a different area of technological development, Rebecca Cline and K. M. Haynes in Chapter 33 discern new possibilities in the ever-expanding world of health information seeking on the Internet. They question the quality of online health information, and argue that future research in this area needs to address the Internet as part of the larger health communication system.

The persistence of major inequalities forms the theme of Chapter 34, where Lesley Doyal, pointing to the 'gender blindness' of decision makers and medical researchers, teases out various levels at which men continue to be regarded as the norm and women as the 'other' (for example, many epidemiological studies relating to coronary heart disease are based on all-male samples). The solution, she concludes, is radical, but in one sense quite simple: if women are to optimize their well-being, men will have to share resources and labour more equally – but whether enough are willing to do so remains an open question.

In Chapter 35, Susan Denman, Alysonn Moon, Carl Parsons and David Stears explore the future for the health-promoting school.

Reviewing local, national and internationally based schemes, they conclude that while implementing the concept of the health promoting school can be fraught with difficulties, if a whole school approach is adopted it can have many positive health-related effects, not only on the school curriculum and ethos but ultimately on young people within the school.

Tackling an even larger canvas, Peter Townsend illustrates and analyses in Chapter 36 growing inequalities between rich and poor at both global and national levels. Acknowledging that the agenda for the achievement of social justice is dauntingly large, he proposes a set of structural remedies. These include democratization of international agencies, a minimum wage, modernized social insurance, and basic income for child and disability support. To both Townsend and Doyal, the way forward is clear: continuing debates and dilemmas reflect a basic lack of commitment to justice.

But where does all this leave visions of Healthy Cities and the project of health promotion in the twenty-first century? Perhaps the imagination has to be re-awakened if the uncomfortable call for greater social justice is to stand a chance of being heard. The final two chapters look back briefly over the achievements of the health promotion movement as provider of new paradigms for a healthier future before launching into two ways of carrying the vision of Health for All into the new century.

Arguing that the concept of Healthy Cities and its underlying philosophical principle of Health for All are simply incomprehensible with conventional discipline-led models of scientific research and rational administration, Michael Kelly and Amanda Killoran, in Chapter 37, examine the shift from postmodern celebration to post-1997 empiricism, where the constant question is 'Did it work?' They argue that while scientific evaluation of health improvement interventions is difficult, it is not a reason for not doing it, or for retreating into a postmodern relativism, but that it is important to derive culturally sensitive and methodological rigorous ways of developing an evidence base.

The closing chapter, Chapter 38, by Lowell Levin and Erio Ziglio has a more sober but equally optimistic flavour. Combining in some measure the perspectives of the previous two chapters, Lowell Levin and Erio Ziglio present twenty-first century health promotion as an investment strategy that will bring about social, economic, ecological and health returns. Turning upside down the notion that expenditure on health means less money for economic development, the argument here is that economic and social development is dependent on investment in health. The World Health Organization's commitment to a vision of equity, empowerment, sustainability and accountability remains buoyant, and new images have surfaced to keep the ship afloat.

31 Lifestyle, public health and paternalism*

Dan Beauchamp

. . . In recent decades it has become a truism that a significant portion (perhaps as much as half) of the disease and early death in industrialized societies stems from personal risk-taking. Dealing with these risks – commonly called lifestyle risks – creates substantial political difficulties in democratic societies.

Questions of what to do about cigarette smoking, alcohol use, or driving without seat-belts arouse great political debate. Policy restrictions for lifestyle choices have in Western democracies been influenced by a strong antipaternalism.

Antipaternalism flourishes in many conditions, but its native soil is political individualism. Political individualism assumes that the political community is an association of self-determining individuals who view the 'purpose of government as confined to enabling individuals' wants to be satisfied, individuals' interests to be pursued and individuals' rights to be protected, with a clear bias toward *laissez-faire* and against the idea that [the government] might legitimately influence or alter their wants, interpret their interests for them or invade or abrogate their rights' . . . (Lukes, 1973)

Moving away from antipaternalism to a democracy that includes some forms of paternalism, especially for public health, does not imply political collectivism or the view that government seeks only to improve the welfare of the community and that the citizenry have only loyalties to the larger interests of society. Democracy that includes some legitimate forms of paternalism is based on the view that government must reconcile two main ends: the rights and interests of the individual taken separately and the good of individuals together – the community – even for lifestyle risks . . .

The case of alcohol problems

What has been the experience of the Western democracies with alcohol problems in the post-war period? With the exception of France, the

---

* From S. Doxiadis (ed.) (1987). *Ethical Dilemmas in Health Promotion*. London: John Wiley, 69–83 © John Wiley & Sons Ltd.

general experience has been that alcohol consumption in the aggregate has increased greatly, reflecting the fundamental increase in economic productivity and personal consumption that occurred in the decades from 1950s to the 1970s (Markela *et al.*, 1981). Alcohol became, during this period, a commodity much like others. Community sanctions over alcohol commerce were gradually but dramatically weakened in many places. Alcohol products like beer became available in general retail outlet chains, which themselves greatly expanded. Regional and local restrictions were relaxed or totally eliminated. The hours of sale expanded. Age limits were often reduced. Drinking patterns became increasingly homogeneous across national and regional boundaries. Advertising and other forms of promotion dramatically increased.

Given these developments, it should come as no surprise that drinking increased – as did alcohol problems. What is surprising is that while alcohol consumption and consequent problems increased, until very recently governments did not strengthen their alcohol control efforts . . .

Just as alcohol problems and drinking were on the rise in Western societies, many governments were abandoning their commitments to alcohol control. The major exception to this pattern has been drunk driving (Markela *et al.*, 1981).

One of the forces countering this trend has been the growing influence of public health agencies and public health interests in society. The new public health, and the 'second epidemiological revolution' (Terris, 1985) that undergirds it, call attention not only to the risks of the motor car, the motor cycle, the dangers of the Western diet high in saturated fats, to cigarette smoking, or to alcohol, but also to how commercial practices exacerbate these risks.

The growth of a new alcohol epidemiology stressed the relation of alcohol availability, in price, advertising, and age limits in the genesis of alcohol problems. Several broad principles underlie this new alcohol epidemiology. Increases in total alcohol consumption are likely to mean increases in the number of heavy consumers; heavy consumption and damage to health are highly correlated; therefore, preventive programmes must seek to limit increase in general consumption (Schmidt and Popham, 1980).

The importance of these findings is that they bring into view damages to the community as a whole that arise from changes in the organization of alcohol commerce – production, availability, price, advertising or promotion of alcoholic beverages. Tax policy is a good example. Cook has reviewed the evidence that tax policy is crucial to preventing alcohol related problems like cirrhosis and even drunk driving, and has statistically verified these relationships for the period 1960–75 in the United States (Cook, 1981) . . .

Tax policy is important not only because of the connection between the price of alcohol, drinking, heavy consumption, and other problems but because tax, along with the number of outlets, the hours of sale, who may sell alcoholic beverages, age restrictions, advertising and the like are part of the structure of alcohol commerce, and commerce is social in nature, a matter of the common life. But tax policy only partly explains shifts in alcohol consumption. Actually, beer sales increased sharply during the 1970s, while sales of distilled beverages levelled off. The reason for this is that beer is taxed very lightly compared to distilled beverages, and beer is also nationally advertised on American television.

There is little doubt that tax policy and other relaxations on alcohol commerce influence the level of aggregate consumption of alcoholic beverages, including many alcohol-related problems (Cook, 1981). Even J. S. Mill admitted that the market was social:

> [T]rade is a social act. Whoever undertakes to sell any description of goods to the public, does what affects the interests of other persons, and of society in general.

Mill admitted that those who sell alcoholic beverages have an interest in intemperance and therefore restrictions on availability may be justified:

> The interest, however, of these dealers in promoting intemperance is a real evil, and justifies the State in imposing restrictions and requiring guarantees which but for that justification would be infringements of real liberty.

Yet he goes on to rule out taxes for discouraging intemperance as restrictions aimed at the drinker and not at the seller.

But price is little different from restricting the numbers of public houses or supermarkets in a district; both affect availability, the one economic, the other social. And it is this organization of alcohol commerce that is central to any scheme of balancing the community's interest in temperance with the individual's interest in spending his money how he chooses.

Mill argued that only the individual can know his own particular good:

> He is the person most interested in his own wellbeing: the interest which any other person, except in cases of strong personal attachment, can have in it, is trifling.

But this is precisely the wrong point. Public health paternalism in regulating alcohol commerce seeks to protect the common good, not the good of any particular person. As Richard Flathman (1966) notes, modern governments rarely can be paternalistic in the strict sense of promoting the good of particular persons. The liberalization of availability of alcoholic beverages affects the broad drinking public. Historically, government has sought to regulate trade when it affects an important community interest.

Two cheers for paternalism

Public health paternalism provides some surprising dividends beyond regulating alcohol commerce and improving the public's health. Strengthening the public health is not only a matter of improving aggregate welfare, it is also encouraging the citizen to share in a group scheme to promote a wider welfare, of which his own welfare is only a part. Seatbelt legislation or signs on the beach restricting swimming when a lifeguard is not present, restrict my liberty for my own good, but only as I am a member of the public and for the general or the common good. From the private viewpoint, the motto for such paternalistic legislation employing the group principle might be, 'The lives we save together might include my own.'

Thus, public health paternalism encourages concern for the wider good, for co-operation, and group solidarity in solving problems. These are community virtues which are needed alongside the individual virtues of self-reliance and autonomy. National pension schemes may be narrowly paternalistic, but more importantly they encourage group co-operation for the good of everyone alike, stimulating group solidarity. While policies to raise the price of alcohol may seem considerably less concerned with group solidarity than government pension schemes, we should not ignore the possibility that paternalism in lifestyle areas also advances group values and group approaches to solving problems.

This is speculation, but public health paternalism may also help to stimulate individual responsibility, at least up to a point. There is often the view that coercion and individual responsibility operate in a zero-sum manner – seat-belt legislation may cause individuals to take less heed for their own safety on the highway. But it may work the other way around. Fluoridation programmes may help stimulate personal dental hygiene, and government pension schemes may establish a secure minimum around which individuals take voluntary actions to purchase annuities. Similarly, and within limits, community restrictions on drinking and smoking may provide a climate that encourages more individual responsibility regarding drinking or smoking, independently of the direct coercive effect on individuals. Indeed, this might be a main way in which many lifestyle limitations work.

Another way in which public health paternalism may help strengthen a sense of group as well as individual welfare is through enlarging the sense that the standards behind regulating commerce and lifestyle choices are based on group norms rather than individual ones. For example, alcohol consumption in most societies for most individuals is far lower than the amount which might be safe for them as private citizens. As a rough yardstick, 'safe drinking' from the individual standpoint is one and a half ounces of absolute alcohol daily, or the equivalent of three glasses of beer. But in the United States, which stands roughly at the mid-point among Western nations in total alcohol consumption, probably less than 15 to 20 per cent of the population drinks that much (Beauchamp, 1980). Community standards are therefore based on solidarity of interest, meant to reduce the number who suffer alcohol problems. Similarly, seat-belt legislation seeks a group level of safety that individuals acting alone find hard to choose.

How do we keep public health paternalism from going too far and threatening individual autonomy? Do we go from regulating alcohol and the promotion of cigarettes to forbidding rock-climbing? The short answer is no. Public health paternalism focuses on the market place and on those areas where private interests can exploit the public interest. This would include limiting commercial corporations who have a stake in low levels of safety and in risk-taking, to also limiting medical practice to protect the common interest in rationing medical care and in controlling medical expenditure. Public health paternalism mixes controls on providers or producers and consumers and does not seem too intrusive. However, requiring each citizen to jog three miles a day, or to maintain an optimum body weight would bring the state far too close to the individual and would threaten personal autonomy. Commercial regulations and regulating public space operate generally and at a distance, not singling out one particular individual or another for moral improvement. Perhaps the key limit to the balance principle is the presumption it usually carries for individual liberty. Liberty is to be preferred unless regulation guarantees a significant gain to the community. The restrictions sought should also be least restrictive measures available consistent with the ends to be achieved. And the burden of proof is on those who desire the restriction of liberty to demonstrate community benefits.

Threatening individual interests

Antipaternalism may actually increase rather than reduce threats to individual interests. It does this in three separate areas: by focusing on blame, by putting undue stress on children and young people otherwise not of legal age, and by raising the risk of prohibition. Policies which balance community and individual interest actually do a better job of protecting individual interests overall by spreading responsibility for prevention more equitably among the affected interests.

Drunk driving has been the main exception to governments' lack of interest in alcohol policy. In the United States, this issue has led the way for increased national and local attention to alcohol policy. The group responsible is Mothers Against Drunk Drivers (. . . [later] renamed Mothers Against Drunk Driving), or MADD, which was founded by the charismatic mother of a young girl who was killed by a drunk driver.

Solving social problems by punishing wrongs or crimes is a principal method of those forms of antipaternalism rooted in a strong political individualism. As Mill put it, 'The preventive function of government . . . is far more liable to be abused, to the prejudice of liberty, than the punitory function.' The primary motive behind drunk-driving campaigns is to punish drunk driving as a way of symbolising the community's repugnance for the practice, and secondly, to deter drunk driving by inflicting stiffer penalties and instituting more effective detection methods. These are legitimate and even important governmental interests.

But increasing the legal penalties and certainty of punishment for drunk driving, taken by itself, is not likely to have permanent and long-term results in reducing this problem. The main reason is the difficulty for police forces in detecting drinking and driving. In the United States the risks of detection in most areas is one in 2000 (Reed, 1981). In England the estimate, even during intense enforcement, is only one in 1,000 (Reed, 1981). As Lawrence Ross (1973) has noted, campaigns against drinking and driving probably have their effect because they alter the subjective assessment by citizens of the risks of detection. Once the initial wave of publicity passes, the public learns that risk of detection has not increased appreciably, and the previous levels of drunk driving are re-established.

The main problem is that many Western societies have made alcohol so widely available and convenient to the car as to actually constitute a licence to drink and drive. In most Western countries, beer is widely available in most retail establishments, with few government personnel to detect sales to intoxicated or under age people. In many states in the United States it is permissible to drink and drive – only *drunk* driving is forbidden. Western societies have put heavy reliance on detection of drunk driving by the police, with the result that the practice of police stopping drivers randomly to administer sobriety tests is on the increase. What starts out as antipaternalism and legal sanctions winds up as a very serious increase in the level of law enforcement in democratic societies.

Another paradoxical outcome of political individualism is the unusual emphasis given to control and protection of young persons. As Mill argued, the restrictions on limiting society's and the government's power over the adult's private conduct do not apply to young people:

> Society has . . . absolute power over [children and youth] during all the early portion of their existence: it has . . . the whole period of childhood and nonage in which to try whether it could make them capable of rational conduct in life. (1961)

Political individualism puts so much stress on leaving the adult free to choose his own ends that, almost of necessity, the young bear the brunt of social control. Defining the community's interest in alcohol policy as principally that of regulating the behaviour of the young can make them the scapegoat for society's policies. Nils Christie (1981) in Markela *et al.* has warned that increased governmental interest in alcohol policy is likely to take the form of extending 'childhood' for longer and longer periods to legitimise the supervision by the state. Certainly, the . . . experience in the United States, with the federal government's endorsement of a uniform national legal drinking age of 21 years, is partial evidence that this is occurring.

The point is not to ignore the young or punishment for drunk drivers but to balance restrictions and legislation aimed at these groups with broader controls on alcohol commerce that affect the entire population. As Michael Grossman *et al.* (1984) argue, a slight increase in the tax on beer might save as many lives as a one year increase in the age limit for drinking. The other advantage of this policy is that it would also help prevent problems among those who are older as well, and would also make the young feel less singled out. Policies against drunk driving – whether aimed at the young or not – might also include limitation on the availability of alcohol in the retail distribution system, an increase in the level of surveillance of that system by state liquor licence personnel, or an increase in the price of alcoholic beverages, especially beer. Better yet, we could do all three things at once. The growing application of civil liability for retail operators who serve under age or drunk patrons or both is also likely to help reduce the problem, and to shift attention away from the criminal justice system.

There is yet another danger to individual interests from the undue focus on blame in many kinds of antipaternalism. This is the danger of what has come to be called 'victim blaming' (Ryan, 1976) . . . Victim blaming begins by noting that smoking and alcohol abuse add significant social costs to society, especially by lost productivity and increased medical and insurance costs. The next step is to argue that these groups should be held accountable for these costs to the others in society. As one American critic has argued, ' [O]ne man's freedom in health is another man's shackle in taxes and insurance premiums' (Knowles, 1977). But where does this principle of individual responsibility to the larger society end? Are the obese, those with large families, those who fail to exercise also to be similarly burdened? Thus, it is a short step from a position of individual autonomy to a position of social responsibility to the larger society, from a position of individual autonomy to social stigmatisation.

This position of making the risk-taker pay his own way ignores the extent to which drinking and smoking as actions are a complex bundle of voluntary and involuntary features, structural as well as individual causal relationships. While we should not ignore the role of choice, alcohol and cigarettes are also powerfully addictive and heavily promoted by commercial interests. The community position would spread the responsibility more broadly, seeing these problems as *both* community and individual problems, using prevention rather than blame and measures aimed at all who smoke or drink, as well as the industries.

Finally, there is the paradox of prohibition itself. It is striking that the country that experienced the longest period of national prohibition, the United States, is the democracy that comes nearer to a public philosophy of political individualism. Prohibition came to the United States for many complex reasons. One of the reasons is surely that, when problems such as alcohol abuse become so severe that society has to take action, the militant antipaternalist is forced either to revise his antipaternalism or to escalate seriously the threat that alcohol itself poses to the individual. This is what seems to have happened with the shift from the early temperance drives which were voluntary in character, and which met with limited success. Prohibition came next, and it came in significant part because the philosophy of political individualism offered no middle ground for balancing regulation of alcohol use with its continued commercial availability. Antipaternalist philosophies nearly always contain room for substances or conditions which are so inherently dangerous that extreme government regulation and even prohibition is justified. When a balancing approach is not popularly embraced or understood, there is a strong temptation to take a newly problematic set of conditions (the rise of the saloon in the nineteenth century) and a substance (alcohol) and reclassify it in the same group that today is reserved for drugs like heroin. Room for compromise and balance is thus lost, because why should a dangerous drug be allowed in the stream of commerce? This experience might serve as a cautionary tale for commercial interests who defend their interests in the name of political individualism.

So, two cheers for paternalism – public health paternalism. Public health paternalism permits a sharing of responsibility for controlling the impulses of one's life, and for strengthening those motives of cooperation and trust that are the cornerstone of the community (Slater, 1970). As with everything else, this principle has its dangers, but societies which ignore the needs of community and mutual dependency are deeply unwise, encouraging the very threats to private interests that they so noisily and blindly seek to protect.

References

Beauchamp, D. (1980). *Beyond Alcoholism: Alcohol and Public Health Policy*. Philadelphia: Temple University Press.

Cook, P. J. (1981). The effect of liquor taxes on drinking, cirrhosis, and auto accidents. In Moore, M. and Gerstein, D. (eds), *Alcohol and Public Policy: Beyond the shadow of prohibition*. Washington, DC: National Academy Press.

Flathman, R. (1966). *The Public Interest: An essay concerning the normative discourse of politics*. New York: Wiley.

Grossman, M., Coate, D. and Arluck, G. (1984). Price sensitivity of alcoholic beverages in the US. Paper presented at the Conference on Control Issues in Alcohol Abuse Prevention: Impacting Communities. South Carolina Commission on Alcohol and Drug Abuse, Charleston, SC, 7–10 October.

Knowles, J. H. (1977). The responsibility of the individual. In Knowles, J. H. (ed.), *Doing Better and Feeling Worse*. New York: Norton.

Lukes, S. (1973). *Individualism*. New York: Harper & Row, 79–87.

Markela, K., Room, R., Single, E., Sulkunen, P. and Walsh, B. (1981). *Alcohol, Society and the State: A comparative study of alcohol control*. Toronto: Addiction Research Foundation, xiv.

Reed, D. S. (1981). Reducing the costs of drinking and driving. In Moore, M. and Gerstein D. (eds), *Alcohol and Public Policy: Beyond the Prohibition*. Washington, DC: National Academy Press, 336–87.

Ross, H. L. (1973). Law, science, and accidents: the British Road Safety Act of 1967, *Journal of Legal Studies*, 2, 1–78.

Ryan, W. (1976). *Blaming the Victim*. New York: Vintage.

Schmidt, W. and Popham, R. (1980). Discussion of paper by Parker and Harman. In Harford, T. C., Parker, D. A. and Light, L., *Normative Approaches to the Prevention of Alcohol Abuse and Alcoholism*, Research Monograph, 3, National Institute on Alcohol Abuse and Alcoholism, Department of Health and Human Services. Washington, DC: United States Government Printing Office.

Slater, P. (1970). *The Pursuit of Loneliness*. Boston: Beacon.

Terris, M. (1985). The changing relationships of epidemiology and society: The Robert Cruikshank lecture, *Journal of Public Health*, 6, 15–36.

32 Surveillance, health promotion and the formation of a risk identity*

Sarah Nettleton

Contemporary forms of surveillance within the context of health promotion and the new public health are characterized by their emphasis on risk. This chapter explores the relationship between surveillance and risk, and suggests that the current emphasis on the construction and monitoring of risk factors has contributed to the formation of a new conceptualization of 'self' – one that is perpetually both cognisant of, and, resistant to, risk.

Administering health

To aspire to be healthy is not just a personal goal, it is also a political one. Governments in liberal democratic societies take action to improve the health of their populations. A feature of governments since the eighteenth century is the way in which they have intensified, developed and refined administrative procedures and technologies to gather data and information on individuals and populations. Data has long been gathered on variables such as levels of morbidity, procreation, life expectancy and mortality (Foucault, 1980). In fact, it was this activity that contributed to the development of the discipline that we now call statistics. Foucault (1980) describes how the body became the prime site of political regulation and surveillance: 'the body of individuals and the body of populations – appears as the bearer of new variables' (p. 172). This is what he famously describes as 'disciplinary power': the mechanisms of discipline which fashion and train bodies. Alongside the development of procedures for monitoring populations emerged another political preoccupation, as Foucault explains:

> This is the emergence of the health and the physical well-being of the population in general as one of the essential objectives of political power. Here it is not a matter of offering support to a particularly fragile, troubled and troublesome margin of the population,

---

* Commissioned for this volume.

but of how to raise the level of health of the social body as a whole. Different power apparatuses are called upon to take charge of 'bodies', . . . *The imperative of health: at once the duty of each and the objective of all.* (Foucault, 1980, pp. 169–70, emphasis mine)

For Foucault, however, such activities constitute only one side of the practical administrative systems by which individuals are governed. Individuals also act upon and govern themselves. Indeed, a liberal democratic society requires the individuals who constitute it to be able to act autonomously as 'good citizens' (Burchell, 1993; Rose, 1993). Thus 'technologies of surveillance' or 'disciplinary power' rely on, and interact with, what Foucault calls 'the technologies of the self'. Here Foucault is referring to the means by which individuals can have an effect on their own bodies, minds, souls and their conduct. If health was to be achieved by government it had to be the goal of *both* administrative programmes and of individuals. The desire to be healthy, from this perspective, is not an innate aspiration but one that is bound up intimately in the processes of governance. Such a desire forms part of a political aspiration. Following this line of argument, the historian Barbara Duden (1991) argues that health as a 'goal of individual well-being' was derived from the 'administrating and objectivising of the "body politic"' (p. 18).

The Enlightenment wrote health onto its banner as a physical–moral category. The concept was politically so effective and so double-edged because the interest of the authorities and the national economy in a self-administered objectification of the self appeared in it as a subjective need of the individual or an act of philanthropy . . . Political medicine cast this desire for a healthy body into a scientifically solid mold of norms and pathologies, thus creating a new image of humankind . . . the human right to the 'pursuit of happiness' (as laid down in the Constitution of the United States) took on concrete form as a right to health. (Duden, 1991, p.19).

Thus the actions we take to improve the health of individuals are bound up with wider political motives and ambitions. The activities, policies and procedures of those authorities who are concerned to promote health reverberate on the activities and desires of individuals. The consequences of public health and health promotion practices should not therefore be underestimated.

The nature of the 'technologies' or administrative mechanisms which Foucault and others write about invariably change over time. For example, within the context of health and medical care, new methods of collecting data are developed, new technologies for observing people's bodies and behaviours are devised, and different aspects of people's social lives are deemed to be relevant. The last few decades of the twentieth century saw a significant change in the mechanisms used to monitor populations, and this has occurred alongside a transformation of the philosophical or ideological base of medicine. Furthermore, as we shall see, it was this revolution in medicine that generated the political and administrative space for the emergence of health promotion.

From 'dangerousness' to 'risk'

The French philosopher, Robert Castel (1991), in a paper entitled 'From Dangerousness to Risk', provides a useful way of conceptualizing this transformation when he argues that we are entering a new paradigm of health care. He suggests that we are moving from a health care system premised on 'dangerousness' to one based on 'risk'. Hitherto, he argues, health professionals have tended to err on the side of caution to prevent the development of disease, and, consequently, the illnesses suffered by patients have been treated as being potentially dangerous. However, the target of health and medical care is now shifting, from the symptoms of an individual *patient* to the social and behavioural characteristics of the *person*. The 'clinic of the subject', Castel (1991, p. 282) suggests, is being replaced by the 'epidemiological clinic'. Thus we are witnessing the advent of a new mode of surveillance, aided by technological advances which make the calculus and possibilities of 'systematic pre-detection' increasingly sophisticated.

Castel suggests that there are two very real consequences of this profound change. First, practitioners' key function will be to assess the social and behavioural characteristics of their clients, and on the basis of these assessments provide guidance and advice. In the United Kingdom, an example of this would be the requirement of general practitioners (GPs) to keep more and more data on their patients 'risk factors', such as their levels of smoking and drinking. A second consequence is that practitioners become subordinate to health care administrators or managers, who are charged with tasks such as the profiling of populations and developing health strategies. While Castel labels this new form of health care the 'epidemiological clinic', the medical sociologist David Armstrong (1995) calls it 'surveillance medicine': 'A cardinal feature of Surveillance Medicine', he writes, 'is its targeting of everyone'. Increasingly, health and medical care are not just concerned with those who are ill but with those who are well, and it is not just orientated towards treating the symptoms of disease but also identifying and monitoring *risk factors* which 'point to' the possibility of a future illness.

A 'risk epidemic'

In the last decades of the twentieth century there has been a proliferation of so called 'risk factors' associated with health. One is sometimes left with the impression that whatever one does carries some form of 'risk' or danger. Eating certain foods, drinking alcohol, coca cola or coffee, not doing enough exercise, doing too much of the wrong type of exercise, being overweight, being underweight, watching too much television, not having enough leisure time, smoking cigarettes – in fact, doing almost anything now seems to have potential connotations for one's health.

A number of sociologists (Douglas, 1986; Beck 1992; Giddens, 1992) have pointed to the fact that we are living in a society that is characterized by a 'politics of anxiety' – indeed, that we are living in a *risk society* (Beck, 1992). A point on which all these authors appear to agree is that the risks associated with modern-day living are person made, they are a product of social organization and human actions. Armstrong (1993) contrasts the health risks of the twenty-first century with the health risks present in the nineteenth century. While in the nineteenth century, health risks were associated with the 'natural' environment and dangers lurked in water, soil, air, food and climate, today the environmental factors that impinge on health, such as acid rain and radiation are the consequence of human actions. Of course, not all contemporary health risks are human products, AIDS, for example, is the consequence of a virus. Nevertheless, the disease has come to be conceptualised within a social matrix; it exists within a wider context of social activities and is envisaged in terms of complex social interactions between gay men, intravenous drug users, and those requiring and administering blood transfusions (Armstrong, 1993). In this respect it has increasingly become articulated in the same terms as human-created risks.

The proliferation of risks is not confined only to popular discourse or sociological debates, it has also occurred within the medical literature. A comprehensive analysis of medical journals in Britain, the United States and Scandinavia found that the increase in the use of the term 'risk' has reached 'epidemic proportions' (Skolbekken, 1995). The study looked at journals published between 1967 and 1991. For the first five years, the number of 'risk articles' published was around 1,000, and for the last five years of the period there were over 80,000. Skolbekken refers to this as a 'risk epidemic' in order to highlight the high prevalence of the term; the fact that there is a degree of contagiousness which 'is indicated by increase in the number of illnesses/disease that are subject to some kind of risk approach' (p. 296) and, finally, to draw attention to the 'side effects' of the current preoccupation with the term.

Skolbekken argues further that health promotion provides 'the ideologoical frame needed to explain the present emphasis on factors regarded as risks to our health . . . Through the ideological frame of health promotion we get a glimpse of some of the functions served by the risk epidemic' (1995, p. 296). He cites these functions as: first, to predict disease and death – in other words, to gain control over disease, which in turn confirms our faith in medical science. Second, it is sometimes assumed that the findings of this type of research may help to save money, as people are less likely to require acute – and therefore expensive – services. Third, it contributes to medicalization. Risk factors which are hypothesized to be linked to disease come to be treated as 'diseases to be cured' (Skolbekken, 1995, p. 299). Certainly, in the public health and health promotion documentation, health related behaviours such as smoking or drinking alcohol come to be treated as variables which need to be explained. Whether or not the first function is legitimate, or the second function is likely, may be undermined by the third point which draws attention to the 'unscientific' nature of much of this research. Even spurious correlations between risk factors and disease may easily come to be treated as causal (Davey Smith *et al.*, 1992). Certainly, there is considerable controversy within the medical journals about the links between, say, diet and coronary heart disease, and the merits and demerits of various interventions – for example, the lowering of cholesterol levels (Oliver, 1992; Ravnskov, 1992; Atrens, 1994).

The techniques deployed in the scrutinization of these 'risk factors' within the context of public health and health promotion are primarily: screening for a range of diseases and symptoms; the collection of information on patients by health professionals; epidemiological studies; social surveys; and qualitative studies. Once a 'factor' such as eating 'fatty foods' is found to be associated statistically with another indicator of ill health (or risk factor) such as cholesterol levels, it is deemed to be a risk. The social aspects of eating this type of food may then be explored by sociologists and anthropologists, who aim to answer questions such as: Why do people eat fat? What does eating fatty foods mean to them? What is the social and symbolic significance of eating fatty foods? This information is considered to be crucial to the development of effective health promotion. The findings of the epidemiologists and the social scientists are drawn upon by health promoters to encourage people to eat less fatty foods. The government will keep an eye on the populations fat consumption and set nutritional targets. For example, the Department of Health (2000) pledged that by April 2002 every local health community would 'have quantitative data no more than 12 months old about the implementation of the policies on: reducing the prevalence of smoking, promotion healthy eating, promoting physical activity [and] reducing overweight and obesity.

Thus surveillance techniques and risk go hand in hand. The techniques deployed to survey and monitor populations contribute simultaneously to the construction of more and more risk factors, and monitor the extent to which individuals, groups and populations possess them.

The social construction of risk factors

As with any area of medical or scientific research (Wright and Treacher, 1982) the selection of 'factors' to be studied cannot be immune from prevailing social values and ideologies. This is perhaps most overt in relation to AIDS, where the sexist, racist and homophobic assumptions which underpin epidemiological research have been identified (Patton, 1990; Bloor *et al.*, 1991). It is also evident that so-called lifestyle or behavioural factors (such as the 'holy trinity' of risks – diet, smoking and exercise) receive a disproportionate amount of attention. As we have seen, the identification and confirmation of risk factors is often subject to controversy, and the evidence about causal links is not unequivocal. However, health promotion interventions are developed on the basis of such evidence, and may often gloss over contradictory research findings (Frankel *et al.*, 1991). The recourse to epidemiology by those involved in public health and health promotion results in a veneer of scientific legitimacy, and as such the findings of epidemiological research are often taken to be politically neutral (Lupton, 1995, p. 67). However, the nature of the dialogue between health promoters and epidemiologists may also be one of 'double standards', as we shall see below.

The individualization of risk

A risk factor associated with health is a characteristic of the given population it concerns. Within the context of epidemiological research, risks are calculated on the basis of *collective* data. Risk factors are therefore not properties possessed by individuals, but refer to probabilities which, by definition, can only be derived from the study of a group of people. Confidence in predictions is enhanced by the size of the sample population studied. This conceptualization of risk is rooted in probability statistics. In fact, as Ewald (1991), writing on the subject of insurance, sociology and risk, has pointed out, there is no such thing as an individual risk:

> Whereas an accident, as damage, misfortune and suffering, is always individual, striking at one and not another, a risk of accident affects a population. Strictly speaking there is no such thing as an individual risk; otherwise insurance would be no more than a wager. Risk only becomes something calculable when it is spread over a population. (p. 203).

In fact, as Lindsay Prior (1995) points out in his paper 'Accidents as a Public Health Problem', it is entirely feasible to predict the number of accidents for any given population. The *rate* of accidents will vary for subpopulations: for example, working-class boys may have more accidents than middle-class girls. However, it is not possible to predict with any certainty for an individual working-class boy that he, in particular, will have an accident. In many respects, this may seem obvious; however, as epidemiological findings become transformed into health promotion discourse; this simple fact appears to be lost. Prior points out that we are encouraged to believe two things. First, that we can prevent ill health, or, in this case, accidents: 'In theory at least, all accidents are preventable' (Department of Health, 1992, cited by Prior, 1995, p. 139).

Second, that the maintenance of health, or the prevention of accidents is something that is largely the responsibility of individuals. Prior (1995, p. 140) draws attention to the document *The Health of the Nation . . . And You* (Department of Health, 1992), which encourages its readers to take pay attention to their own households and to: 'fit a smoke detector', 'beware of the chip pan', 'beware of damaged carpets', 'make sure that there is good lighting in hallways and stairs'. The key point that Prior is making is that there is something of a double standard here. Epidemiological research confirms the fact that accidents are a *collective* phenomenon and the accident rate remains fairly constant for given populations; however, *individual* and technical solutions are proposed to alleviate the problem.

The interpretation and communication of the results of research is clearly affected by the prevailing political and ideological context. We live in an ideological environment which privileges the individual, and in particular an individual who is able to manage and negotiate her or his own risks. Within clinical practice, health professionals have to inform patients about the results of various screening procedures, tests and measurements. They are also required to counsel individuals about any current and future threats to their health. A study by Lauritzen and Sachs (2001) carried out in Sweden explored the ways in which the 'language of risk' is employed in two types of health surveillance: a child health programme and a surveillance programme of 40-year-old men. They found that nurses who communicate the 'results' to individuals have to deal with the tension that 'health risks' are a property of the population, but in the context of the clinical consultation the risk becomes a property of an individual. Hence, 'awareness of risk has to be balanced against undue anxiety' (p. 514). This balance is not easy to achieve, and the study found that any slight deviations from the norm did engender anxiety among both the parents (usually mothers) and the men. Mechanisms of surveillance which focus on individual risk factors may contribute to the formation of a new individual identity. As Armstrong (1995) has put it, the:

> real significance [of surveillance medicine] lies in the way in which a surveillance machinery deployed throughout a population to

monitor a precarious normality delineates a new temporalised risk identity. (1995, p. 404)

The formation of the 'risky self'

In recent decades, there have been transformations in the 'technologies of self' – the means by which human beings fashion their thoughts and conduct. Contemporary forms of governance encourage individuals to be enterprising; to make choices; to seek out and make use of information; to be discerning consumers; and to be accountable. Individuals are encouraged to take care of their own welfare needs and manage their own risks, be it in relation to housing, education, pensions or health. Welfare is no longer provided by the government for citizens 'as of right'; it is targeted increasingly at those who are deemed to be in 'real need', and everyone else has to insure against, or invest in, their own futures. Contemporary forms of government involve a greater emphasis on self-governance and, associated with this, there has been a proliferation of diverse activities and resources in both the public and the commercial sectors to support individual consumers. Hence the notion of self-governance implies an ongoing project whereby individuals are constantly assessing information and expertise in relation to themselves.

The sociologist, Anthony Giddens, has labelled this 'project', which he considers to be a key feature of late modern society, as *reflexivity*: 'It is a project carried on amid a profusion of reflexive resources: therapy and self help manuals of all kind, television programmes and magazine articles' (Giddens, 1992, p. 30). Few people could be unaware of the explosion of information and advice about health. Barbara Duden was struck by this in the United States some years ago:

> in a bookstore in Dallas I found about 130 manuals that would teach me 'how to be an active partner in my own health.' For many years now the self-care budget in the United States has been growing at three times the rate of all medical expenses combined. (Duden, 1991, p. 20).

Exhortations about healthy living do not only originate in the activities of state-sponsored health professionals – public health consultants, health promoters. GPs, nurses, etc. – but also a myriad of other sources such as schoolteachers, community group leaders, supermarkets, TV, radio, magazines and so on. There has also been an explosion of health 'resources', be it goods, such as healthy foods, exercise bikes or services, such as fitness clubs and therapies, of every kind within the commercial sector. They can all be used by consumers in the construction of their identities. As Lupton puts it succinctly:

> All are directed at constructing and normalising a certain kind of subject; a subject who is autonomous, directed at self improvement, self-regulated, desirous of self-knowledge, a subject who is seeking happiness and healthiness. (Lupton, 1995, p. 11)

Indeed, as we have seen, those health risks that are identified in the epidemiological literature, and perhaps more importantly those taken up by those involved in 'promoting health', are those that are taken to be within the control of the individual. This, in concert with transformations that have occurred in the psychological and therapeutic sciences, has contributed to the construction of what Jane Ogden (1995) has called the 'risky self':

> In the last decades of the twentieth century, the surveillance machinery, which finds reflection in the individualistic and self reliance ethic of the New Right, has successfully penetrated the spaces of the body to reconstruct an intra-active identity which is increasingly compartmentalised into the controlling self and the risky self. (1995, p. 413–14)

Within the context of the 'epidemiological clinic' disease or illness is something the individual can work to prevent, be it through a positive mental attitude or 'healthy lifestyles'. Certain moral and ethical considerations emerge from this. Monica Greco (1993) points out that health which can be 'chosen' represents a very different value and moral dimension to a health which one simply enjoys or has. She writes:

> It testifies to more than just a physical capacity; it is the visible sign of initiative, adaptability, balance and strength of will. In this sense, physical health has come to represent, for the neo-liberal individual who has 'chosen' it an 'objective' witness to his or her suitability to function as a free and rational agent. (Greco, 1993, pp. 369–70)

Help is at hand for those individuals who are not able to pursue healthy lifestyles. Health promoters may draw on a range of activities orientated towards 'empowering' people to lead healthier lives. For example, those people who do not appear to have a capacity for health can be equipped with all sorts of psycho-social and practical skills to overcome their difficulties.

We have seen that contemporary surveillance techniques and the current proliferation of discourses on risk are mutually constitutive. We have also seen that these processes have helped to forge a new risk identity or risky self. We must however be careful here. This is not the same as saying that humans are simply dupes, shaped by the dominant discourses or ideologies of the day. On the contrary, as we have seen, within the context of liberal democratic societies, governance requires that individuals are autonomous and free to question the policies and practices of government. This is, of course, obvious. Lots of people (including those involved in the dissemination of information about health) resist the advice of the health experts – actively, openly and willingly indulging in 'risky health behaviours'. But such resistance is a necessary prerequisite for the effective functioning of forms of governance which rely on techniques of surveillance or 'disciplinary power'.

References

Armstrong, D. (1993). Public health spaces and the fabrication of identity, *Sociology*, 27(3), 393–410.

Armstrong, D. (1995). The rise of surveillance medicine, *Sociology of Health and Illness*, 17(3), 343–404.

Atrens, D. (1994). The questionable wisdom of a low-fat diet and cholesterol reduction, *Social Science and Medicine*, 39(3), 433–47.

Beck, U. (1992). *Risk Society: Towards a new modernity*. London: Sage.

Bloor, M., Goldberg, D. and Emslie, J. (1991). Ethnostatistics and the AIDS epidemic, *British Journal of Sociology*, 42(1), 131–9.

Burchell, G. (1993). Liberal governments and techniques of the self, *Economy and Society*, 22(3), 267–81.

Castel, R. (1991). From dangerousness to risk. In Burchell, G., Gordon, C. and Miller, P. (eds), *The Foucault Effect: Studies in governmentality*. Brighton: Harvester Wheatsheaf.

Davey Smith, G., Phillips, A. and Neaton, J. (1992). Smoking as an 'Independent' risk factor for suicide: illustration of an artifact from observational epidemiology?, *The Lancet*, 340, 709–12.

Department of Health (1992). *The Health of the Nation . . . And You*. London: HMSO.

Department of Health (1993). *The Health of the Nation*. London: HMSO.

Department of Health (2000). National Service Framework for Coronary Heart Disease. London: HMSO.

Douglas, M. (1986). *Risk Acceptability According to the Social Sciences*. London: Routledge.

Duden, B. (1991). *The Woman Beneath the Skin: A doctor's patients in eighteenth century Germany*. London: Harvard University Press.

Ewald, F. (1991). Insurance and risk. In Burchell, G., Gordon, C. and Miller, P. (eds), *The Foucault Effect: Studies in governmentality*. London: Harvester Wheatsheaf.

Foucault, M. (1980). The politics of health in the eighteenth century. In Gordon, C. (ed.), *Michel Foucault, Power/Knowledge: Selected interviews and other writings 1972–1977 by Michel Foucault*. Brighton: Harvester Press.

Frankel, S., Davison, C. and Davey Smith, G. (1991). Lay epidemiology and the rationality of responses to health education, *British Journal of GPs*, 41(351), 28–30.

Giddens, A. (1992). *The Transformation of Intimacy*. Cambridge: Polity Press.

Greco, M. (1993). Psychosomatic subjects and the 'duty to be well': personal agency within medical rationality, *Economy and Society*, 22(3), 357–72.

Lauritzen, S. O. and Sachs, L. (2001). Normality, risk and the future: implicit communication of threat in health surveillance. *Sociology of Health and Illness*, 23(4) 497–516.

Lupton, D. (1995). *The Imperative of Health: Public health and the regulated body*. London: Sage.

Nettleton, S. (1996). Women and the new paradigm of health and medicine, *Critical Social Policy*, 16(3), 33–53.

Nettleton, S. (1997). Governing the risky self: how to be healthy wealthy and wise. In Bunton, R. and Petersen, A. (eds), *Foucault, Health and Medicine*. London: Routledge.

Ogden, J. (1995). Psychosocial theory and the creation of the risky self, *Social Science and Medicine*, 40(3), 409–15.

Oliver, M. (1992). Doubts about preventing coronary heart disease, *British Medical Journal*, 304, 393–4.

Patton, C. (1990). *Inventing AIDS*. London: Routledge.

Plummer, K. (1988). Organising AIDS. In Aggleton, P. and Homans, H. (eds), *Social Aspects of AIDS*. London: Falmer Press.

Prior, L. (1995). Chance and modernity: accidents as a public health problem. In Bunton, R., Nettleton, S. and Burrows, R. (eds), *The Sociology of Health Promotion: Critical analysis of consumption lifestyle and risk*. London: Routledge.

Ravnskov, U. (1992). Cholesterol lowering trials in coronary heart disease: frequency of citation and outcome, *British Medical Journal*, 305, 15–19.

Rose, N. (1993). Government, authority and expertise in advanced liberalism, *Economy and Society*, 22(3), 283–99.

Skolbekken, J. (1995). The risk epidemic in medical journals, *Social Science and Medicine*, 40(3), 291–305.

Turner, B. S. (1992). *Regulating Bodies: Essays in medical sociology*. London: Routledge.

Wright, P. and Treacher, A. (eds) (1982). *The Problem of Medical Knowledge: Examining the social construction of medicine*. Edinburgh: Edinburgh University Press.

33 Consumer health information-seeking on the Internet: the state of the art*

R. J. W. Cline and K. M. Haynes

Introduction

. . . Increasingly, professionals and consumers engage in interactive health communication. Robinson *et al.* (1988) define 'interactive health communication' as 'the interaction of an individual – consumer, patient, caregiver or professional – with or through an electronic device or communication technology to access or transmit health information or to receive guidance and support on a health-related issue' (Robinson *et al.*, 1998, p. 1264). Perhaps the most common and influential function of interactive health communication today is health-information seeking by consumers . . .

Public health interest in consumer health-information seeking via the Internet

Public health professionals need to focus on health-information seeking via the Internet for a variety of reasons. These include magnitude and diversity of use, diversity of users; and, ultimately, implications for the health care system, in terms of structure, health care interaction and quality of medical outcomes.

As the Internet has grown, so too have health-related purposes. Perhaps most common is consumer health-information seeking . . .

Consumer use of the Internet for health information is large and growing; more than 70,000 websites provide health information (Grandinetti, 2000) . . .

Reasons for the growth of consumers' online health-information seeking include the development of participative or consumer-orientated health care models, the growth of health information that makes any one clinician incapable of keeping pace, cost-containment efforts that

* From Cline, R. J. W. and Haynes, K. M., 'Consumer Health Information Seeking on the Internet: the state of the art' (2001), *Health Education Research*, vol. 16, no. 6, pp. 671–45, Oxford University Press.

reduce clinicians' time with patients and raise concern about access to 'best' care, emphasis on self-care and prevention, an ageing population with increased health-care needs, and increased interest in alternative approaches to health care (Eng *et al.*, 1998; Gallagher, 1999). In addition, consumers report convenience, anonymity and diversity of information sources as attractions (Pew Internet and American Life Project, 2000c).

Diverse purposes

The scope of the health-related Internet applications is 'as broad as medicine itself' (Sonneriberg, 1997, p. 151). Consumers access online health information in three primary ways: searching directly for health information, participating in support groups and consulting with health professionals . . .

Diverse users

Early Internet users were likely to be white male Professionals. Today's health-related use tends to defy stereotypes and increasingly reflects the population's composition.

Initially, men tended to use the Internet more than women. but women constituted 50 per cent of Internet users for the first time in 1999 (Reuters, 2000). The number of women using the Internet grew by 32 per cent in 1999, compared to 20 per cent among men. However, any gender difference may be mediated by race. One study found that women make up 56 per cent of the black population using the Internet, compared to an even gender split among whites (Associated Press, 2000b). Women, more than men, tend to prefer health sites, in part because of care-taking roles. A Health on the Net Foundation (HON) survey (Health on the Net Foundation, 1999a) found that 60 per cent of respondents using the net to locate health information were women (see also Pennbridge *et al.*, 1999; Pew Internet and American Life Project, 2000b) . . .

Collaborations or collisions ahead? Implications for the health care system

Increased consumer participation in interactive health communication is likely to influence the health care system because of its information dissemination, health promotion, social support and health services functions (Robinson *et al.*, 1998) . . .

However, critics disagree about the valence of consequences. Optimists anticipate better-informed decisions by consumers, better and more tailored treatment decisions, stronger provider–client relationships, and increased patient compliance and satisfaction (Ayonrinde, 1998:

Wilkins, 1999), resulting in better medical outcomes (Bader and Braude, 1998: Wilkins, 1999) and more efficient service (Pricewater-houseCoopers, 1999). Pessimists contend that interactive health communication will not enhance physician–patient communication, with physicians likely to balk at the added responsibilities (Appleby, 1999; Baur, 2000). Medical outcomes could be diminished by consumers who lack technical background, interpret information incorrectly and try inappropriate treatments (LaPerriére *et al.*, 1998).

Among the ways that interactive health communication is forecast to affect health care include: replacing traditional information, care and community resources with online information, consultations and social support networks (Simpson, 1996; LaPerriére *et al.*, 1998; Gregory-Head, 1999; Oravec, 2000). As consumers use the Internet increasingly to manage their health care more actively and independently, they are likely to take this active role into encounters with providers. One survey found that 67 per cent of physicians report having patients who discuss with them information retrieved from the Internet (Neff, 1999).

This emerging consumer role has implications for healthcare relationships. Consumers may confront providers who are unprepared to deal with the magnitude of available information (Coiera, 1996), with patients sometimes having greater information access than their providers. Providers may be stressed by added responsibilities for information seeking and clarification, and become frustrated and resistant because of time costs in correcting inaccuracies (Ayonrinde, 1998; Appleby, 1999; Lincoln and Builder, 1999). Conflicts between provider and client may be likely as consumers locate information that leads them to challenge, question or 'second-guess' providers, indicating diminished trust in their physicians (Robinson, *et al.*, 1998; Bader and Braude, 1998; Pereira and Bruera, 1998; Eng and Gustafson, 1999; Lamp and Howard, 1999).

The shifting balance of informational power functions to erase prior exclusivity of access to information (Coiera, 1996; Wilkins, 1999), treating everyone as a 'peer' (Buhle, 1996, p. 624). Some applaud this shift as an opportunity for partnerships in health care (Thomas, 1998) and greater use of the consumer as a resource (Wilkins, 1999). while others see a Pandora's Box of 'unmanageable problems' (Mayer and Till, 1996, p. 568). Many providers are threatened by their loss of power and fear damage to physician–patient communication (Anonymous, 2000). Anticipated changes highlight the need to integrate interactive health communication into medical and health professional curricula (Aschenbrener, 1996; Kaufman *et al.*, 1997; Khonsari and Fabri, 1997; Lunik, 1998), continuing medical education (Dovle *et al.*, 1996), and patient education and provider–client interactions. in order to facilitate clients' access to information they trust (Lamp and Howard, 1999; Grandinetti, 2000).

Potential benefits of consumer online health-information seeking

From the Internet's inception. health care was understood to be 'a major potential beneficiary' (Lindberg and Humphreys, 1995, p. 158). *Potential* benefits to consumers are many.

Widespread access to health information

The Internet 'created an avalanche of easily accessible information' (Appleby, 1999, p. 21). Exponential growth of access to health information offers, 'seemingly endless opportunities to inform, teach, and connect professionals and patients alike' (Silberg *et al.*, 1997, p. 1244). Breaking the space and time barriers of traditional information seeking processes, the Internet offers widespread dissemination, high volume and currency (Eng and Gustafson, 1999; Gregory-Head, 1999; McKinley *et al.*, 1999). Theoretically available worldwide at the price of a local telephone call, 24 hours a day (LaPerriére *et al.*, 1998; McKinley *et al.*, 1999), the Internet has the potential to increase health information access in remote areas and to otherwise under-served populations (LaPerriére *et al.* 1998; McGrath, 1997). As a result, the Internet offers the potential for greater equity in access to health information (Morris *et al.*, 1997). In some cases, websites are developed specifically for otherwise hard-to-reach audiences (e.g. NetWellness, a consumer health library developed for a rural population) (Guard *et al.*, 1996).

Interactivity

A major potential benefit of the Internet is its capacity for interactivity, emphasizing transactional rather than linear communication processes (Pereira and Bruera, 1998; McMillan, 1999). Interactivity is reflected in complexity of choice, responsiveness or conversationality and interpersonal communication (McMillan, 1999). Interactivity further promotes tailoring of messages and facilitates interpersonal interaction.

Tailoring of information

In contrast to traditional sources of health information (e.g. print), interactive health communication offers the potential for more individually tailored messages in a variety of formats (Robinson *et al.*, 1998; Eng and Gustafson, 1999). Consumers can select sites, links and specific messages based on knowledge, educational or language level, need, and preferences for format and learning style, often at lower cost than conventional methods (Pereira and Bruera, 1998). At the same time, traditional health information and patient education materials and messages can be placed on the Internet inexpensively (Richards *et al.*, 1998).

Potential to facilitate interpersonal interaction and social support

The Internet offers opportunities for consumers to interact interperson-ally with health professionals and peers. Research consistently indicates that health behaviour change typically results more from interpersonal than from mass communication (e.g. Piotrow *et al.*, 1997); thus the Internet may be used to promote health behaviour change.

Potential for anonymity

Relative to face-to-face interaction, interactive health communication offers potential anonymity (Robinson *et al.*, 1998). Consumers may access information on sensitive topics, and the stigmatized may interact without the predictable disconfirmation of face-to-face interaction. Those who have difficulty in communicating face-to-face may be able to engage in interactive health communication (LaPerriére *et al.*, 1998).

Roadblocks, bumpy roads and hazards on the information superhighway

Despite potential benefits of interactive health communication, limita-tions and cautions abound. Roadblocks to access, navigational difficul-ties and quality concerns constitute potential downfalls of relying on the Internet for health-related information.

Roadblocks to access

Claims that 'the Internet is inherently democratic' by having informa-tion for everyone (Wootton, 1997, p. 576) are countered by evidence of inequitable access. Those in greatest need are least likely to have Internet access (Eng *et al.*, 1998). Havenots include rural, isolated and tradition-ally underserved populations (e.g. inner city and low socio-economic status neighbourhoods; the elderly) (Eng and Gustafson, 1999; Gallagher, 1999). Barriers to online health information include cost, geo-graphic location, literacy, computer skills and institutional policies (Eng *et al.*, 1998; LaPerriére *et al.*, 1998; Gallagher, 1999).

Disparities in access to both computers and the Internet are growing (Chapman, 1999). A Department of Commerce study reported that 40 per cent of US households have personal computers (Chapman, 1999); however, data indicate a growing divide based on both education and income levels. Although 82 per cent of US households with incomes in excess of $75,000 have Internet access, only 38 per cent of those with incomes below $30,000 do so (Pew Internet and American Life Project, 2001), figures that translate to about twenty times greater likelihood of access among the higher than the lower income group (Chapman, 1999). Both consumers' and professionals' (e.g. rural and urban community health providers) access can be bounded by cost (Martin *et al.*, 1997). Access is defined not simply as having a computer,. but also in terms of 'affordability, accessibility, availability, acceptability and accommodation of Internet connections' (Wilkins, 1999, p. 31).

Cost often correlates with geography. The worldwide picture is dismal. Only 10 per cent of the US$55 billion spent globally on health research addresses the needs of poor countries (World Health Organization, 1995). In the US, one in six people use the Internet, but in Africa (excluding South Africa), one in 5000 uses the Internet (Lown, *et al.*, 1998). In Africa, Internet service providers are increasing, but most health professionals and hospitals cannot afford hook-up and access fees. These same countries often lack textbooks for medical and nursing students and have little access to medical journals (Lown *et al.*, 1998). Internet access is prohibitively expensive for many developing countries (Pereira and Bruera, 1998). The role of poverty versus affluence in accessing the Internet is obvious: 'While the affluent travel at greater speed on the information superhighway, a majority of the world's population has never even made a telephone call' (Lown *et al.*, 1998, p. SII36). At the same time that analysts fear information overload regarding HIV treatments (e.g. Green, 1999), 95 per cent of HIV cases occur in the developing world where few doctors can access the Internet and for whom few sites exist in local languages. Thus little attention is paid to making information accessible to those in greatest need.

Computer and health literacy, and English language constrain Internet use. People may not know how to access the Internet, or be afraid of the technology (Wilkins, 1999). People unable to speak, read or understand English are disadvantaged, because English is the dominant online language (Pereira and Bruera, 1998). NOAH (New York Online Access to Health) was one of the first websites developed to address consumer health information needs in both English and Spanish (Voge, 1998). People with the greatest health care needs often have low information access because of lower health literacy levels (American Medical Association, 1999).

Eng *et al.* advocate universal access to health information (Eng *et al.*, 1998). They challenge both public and private stakeholders to collaborate to reduce the gap between 'haves' and 'have-nots', by supporting access in homes and public places (e.g. public libraries. schools, malls, community centres, healthcare facilities. places of worship), developing applications for diverse users, supporting access-related research, addressing quality of information issues and training health information specialists to function as intermediaries (Eng *et al.*, 1998).

Arguments for universal access are three-fold: philosophical, public health and economic. Philosophically, the majority of health information was developed from publicly funded research and should be accessible to all. The authors' views parallel the egalitarian philosophy about public libraries, i.e. 'encouraging an informed citizenry and a vibrant democracy' (Eng *et al.*, 1998, p. 1373). Greater access to health information may improve health status by enhancing the quality of health-related decisions: in turn, health care costs may be reduced.

Bumpy roads: navigational difficulties

Internet users may find health information functionally inaccessible because of design features resulting in difficulty of use.

Information overload

Analysts recognize online health information overload as a problem (e.g. LaPerriére *et al.*, 1998), characterizing it as a 'disease' (Morris, 1998, p. 1866) or a 'traffic jam' (McGrath, 1997, p. 90). Wootton likens the Internet to a vast library in conjunction with a giant set of Yellow Pages (Wootton, 1997). A spokesperson for the US Department of Health and Human Services warned, 'Trying to get information from the Internet is like drinking from a firehose, and you don't even know what the source of the water is' (McLellan, 1998, p. SII39). One physician complained of 'an information glut to the point that people get all balled up' (Appleby, 1999, p. 211). The speed and uncontrolled manner of Internet growth and information accumulation make locating, valid information more difficult (Jadad and Gagliari, 1998).

Disorganization

Not only is the Internet overloaded, it is also disorganized (McKinley *et al.*, 1999). The Internet is like (Jacobson, 1995, pp. A29–A301):

> a library where all the books have been donated by patrons and placed randomly on shelves. There are no call numbers or other classification schemes, and people can move books around from shelf to shelf whenever they wish. Moreover the library is expanding rapidly, with new collections arriving every day and thousands of additional people signing up every week to roam through the stacks . . . It is an unorganized mass of material – some of it wonderful, some of it awful.

Searching difficulties

Even Internet literate users may not be skilled in locating health information. Searching can be difficult for both consumers and professionals (DeGeorges, 1998; Pereira and Bruera, 1998). Users may find that search engines locate too many or too few sites (Chi-Lum, 1999); target audiences are often unspecified. Availability of information on the web is subject to the same disparities as traditional sources. For example, although many sites contain HIV/AIDS information, few are designed for women (Mallory, 1997), mirroring offline discriminating factors in attending to the disease (see, e.g., Cline and McKenzie, 1996).

Inaccessible or overly technical language

Beyond inaccessibility to material in one's native language, users may find much health information presented in jargon or highly technical language. Despite their training, 48 per cent of nurses studied indicated that they found Internet-based health information unclear (AWHONN, 1997). Much health information is presented at a high reading level; overuse of textual formats may exacerbate language problems (McGrath, 1997). However, graphic formats pose their own problems, often in the form of slowness in downloading graphics (McGrath. 1997).

Lack of user friendliness

Once located, health sites may be difficult to use because of confusing layering, difficult-to-follow linkages and lack of searchability. Difficult to use or weak browsers and search engine technologies may challenge users (Pennbridge *et al.*, 1999). Consumers unfamiliar with the technology may be intimidated and retreat both from the Internet and from the healthcare system (Gallagher, 1999).

Lack of permanence

The Internet is fluid rather than permanent. Inconsistent updating means that information may be out of date (Gallagher, 1999). Sites disappear, change and move without warning, because of the 'evanescent' nature of the Internet (Pereira and Bruera, 1998, p. 621).

O'Mahoney's review of Irish health care websites summarizes navigational difficulties (O'Mahoney, 1999). O'Mahoney judged these sites 'disappointing' (O'Mahoney, 1999, p. 334) because of little dating, unspecified target audiences, poor design, lack of e-mail contact addresses, high readability levels, lack of interactivity, little maintenance and being static or out of date.

Hazardous conditions

Increasingly, medical professionals and Internet users voice concerns about the *quality* of online health information (e.g. Maugans *et al.*, 1998; McLeod, 1998; Boyer *et al.*, 1999). Concerns persist, although evidence finds more than 90 per cent of Internet users satisfied, having found 'the information they were looking for' (Louis Harris and Associates, 1999) or 'useful' information (Health on the Net Foundation, 1999a; Associated Press, 2000b). Despite consumer satisfaction, 'incorrect information could . . . be life-threatening' (Lunik, 1998), p. 40). Well-reasoned criticism identifies why the information consumers find may be harmful.

Lack of peer review or regulation
'There is no "arbiter" of truth on the Internet' (Lunik, 1998, p. 40), no 'quality filter' (Lacroix *et al.*, 1994, p. 417). Anyone can develop an Internet site, thus, 'the Web has become the world's largest vanity press allowing anyone with Internet access to act as an author and publisher of material on any subject' (Richards *et al.*, 1998, p. 281). The Internet is characterized by uncontrolled and unmonitored publishing with little peer review (Marra *et al.*, 1996; Pereira and Bruera, 1998). Authorship can be misleading, as anyone can claim medical expertise; pages may be 'official looking' and mislead consumers into believing they are authoritative (Pereira and Bruera, 1998, p. 61).

A variety of types of unreviewed sources are available to consumers, including quacks, cranks and charlatans (Gregory-Head. 1999), leading one observer to complain, 'Finding anything means there is a huge pile of rubbish' (Machles, 1998a, p. 410). Well-intentioned individuals may provide information based on personal experience, quacks promote unproven remedies, giving false hope and inaccurate information about outcomes: cranks have some scientific background but are disenchanted with traditional science: most alarming are charlatans who 'engage in fraudulent practices with the intent to deceive' (Pereira and Bruera, 1998, p. 48). Because the Internet is unregulated, accuracy, currency and bias vary (McGrath, 1997; Lamp and Howard, 1999); inaccurate information is disseminated widely (Richards *et al.*, 1998).

Inaccurate, misleading and dangerous information
Typical criticisms find health information on the Internet 'bad, and even dangerous' (McKinley *et al.*, 1999, p. 265), 'inaccurate, erroneous, misleading, or fraudulent' (McLeod, 1998, p. 1663), 'incomplete. misleading and inaccurate' (Silberg *et al.*, 1997, p. 1244) and 'incomplete, contradictory or based on insufficient scientific evidence' (Adelhard and Obst, 1999, p. 75). Not only is information incomplete, often it is not evidence based (Pereira and Bruera, 1998; Pandolfini *et al.*, 2000). 'Science and snake oil may not always look all that different on the Net' (Silberg *et al.*, 1997, p. 1244). Dow *et al.* warned that 'fringe, nonscientific therapies may be touted . . . as valid' (Dow *et al.*, 1996, p. 152). Thus concern exists for both fraudulent and unsubstantiated information on the Internet (Marra *et al.*, 1996).

More experienced users of the Internet for health information seeking are more critical of its quality than less experienced users (Health on the Net Foundation, 1999b). A large and growing majority (69 per cent up from 53 per cent in a May/June 1998 survey) of Internet users are concerned about quality of online health information (Health on the Net Foundation, 1999a).

Coiera characterizes the potential for harm caused by inaccurate online health information as an 'information epidemic' (Coiera, 1998, p.

1469). Although limited in quantity, evidence of potential harm caused by low-quality online information is emerging (e.g. Weisbord *et al.*, 1997). One study shows that more than half of health information websites offer unreliable information (Adelhard and Obst, 1999) . . .

Internet searches may yield false and deceptive service, product and treatment claims without providing supporting evidence or sources permitting verification (Dow *et al.*, 1996). Even savvy Internet users 'can have trouble distinguishing the wheat from the chaff' (Rudin and Littleton, 1997, p. 934). Sonnenberg claims 'Most people will be unable to determine the qualifications of Web authors and separate truth from opinion' and 'even well-educated users are unlikely to have the background required to critically evaluate medical information' (Sonnenberg, 1997, p. 152). As a result, consumers lacking evaluation skills are particularly vulnerable.

Consumers' evaluation skills

Quality concerns include the public's ability to select valid information (Pereira and Bruera, 1998; Adelhard and Obst, 1999). Sonnenberg questions whether consumers 'can make good selections when more than one site is available to address their concerns' (Sonnenberg, 1997, p. 151).

'In medicine, the ability to review scientific literature critically, to identify major research flaws, and to interpret correctly the clinical implications of research findings, are skills acquired through training' (Avonrinde, 1998, p. 449). Consumers may misjudge information, become information-overloaded and thereby easily confused, misinformed or misled. Without skills needed to discern validity and familiarity with the scientific review process (Pereira and Bruera, 1998), consumers may: (1) fail to recognize that key information is missing, (e.g. Sacchetti *et al.*, 1999); (2) fail to distinguish between biased and unbiased information (Sachetti *et al.*, 1999); (3) fail to distinguish between evidence-based and non-evidenced-based claims (Ayonrinde, 1998), and (4) misunderstand health information intended for health professionals (Ayonrinde, 1998). These limitations are particularly salient given evidence that people may give greater credibility to information from computers than from other media (Hawkins *et al.*, 1987; Rudin and Littleton, 1997; Bader and Braude, 1998).

Risk-promoting messages abound

The Internet is a reservoir of potentially influential risk-promoting as well as health information and messages. For example, the Internet is a source of information about suicide methods (Alao *et al.*, 1999). Some evidence indicates that Internet use may promote sexual risk-taking. A recent survey of youth (ages 10–17 years) found that among those who used the Internet regularly, 19 per cent were the targets of unwanted sexual solicitation during the previous year, resulting in high levels of distress among 25 per cent of those solicited (Mitchell *et al.*, 2001). Further, people who choose to use the Internet to find real-life sex partners are more likely to contract sexually transmitted diseases or to engage in risky behavior (e.g. have anal sex, more partners or partners known to be HIV positive) than those who become acquainted offline (McFarlane *et al.*, 2000). Toomey and Rothenberg criticized the public health establishment for failing to anticipate this Internet consequence, a foreseeable result of the anonymity of sex facilitated by the Internet (Toomey and Rothenberg, 2000, p. 486): 'For populations with levels of education and income sufficient to support computer use, the Internet has become an efficient facilitator of behaviors and practices that have been taking place for many years among certain high-risk individuals.' Thus the Internet represents new challenges to public health professionals . . .

Evaluating health information on the Internet

The problem

The uneven and often indeterminate quality of online health information raises concerns (McLeod, 1998). The Internet is composed of over 30 million pages lacking consistent peer review, editorial systems or safeguards, placing consumers and professionals in need of quality assessment standards (McGrath, 1997; Rudin and Littleton, 1997; McKinley *et al.*, 1999). Silberg *et al.*'s warning captures the problem: *'caveat lector et viewor* – let the reader and viewer beware' (Silberg *et al.*, 1997, p. 1244). A 'pressing need' exists for tools to evaluate health information found on the Internet (Lamp and Howard, 1999, p. 34). Little scholarship addresses Internet health information quality in depth (e.g. Ambre *et al.*, 1997; Garrison, 1998; Robinson *et al.*, 1998; Adelhard and Obst, 1999; Rippen, 1999); many authors address quality briefly in the contexts of particular health professions (e.g. dentists, ophthalmologists, pharmacists) or topics (e.g. ageing, women's health, health of newborns), for example, Post, 1996; Rudin and Littleton, 1997; Wootton, 1997; Lunik, 1998; McLeod, 1998; Lamp and Howard, 1999.

Criteria for evaluating health information websites

Numerous authors bemoan the difficulty and limitations of establishing quality standards (e.g. McLeod, 1998), yet a review of the literature yields substantial consensus regarding such criteria. Health-related websites should be judged by the quality of health information found on them and by design features that may facilitate or impede use. Quality should be based on a comprehensive assessment rather than any single criterion. A readily navigable or updated site may contain inaccurate information (Ambre *et al.*, 1997; McLeod, 1998: Rippen, 1999).

Quality of health information

Quality of health information found on the Internet should be subjected to the same standards as traditional information, including source and message characteristics, as well as adaptability to targeted audiences.

Internet *sources* include both site sponsors and sources of specific information. Credible Internet sources mirror tradition, including journals, universities and recognized research centres, libraries, government agencies and professional organizations (Silberg *et al.*, 1997; Lamp and Howard, 1999). However, health information may be found on sites sponsored by little known but credible organizations (e.g. organizations of providers, consumer advocacy groups, voluntary health-related organizations), as well as organizations whose names only *sound* credible, commercial sponsors, and individuals (both professionals and members of the public). Credibility constitutes the 'premier criterion' for evaluating online health information (Rippen, 1999, p. 4). *Credibility* is defined as in terms of judgements regarding believability of sources of messages, reflected in two dimensions: *authoritativeness* and *trustworthiness* (O'Keefe, 1990).

Authoritativeness (also termed competence or expertise) involves judgements of whether the source is in a position to know what is truthful or correct (O'Keefe, 1990). Consumers should seek evidenced-based information and advice from expert sources (Wyatt, 1997; Appleby, 1999). Typically, physicians and healthcare organizations are perceived as authoritative (Ambre *et al.*, 1997); however, those associated with medical schools are deemed more credible by their research involvement. Evidence of authoritativeness includes:

- Clearly identified authorship and/or source. Websites should identify the qualifications and credentials (e.g. educational backgrounds, board certifications, and affiliations with organizations) of their own and cited authors (Kibbe *et al.*, 1997; Silberg *et al.*, 1997; Adelhard and Obst, 1999; Lamp and Howard, 1999).
- Attribution. References to other publications, particularly clinical studies, permit users to verify information independently (Silberg *et al.*, 1997; Adelhard and Obst, 1999; Rippen, 1999).
- Clearly identified editorial practices and/or seals of approval. Sites should specify editorial review processes and identify reviewers (Rudin and Littleton, 1997; Rippen, 1999). The HON seal of approval signifies ostensible compliance with HON quality standards (described below) (Boyer *et al.*, 1998).
- Opportunities for feedback and interactivity. The potential for e-mail with a site and associated health professionals permits consumers to clarify technical information and misunderstandings (Silberg *et al.*, 1997; Adelhard and Obst, 1999; Essex, 1999).
- Evidence of monitoring links to other sites (Silberg *et al.*, 1997). A

site's own authoritativeness is limited by the credibility of the sites to which it is linked.

Trustworthiness refers to judgements regarding the character or integrity of a source in terms of motivation to be truthful (O'Keefe, 1990). Even authoritative sources may be biased (Ambre *et al.*, 1997; Wyatt, 1997). Evidence to assess trustworthiness includes:

- Disclosure of mission, purpose and processes and standards for posting information (Wootton, 1997; Rippen, 1999).
- Disclosure of potential conflicts of interest by the site's sponsors. Conflicts of interest may be based on financial dependence, theoretical preference, or intellectual investment (Rippen, 1999), and may indicate bias (Kibbe *et al.*, 1997; Silberg *et al.*, 1997; Wyatt, 1997; Adelhard and Obst, 1999). Information embedded in advertisements needs to be labelled as such (Ambre *et al.*, 1997).
- Disclosure of the collection process, use and final destination of information gathered (either explicitly or via tracking mechanisms) about users (Rippen, 1999).
- Warning signs. Untrustworthy sites often include 'sounds too good to be true' claims (Federal Trade Commission. 1997, p. 1), products advertised as cure-alls, and phrases like scientific breakthrough', 'exclusive product', 'miraculous cure' or 'secret ingredient' (Ambre *et al.*, 1997, pp. 2–7; Federal Trade Commission, p. 1). Plagiarizing or failing to identify sources may tarnish trustworthiness (Ambre *et al.*, 1997).
- Disclaimers. Disclaimers address a site's limitations, scope, purpose, reporting errors and information currency (Ambre *et al.*, 1997). A disclaimer may disclose a site's viewpoint (e.g. advancing surgical interventions). A common disclaimer warns users not to use a site to replace traditional health care, representing itself as an information source rather than one for medical advice, thus facilitating rather than replacing provider–client interaction (Silberg *et al.*, 1997; Rippen, 1999).

Message characteristics

Internet content or information may be judged as 'messages', subject to the same evaluation standards as traditional print sources (Garrison, 1998). Evidence of valid messages includes:

- Currency of information. Evidence includes: the date of the last site updating, policies and methods regarding updating, and site development date (Silberg *et al.*, 1997; Adelhard and Obst, 1999; Rippen, 1999).
- Accuracy of information. Judging accuracy independent of other cri-

teria is difficult (Ambre *et al.*, 1997). Users should be wary of information conflicting with commonly agreed upon medical or scientific positions (Ambre *et al.*, 1997). Substance and depth of content may enhance accuracy (Post, 1996).

- Organization. Information should be presented in a logically organized fashion (Adelhard and Obst, 1999).
- Readability and intelligibility (Appleby, 1999). Health information may be presented in varied formats, including text, graphics and animation: regardless of format, content needs to be understandable to users (Ambre *et al.*, 1997; Wyatt, 1997). However, text on many health websites exceeds the reading level of the typical consumer (O'Mahoney, 1999). Design features may enhance or detract from intelligibility. For example, large and bold print may enhance readability (Essex, 1999); graphics may clarify by illustrating or confuse if too complex.

Audience characteristics

A site's audience and context should be identified clearly and the site adapted accordingly. Audience refers to targeted users (e.g. consumers or health professionals), while context refers to a site's topic and intended users (e.g. informational, advisory, commercial) (Adelhard and Obst, 1999). A site's appropriateness, relevance and usefulness should be readily discernable; content and design should match targeted audiences (e.g. reading and language levels) and contexts (Adelhard and Obst, 1999).

Design features

Format characteristics may enhance delivery of information, but do not affect the quality of message content (Ambre *et al.*, 1997). Design features vary widely, making sites more or less facilitative when seeking particular information or locating specific sites. Facilitative design features include:

- Accessibility. Websites should facilitate navigation through large quantities of information while maintaining simplicity of technology, operation, and format. Complex sites with highend technology may enhance aesthetic value but reduce access (Lamp and Howard, 1999; Rippen, 1999). Access is enhanced by relatively simple browser technology, providing options when multimedia browsers are unavailable, and offering options for the hearing- and sight-impaired (Ambre *et al.*, 1997; Rippen, 1999; W3C, 1999). Such options include text equivalents for visual and auditory images, avoiding reliance on colour alone to clarify images or messages, and the capacity for activating site elements from a variety of devices (W3C, 1999).
- Ease of use. Logical organization, essential to locating information quickly, underlies a site's usability or ease of use (Post, 1996; Adelhard

and Obst, 1999; McKinley *et al.*, 1999). Put simply, the number of steps needed to locate a site or specific information constitutes one operational definition of navigability (Wyatt, 1997). The basic premise behind ease of use is designing a website that builds on the *user's perspective*; formative research can facilitate the creation of a consumer-oriented organizational architecture (e.g. W3C, 1999; Nielsen and Norman, 2000; Petersen, 2000; Farrell, 2000). Navigability is facilitated by organizing and grouping ideas and information by categories that make sense from the consumer's perspective, clarifying that organization by grouping links on a navigation bar or menu while avoiding irrelevant links; labeling links in comprehensible and accurate terms; using consistent page layouts with recognizable graphics, and providing a help or search tool.

- Links between sites. Links between sites help in locating specific information. Useful links match the original site's audience or context, reflect an architecture that permits free movement forward and backward, and contain content meeting the criteria described here (Rippen, 1999). Sites should seek to avoid 'dead-end' links (Post, 1996) and overloading users with links (McGrath, 1997; Wootton, 1997).

- Aesthetic and format characteristics. Websites combining text, audio and visual formats afford adaptability to consumer preferences and learning styles. Aesthetic qualities should contribute to comfort and use. Colour co-ordination, lack of clutter, unobtrusive backgrounds and legibility of text contribute to quality (Post, 1996). Technical materials may be simplified by translation into pictorial format (Essex, 1999). However, too many graphics may slow access (McGrath, 1997).

Mechanisms for evaluating websites

Access to peer-reviewed resources, user surveys and codes of conduct may facilitate the consumers' task of evaluating online health information.

Peer review
Unlike medical literature, much online health information lacks peer review (Ambre *et al.*, 1997; Rippen, 1999). However, informed consumers increasingly can access peer-reviewed health information (via sites that provide abstracts and full-text journal articles, often with extensive archives), e.g. consumers' access to Medline equals that of professionals. Beyond scientific research articles, consumers can access websites developed specifically to assure high quality evidenced-based information (e.g. Healthfinder, MedlinePlus) to search for information or verify that found elsewhere (Wootton, 1997).

Rating systems
Few websites feature user-rating systems (Ambre *et al.*, 1997). Some post

unofficial reviews, ratings and standards for evaluating sites (Essex, 1999). For example, Quackwatch.com was designed to combat health-related fraud both online and offline (Barrett, 2001). A review of 'best' attempts to develop systematic rating systems questioned both their validity and benefits, and concluded that they may do more harm than good (Jadad and Gagliari, 1998). As Berland *et al.* point out, when sites or systems rely on voluntary self-assessments, reliability and validity are unknown (Berland *et al.*, 2001). Numerous organizations offer criteria for assessing websites (e.g. Eng and Gustafson, 1999), but such assessments are for personal use rather than formal site evaluation.

HON code of conduct
At present, the most widespread attempt to apply a code of conduct to online health information was developed by HON. HON is a self-governing body promoting eight ethical standards for online health information online: (1) advice provided by qualified professionals, unless otherwise indicated; (2) support versus replace existing provider–client relationships; (3) confidentiality of user data; (4) clear referencing with links to sources where possible and dates of modification noted; (5) balanced evidence for claims; (6) information clear, with contact addresses to facilitate clarification; (7) sources of funding indicated clearly; and (8) any advertising (as funding) acknowledged and clearly differentiated from the site's content (Boyer *et al.*, 1998). Websites that comply with the HON code contain the HON logo (Health on the Net Foundation, 1997; Boyer, *et al.*, 1998). As of January 2000 HON registered connections to its code from more than 5,000 external servers and more than 20,000 external web pages (Health on the Net Foundation, 2000). However, HON encourages use of their verification system to determine if sites are bonafide HON subscribers (versus simply displaying the logo) (Health on the Net Foundation, 2000).

In summary, increasing quality concerns mandate evaluation standards. Despite relative consensus on evaluation criteria, they have not been widely disseminated to the public nor are they a fail-safe method for assuring quality.

Research and the Internet as a source of health information: the vast wasteland or the new frontier?

Extant Internet health-information literature is characterized by basic 'how to' presentations, speculative and anecdotal accounts, and reporting little empirical research. Articles educate readers about Internet use, speculate on the impact of online health information and report or project innovations. Little literature reports research regarding Internet use or its effects.

Just five years ago, journal articles commonly explained what the Internet *is* to health professionals (e.g. Guay, 1994; Dow *et al.*, 1996; Huang and Alessi, 1996). Much early writing (1993–6) simply defined key terms, explained the use and projected impact on a profession (e.g. McKinney and Bunton, 1993, Frisse *et al.*, 1994; Tomaiuolo, 1995; Steiner *et al.*, 1996; Weiler, 1996). Even more recently, numerous articles explain the Internet and summarize basic use (e.g. Gagel, 1998; Littleton, 1998, Lunik, 1998; Machles, 1998a, 1998b). Many articles address best sites, in general (e.g. Judkins, 1996), or based on profession, specialization or disease or disorder (e.g. Korn, 1998; Bell, 1999; Mann, 1999), including articles for consumers (e.g. Stemmer-Frumento, 1998; Tomlin, 1998).

Second-generation health-related Internet uses go beyond disseminating information. Numerous authors project what the Internet will offer consumers in the future; often reality is not far behind. Only a few years ago, authors 'predicted innovations' that are now in practice, such as hospital telephone directories online, patients searching for information about upcoming surgical procedures, newly diagnosed patients using the web for patient education (Doyle *et al.*, 1996), e-mailing physicians (Bazzoli, 1999) and cyberspace visits replacing live visits (e.g. for prison populations; in rural areas) (Keen, 1997). The rate of Internet development quickly renders projections out of date, blurring a sense of present and future. Some 'projections' include: hospital online nurseries to allow friends and family to see newborns (Bazzoli, 1998), physicians using the Internet for patients to review diagnostic information on depression in order to convince the patient of the diagnosis and printing this information as a fact sheet (Stevens, 1998), providers creating customized pages to meet patients' specific needs (Flory, 1998; Stevens, 1998), and patients storing electrocardiogram records on secret web pages for emergency access (Doyle *et al.*, 1996).

Directions for future research: challenges and opportunities

This review of literature regarding consumer online health-information seeking mirrors health information on the Internet; the literature often has little evidence base for its claims. Challenges to consumers, public health professionals and researchers alike include the rapidity of change of content, structure and technology embedded in the Internet. Sometimes analysts are challenged to research and publish findings before they are obsolete! The challenge of future research is to devise methods and conceptual frameworks appropriate for investigating the richness of the Internet's dynamics relative to health issues.

Adelhard and Obst, in grappling with research challenges, indicate that new methods may be required with regard to sampling (as users may vary with amount of use, expertise, nature of use) (Adelhard and Obst, 1999). Researchers will be challenged to discriminate effects due to the Internet versus other highly accessible health-information sources (e.g. television, direct-to-consumer prescription drug advertising). Controlled studies may include longitudinal investigations (as use and influence may vary over time), retrospective cohort studies and case control studies, as alternatives to traditional studies using control groups (Adelhard and Obst, 1999).

In response to now-common criticisms and concerns regarding health-information seeking on the Internet, future research needs to assess the 'net gap' as well as the quality of information (message content). Research needs to address the demographic characteristics of participants, to identify more precisely the underserved, as well as the kinds of information consumers are seeking, what they locate, how they judge the quality of information found, what they learn (Wyatt, 1997), and how they are influenced behaviourally. Researchers need to compare the processes, outcomes and cost-effectiveness of traditional versus online health-information seeking, as well as various types of online information seeking (e.g. direct searching compared to interactions with support groups or professionals). Future research, practice and public policy need to focus on reducing the 'net gap' in terms of both accessibility and evaluation skills.

Despite abundant speculation regarding the consequences of consumer participation in interactive health communication, little research has investigated these issues; a lack of compelling evidence exists regarding relative *effectiveness*; perhaps more importantly, little evidence exists regarding *effects*. Critics bemoan absence of research regarding the Internet's effectiveness (e.g. Eng and Gustafson, 1999). However, assessing effectiveness presumes a consensus regarding websites' goals and objectives. Public health professionals' goals involve enhancing health knowledge, beliefs and behaviour. However, taken collectively, health websites do not reflect a monolithic objective: some are created for profit, others for personal benefit, and still others to 'validate' views that lack an evidence base. Thus, from the perspective of their creators, some websites may be deemed effective if they are commercially successful, personally confirming, or succeed in disseminating information and gathering support for risk-promoting or unhealthy functions. Moreover, given the potential for health websites to 'promote disease' as well as health and to disseminate fiction as well as fact (including those designed for health-promotion goals), researchers may do well to think in terms of assessing 'effects' rather than 'effectiveness'.

Ultimately, interest and research on *effects* should focus on quality of health and health care. Despite observers' contentions, little research has assessed the impact of interactive health communication on the health care system (Wyatt, 1997; Adelhard and Obst, 1999), although health care (Sonnenberg, 1997), health care interaction, and health and medical outcomes (Adelhard and Obst, 1999) are probably affected.

This article begins by defining health information seeking on the Internet in terms of 'interactive health communication' and focuses on the information seeking function. That terminology, and this review, suggest a conceptual framework for future research and practice: *we may improve our understanding, investigation, and ability to influence processes of health-information seeking on the Internet by framing them as communication processes rather than information dissemination or educational processes.* Much of the literature reviewed here focuses on the Internet as a high-tech conveyor in the rapid diffusion of information or health lessons. However, to do so is to ignore the very nature of the Internet. Compared to traditional planned information dissemination phenomena, the Internet reflects a paradigm shift by offering interactivity and reciprocal influence, pointing towards transactional rather than one-way processes, and blending inter-personal and mass communication processes. Framing Internet use as health communication invites social systems and social influence theoretical frameworks. These frameworks suggest additional avenues for research.

The present review clarifies the inter-dependence of the Internet with other components of health communication systems, including health care, health promotion, risk-inducing communication, and the roles of everyday inter-personal communication and mass media in health. Understanding the opportunities and influences posed by the Internet as *one component of the larger health communication system* offers directions for research as well as practice. For example, research needs to address (i) the impact of interactive health communication on the physician–patient relationship, as well as how healthcare providers might influence consumers' use of the Internet; (ii) the implications of the Internet for the larger health care system, including medical outcomes and health-care costs; and (iii) how the Internet influences and is influenced by a managed care environment.

To view Internet use as a communication process activating social influence suggests the shifting of focus from information to messages and meanings. Although the issue of quality of health information is significant, understanding the Internet's impact (both positively and negatively) defies simply considering information and its accuracy. How and why Internet use validates and promotes functional as well as dysfunctional outcomes (e.g. desire to be an amputee) may be understood in terms of types of messages shared and meanings invoked by those messages for participants. Inter-personal communication concepts, such as empathy, confirmation, validation, self-disclosure and immediacy, shift attention from the content of messages (information) to their meta-communicative functions (Wilmot, 1980), including sustaining identities and relationships (i.e. matters of social influence). (For further discussion, see Lewis, 1994; Cline, 2002). Concepts traditionally employed for understanding planned change messages and campaigns may also illuminate the dynamics and effects of interactive health communication (e.g. audience analysis and segmentation, credibility, homophily message design, language personalness and intensity, affect, metaphor. one-sided versus two-sided messages, central versus peripheral message cues and processing, message sequencing, evidence, exposure, tailoring, and an array of persuasion strategies) (see, e.g., Maibach and Parrott, 1995; Rice and Atkin, 2001).

The challenge to public health practice is to facilitate health-promoting use of the web among consumers in conjunction with their health care providers. Meeting that challenge requires developing discerning and critical usership among consumers, persuading health care professionals of the importance of collaborating in that facilitation and use, and providing both parties with the strategies, skills, programs, and systems to do so. Meeting that public health challenge requires an evidence base that matches the nature of the phenomenon. Thus, we join Deering in calling for research on the 'optimum' use of the web for communicating about health and medicine, particularly research with an emphasis on communication (Deering, 1998, p. 136).

References

Adelhard, K. and Obst, O. (1999). Evaluation of medical Internet sites, *Methods of Information in Medicine*, 39, 75–9.

Alao, A. O., Yolles, J. C. and Airmenta. W. (1999). Cybersuicide: the Internet and suicide. *American Journal of Psychiatry*, 156, 1836–7.

Ambre, J., Guard, R., Perveila, F. M., Renner, J. and Rippen, H. (1997). White Paper: Criteria for assessing the quality of health information on the internet (working draft). Available at http://www.niitretek.org/hiti/showcase/documents/criteria.html. Accessed: 24 July 2000.

American Medical Association, Ad Hoc Committee on Health Literacy for the Council on Scientific Affairs (1999). Health literacy: report of the Council on Scientific Affairs, *Journal of the American Medical Association*, 281, 552–7.

Anonymous (1997). Coalition expands to help consumers: HealthPartners' Internet data provide hospital comparisons, *Profiles in Healthcare Marketing*, 13(6), 2.

Anonymous (1998). Thirty million to go online for health information. In Susman, E. S. (ed.), *Telemedicine and Virtual Reality*, 3(12), 134.

Anonymous (2000). E-health spending fails to spur physician use, *Advance for Speech-Language-Pathologists and Audiologists*, 24 July, 18.

Appleby, C. (1999). Net gain or net loss? Health care consumers become Internet savvy, *Trustee*, 52(2), 20–3.

Aschenbrener, C. A. (1996). News from the future: health care summit caps decade of transformation, 1996–2005, *Academic Medicine*, 71. 323–7.

Associated Press, The (1999). Elderly caught up in net, *The Gainesville Sun*, 22 November, 2A.

Associated Press, The (2000a). Post office heads off erosion from e-mail, *The Gainesville Sun*, 2 August, 3A.

Associated Press, The (2000b). Study: Internet value appreciated by blacks, *The Gainesville Sun*, 13 October, 3A.

AWHONN (1997). Nurses speak out: are you using the Internet for nursing?, *Association of Women's Health, Obstetric, and Neonatal Services*, 1(4), 17.

Ayonrinde. O. (1998). Patients in cyberspace: information or confusion?, *Postgraduate Medical Journal*, 74, 449–50.

Bader, S. S. and Braude, R. M. (1998). 'Patient informatics': creating new partnerships in medical decision making, *Academic Medicine*, 73, 408–11.

Barrett, S. (2001). Quackwatch: your guide to health fraud. quackery and intelligent decisions. Available at http://www.quackwatch.com. Accessed: 21 January 1001.

Baur, C. (2000). Limiting factors on the transformative powers of e-mail in patient–physician relationships: a critical analysis, *Health Communication*, 12, 239–59.

Bazzoli, F (1998). Inside health care's innovative websites, *Health Data Management*, 7(7), 40–2, 44, 46–9

Bell, C. S. (1999). The best web sites for doctors, *Medical Economics*, 76(9). 81–2, 87–8, 93.

Berland, G. K., Elliott, M. N., Morales, L. S., Alizazy. J. I., Kravitz, R. L., Broder, M. S., Kanouse, D. E., Munoz, J. A., Puyol, J.-A., Lara, M., Watkins, K. E., Yang, H. and McGlynn, E. A. (2001). Health information on the Internet: accessibility, quality and readability in English and Spanish, *Journal of the American Medical Association*, 285. 2612–37.

Biermann, J., Golladay, G., Greenfield, M. and Baker, L. (1999). Evaluation of cancer information on the Internet, *Cancer*, 86, 381-390.

Boyer, C., Selby, M. and Appel, R. D. (1998). The Health on the Net Code of Conduct for medical and health web sites, *Medinfo*, 9 (part 2), 1163–6.

Buhle, E. L., Jr (1996). Medicine and the Internet: what can I learn from the Internet?, *Journal of the Florida Medical Association*, 83, 624–7.

Chapman, G. (1999). The cutting edge; digital nation; inequality runs deeper than skills gap, *Los Angeles Times*, 19 July, C1.

Chi-Lum, B. (1999). Friend or foe: consumers using the Internet for medical information, *Journal of Medical Practice Management*, 14, 196–8.

Cline, R. J. W. (1999). Communication in social support groups. In Frey, L., Gouran, D. and Poole, S. (eds), *Handbook of Small Group Communication*. Thousand Oaks, Calif.: Sage, 516–38.

Cline, R. J. W. (2002). Everyday interpersonal communication and health. In Thompson, T., Dorsey, A., Miller. K, and Parrott, R. L. (eds), *Handbook of Health Communication*, Mahwah, NJ: Lawrence Erlbaum.

Cline, R. J. W. and McKenzie. N. J. (1996). Women and AIDS: the lost population. In Parrott, R. L. and Condit. C. M. (eds), *Evaluating Women's Health Messages: A Resource Book*. Thousand Oaks, Calif.: Sage, 382–401.

Coiera, E. (1996). The Internet's challenge to health care provision, *British Medical Journal*, 312. 3–4.

Coiera. E. (1998) Information epidemics, economics, and immunity on the Internet: we still know so little about the effects of information on public health, *British Medical Journal*, 317, 1469–70.

Coile. R. C., Jr and Howe, R. C. (1999). The Internet: changing the way consumers receive health care. *Russ Cloies Health Trends*, 11(9), 9–12.

Cox, C. G. (1998). Highway to health: online health education. *Journal of School Nursing*, 14(5), 48–51.

Cronin, C. (1998). Using the Internet to educate consumers about health care choices, *Mana ged Care Quarterly*, 6. 29–33.

Culver, J. D., Gerr, F. and Frumkin, H. (1997). Medical information on the Internet: a study of an electronic bulletin board, *Journal of General Internal Medicine*, 12. 466–70.

Cyber Dialogue (1998). Online health reaches critical mass; Nua Internet Surveys. Available at http://www.nua.net.surveys/?f=VS&art_id=905354453&rel=true. Accessed: 10 October 2001.

Cyber Dialogue (2000a). Doctors keep work offline; Nua Internet Surveys. Available at http://wwwnua.net/surveys. Accessed: 15 January 2001.

Cyber Dialogue (2000b). The future's bright for online health industry. Nua Internet Surveys. Available at http://www.nua.net/surveys. Accessed: 15 January 2001.

Deering, M. J. (1998). Health communication and health policy. In Jackson. L. D. and Duffy, B. K. (eds), *Health Communication Research*. Westport, Conn.: Greenwood Press, 125–37.

DeGeorges, K. M. (1998). Taming the World Wide Web: if everything is on the Web. why can't I find anything?, *AWHONN Lifelines*, 2(4), 50–2.

Dow, M. G., Kearns, W. and Thornton, D. H. (1996). The Internet II: future effects on cognitive behavioral practice, *Cognitive and Behavioral Practice*, 3, 137–57.

Doyle, D. J., Ruskin, K. J. and Engel, T P. (1996). The Internet and medicine: past. present, and future, *Yale Journal of Biology and Medicine*, 69, 429–37.

Elliott, C. (2000). A new way to be mad, *The Atlantic Monthly*, 286 (December), 72–84.

Eng, T R. and Gustafson, D. H. (eds) (1999). *Wired for Health and Well-Being: The Emergence of Interactive Health Communication*. Washington, DC: Science Panel on Interactive Communication and Health, US Department of Health and Human Services. Office of Disease Prevention and Health Promotion.

Essex, D. (1999). Life line: consumer informatics has gone beyond patient education on the Web. *Healthcare Informatics*, 16(2), 119–120, 124, 128–9.

Farrell, T. (2001). Some tips on navigation. Frontend Usability InfoCentre. Available at http://infocentre.frontend.com. Accessed 10 July 200 1.

Federal Trade Commission (1997). North American Health claim Surf Day targets Internet ads. hundreds of e-mafls messages sent (Press release). Available at http://www.ftc.gov/opa/1997/9711/hlthsurf.htm. Accessed: 1 September 2000.

Find/SVP (1998). *Profiles of Consumers Using Online Health and Medical Information*. New York: The HealthMed Retrievers.

Flory, J. (1998). Patient and physician satisfaction is aim of new program, *The Healthcare Strategist*, 29(12), 9.

Frisse, M. E., Kelly, E. A. and Metcalfe, E. S. (1994). An Internet primer: resources and responsibilities, *Academic Medicine*, 69, 20–4.

Gagel, M. P. (1998). The Internet – a new information medium for nurses – part 1, *Canadian Oncology Nursing Journal*, 8. 216–221.

Gallagher. S. M. (1999). Rethinking access in an information age, *Ostomy Wound Management*, 45(9), 12–14, 16.

Garrison, S. (1998). Evaluating health Internet sites: a White Paper's criteria, *Medical Reference Services Quarterly*, 17(13), 41–7.

Grandinetti, D. A. (2000). Doctors and the Web: help your patients surf the Net safely.Medical Economics, April, 28–34.

Green, C. W. (1999). HIV/AIDS information overload, *Lancet*, 352, 412.

Green, J. (1996). Joint Commission to post quality reports on the Internet, *Materials Management in Health Care*, 5(11), 16.

Gregory-Head. B. (1999). Patients and the Internet: guidance for evidence-based choices. *Journal of the American College of Dentists*, 66(2), 46–50.

Griffiths, M. (1998). Internet addiction: does it really exist' In Gackenbach, J. (ed.), *Psychology and the Internet: Intrapersonal. interpersonal. and transpersonal implications*, San Diego, Calif.: Academic Press, 61–75.

Grohol, J. M. (1998). Future clinical directions: professional development. pathology, and psychotherapy online. In Gackenbach, J. (ed.), *Psychology and the Internet: Intrapersonal. interpersonal, and transpersonal implications*. San Diego, Calif.: Academic Press, 111–40.

Guard, R., Haag, D., Marine, S., Morris, T. and Sckick, L. (1996). An electronic consumer health library: NetWellness, *Bulletin of the Medical Library Association*, 84, 468–77.

Guay, T. (1994). An introduction to INTERNET for medical professionals, *Physician Assistant*, 18(6), 69–74.

Harris Interactive (2001). 100 million US Net users are 'cyberchondriacs'. Nua Internet Surveys. Available at http://www.nua.net.surveys/?f=VS&art_id=905356697&rel=true. Accessed: 10 October 2001.

Hatfield, C. L., May, S. K. and Markoff, J. S. (1999). Quality of consumer drug information provided by four Web sites. *American Journal of Health-Systems Pharmacists*. 56, 2308–11.

Hawkins, R., Gustafson, D. H., Chewning, B., Bosworth. K. and Day, P. (1987). Interactive computer programs as public information campaigns for hard-to-reach populations: the BARN Project example, *Journal of Communication*, 37, 8–28.

Haythomwaite, C., Wellman, B. and Garton, L. (1998). Work and community via computer-mediated communication. In Gackenbach, J. (ed.), *Psychology and the Internet: Intrapersonal. interpersonal, and transpersonal implications*. San Diego, Calif.: Academic Press, 199–226.

Health on the Net Foundation (1997). HON Code of Conduct (HONcode) for medical and health web sites. Available at http://www.hon.ch/HONcode/Conduct.html. Accessed: 19 January 2001.

Health on the Net Foundation (1999a). HON's fourth survey on the use of the Internet for medical and health purposes. Available at http://www.hon.ch/Survey/ResumeApr99.html. Accessed: 10 October 2001.

Health on the Net Foundation (1999b), Report Ids trends in online health sector. Nua Internet Surveys. Available at http://www.nua.net.surveys/?f=VS&art_id=905354985&rel=true. Accessed: 10 October 2001.

Health on the Net Foundation (2000) Our users. Available at http://www.hon.ch/HONcode/audience.html. Accessed: 19 January 2001.

Huang, M. P. and Alessi, N. E. (1996). The Internet and the future of psychiatry, *American Journal of Psychiatry*, 153. 861–9.

Impicciatore, P., Pandolfini, C., Casella, N. and Bonati, M. (1997). Reliability of health information for the public on the World Wide Web: systematic survey of advice on managing fever in children at home, *British Medical Journal*, 314, 1875–9.

Izenberg, N. and Lieberman. D. A. (1998). The Web. communication trends, and children's health: part 4: how children use the Web, *Clinical Pediatrics*, 37, 335–40.

Jacobson, R. L. (1995). Tarning the Internet, *The Chronicle of Higher Education*, 41(32). A29–30.

Jadad, A. R. and Gagliari, A. (1998). Rating health information on the Internet: navigating to knowledge or to Babel? *Journal of the American Medical Association*, 279, 611–14.

Joinson, A. (1998). Causes and implications of disinhibited behavior on the Internet. In Gackenbach, J. (ed.), *Psychology and the Internet: Intrapersonal. interpersonal, and transpersonal implications*. San Diego, Calif.: Academic Press, 43–60.

Judkins, D. Z. (1996). Health resources on the Internet: a basic list, *Medical Reference Services Quarterly*, 15(4), 13–20.

Kaufman, D. M., Eng, M. and Jennett, P. A. (1997). Preparing our future physicians: integrating medical informatics into the undergraduate medical education curriculum. In Morgan, K. S., Hoffman, H. M., Stredney, D. and Sweghorst, S. J. (eds), *Medicine Meets Virtual Reality*. Amsterdam: IOS Press, 52–5.

Keen, C. (1997). Doctors soon may make Internet calls, *The Gainesville Sun*, 2 1 January, B1, B2.

Khonsari, L. S. and Fabri. P. J. (1997). Integrating medical informatics into the medical undergraduate curriculum. In Morgan, K. S., Hoffman, H. M., Stredney, D. and Sweghorst, S, J. (eds), *Medicine Meets Virtual Reality*, Amsterdam: IOS Press, 547–51.

Kibbe, D. C., Smith, P. P., LaVallee, R., Bailey, D. and Bard, .M. (1997). A guide to finding and evaluating best practices health care information on the Internet: the truth is out there? *Joint Commission Journal on Quality Improvement*, 23, 678–89.

King, S. A. and Moreggi, D. (1998). Internet therapy and self-help groups – the pros and the cons. In Gackenbach, J. (ed.), *Psychology and the Internet: Intrapersonal. interpersonal, and transpersonal implications*. San Diego, Calif.: Academic Press, 77–109.

Korn, K. (1998). Mental health information on the Internet, *Journal of American Academy of Nurse Practitioners*, 10, 267–8.

Lacroix, E. M., Backus, J. E. and Lyon, B. J. (1994). Service providers and users discover the Internet, *Bulletin of the Medical Library Association*, 82, 412–18.

Lamp, J. M. and Howard, P. A. (1999). Guiding parents' use of the Internet for newborn education, *MCN, American Journal of Maternal Child Nursing*, 24(l), 33–6.

LaPerriére. B., Edwards, P. Romeder, J. M. and Maxwell-Young, L. (1998). Using the Internet to support self-care, *Canadian Nurse*, 94(5), 47–8.

Lewis, L. K. (1994). A challenge for health education: the enactment problem and a communication-related solution, *Health Communication*, 6, 205–24.

Lincoln, T. L. and Builder, C. (1999). Global healthcare and the flux of technology, *International Journal of Medical Informatics*, 53, 213–24.

Lindberg, D. A. and Humphreys, B. L. (1995). The High Performance Computing and Communications program, the national information infrastructure and health care, *Journal of the American Medical Informatics Association*, 2, 156–59.

Littleton, D. (1998). A review of strategies for finding health information the World-Wide Web. *Medical Reference Services Quarterly*, 17(2), 51–5.

Louis Harris and Associates (1999). Sixty million seek health information online in the US. Nua Internet Surveys. Available at http://www.nua.nei.surveys/?f=VS&art_id=905354697&rel=true. Accessed: 10 October 2001.

Lown, B., Bukachi, F. and Xavier, R. (1998). Health information in the developing world, *Lancet*, 352, SII34–8.

Lunik, M. C. (1998). What's there for me? The Internet for pharmacists. *Pharmacy Practice Management Quarrerly*, 17(4), 37–47.

Machles, D. (1998a). Finding information on the Internet, *AAOHN Journal*, 46. 410–11.

Machles, D. (1998b). Using basic search tools on the Internet, *AAOHN Journal*, 46, 557–8.

Maibach, E. and Parrott, R. L. (1995). *Designing Health Messages: Approaches from Communication Theory and Public Health Practice*, Thousand Oaks, Calif.: Sage.

Mallory C. (1997). What's on the Internet? Services for women affected by HIV and AIDS, *Health Care for Women International*, 18, 315–22.

Mann, C. E. (1999). Searching for HIV/AIDS information on the World Wide Web. *Journal of the Association of Nurses in AIDS Care*, 10, 79–81.

Marra, C. A., Carleton, B. C., Lynd, L. D., Marra, F., McDougal, A. R., Chow, D. and McKerrow, R. (1996). Drug and poison information on the Internet, part 2: identification and evaluation, *Pharmacotherapy*, 16, 806–18.

Martin, E. R., McDamiels, C., Crespo, J. and Lanier, D. (1997). Delivering health information services and technologies to urban community health centers: the Chicago AIDS Outreach Project, *Bulletin of the American Medical Library Association*. 85. 356–61.

Maugans, T. A., McComb, J. G. and Levy, M. L. (1998). The internet as a pediatric neurosurgery information resource, *Pediatric Neurosurgery*, 28, 186–90.

Mayer, M. and Till, J. E. (1996). The Internet: a modem Pandora's Box?, *Quality of Life Research*, 5, 568–71.

McClung, H. J., Murray, R. D. and Heitlinger, L. A. (1998). The Internet as a source of current patient information, *Pediatrics*, 101, E2.

McFarlane, M., Bull, A. A. and Rietmeiier, C. A. (2000). The Internet as a newly emerging risk environment for sexually transmitted disease. *Journal of the American Medical Association*, 284. 443–6.

McGrath, I. (1997). Information superhighway or information traffic jam for health-care consumers? *Clinical Performance and Quality Health Care*, 5(2), 90–3.

McKinley, J., Cattermole, H. and Oliver, C. W. (1999). The quality of surgical information on the Internet. *Journal of the Royal College of Surgeons of Edinburgh*, 44. 265–8.

McKinney, W. P. and Bunton. G. (1993). Exploring the medical applications of the Internet: A guide for beginning users, *American Journal of the Medical Sciences*, 306, 141–4.

McLellan, F. (1998). 'Like hunger, like thirst': patients, journals, and the Internet, *Lancet*, 352, SII39–43.

McLeod, S. D. (1998). The quality of medical information on the Internet: a new public health concern, *Archives of Ophthamology*, 116. 1663–5.

McMillan, S. J. (1999). Health communication and the Internet: relations between interactive characteristics of the medium and site creators, content, and purpose, *Health Communication*, 11, 375–90.

Mitchell, J. J., Finkhelhor, D. and Wolak, J. (2001). Risk factors for and impact of online sexual solicitation of youth, *Journal of the American Medical Association*, 285, 3011–14.

Morris, K. (1998). Treating HIV/AIDS information overload, *Lancet*, 352, 1866.

Morris, T. A., Guard. J. R., Marine, S. A., Schick, L., Haag, D., Tsipis, G., Kaya. B. and Shoemaker. S. (1997). Approaching equity in consumer health information delivery: NetWellness, *Journal of the American Medical Informatics Association*, 4(l), 6–13.

Neff, J. (1999). Internet could see more web site sponsorships, *Advertising Age*, 70(11), s6–7.

Nielsen, J. and Norman, D. A. (2000). Web-site usability: usability on the web isn't a luxury. Available at http://www.informationweek.com. Accessed: 10 July 2001.

Nochi, M. (1998). Struggling with the labeled self: people with traumatic brain injuries in social settings, *Qualitative Health Research*, 8, 665–81.

O'Keefe, D. J. (1990). *Persuasion: Theory and Research*. Newbury Park, Calif.: Sage.

O'Mahoney, B. (1999). Irish health web sites: a review, *Irish Medical Journal*, 92, 334–7.

Oravec, J. A. (2000). On-line medical information and service delivery: implications for health education, *Journal of Health Education*, 31, 105–10.

Pandolfini, C., Impicciatore, P. and Bonati, M. (2000). Parents on the web: risks for quality management of cough in children, *Pediatrics*, 105. e1.

Pathfinder (1998). DIY diagnosis on the web. Nua Internet surveys. Available at http://www.nua.net.surveys. Accessed: 2 February 2000.

Pennbridge, J., Moya, R. and Rodrigues, L. (1999). Questionnaire survey of Califomia consumers' use and rating of sources of health care information including the Internet. *Western Journal of Medicine*, 171, 302–5.

Pereira, J. and Bruera, E. (1998). The Internet as a resource for palliative care and hospice: a review and proposals. *Journal of Pain and Symptom Management*, 16(l.), 59–68.

Petersen, C. (2000). Seven steps to easier web navigation. Enterprise Development. Available at http://www.enterprisedev.com. Accessed: 10 July 2001.

Pew Internet and American Life Project (2000a). Who's not online: 57% of those without Internet access say they do not plan to log on. Available at http://www.pewinternet,org. Accessed: 10 July 2001.

Pew Internet and American Life Project (2000b). African-Americans and the Internet. Available at hitp://www.pewintemet.org. Accessed: 10 July 2001.

Pew Internet and American Life Project (2000c). The online health care revolution:

how the Web helps Americans take better care of themselves. Available at http://www.pewinternet.org. Accessed: 10 July 2001.

Pew Internet and American Life Project and American Life Project (2001). More online, doing more: 16 million newcomers gain Internet access in the last half of 2000 as women, minorities, and families with modest incomes continue to surge online. Available at http://www.pewinternet.org. Accessed: 10 July 2001.

Piotrow, P. T., Kincaid, D. L., Rimon, J. G., II and Rinehart, W. (1997). *Health Communication: Lessons from Family Planning and Reproductive Health*, Westport. Conn.: Praeger.

Post, J. A. (1996). Internet resources on aging: ten top web sites, *The Gerontologist*, 36. 728–33.

PricewaterhouseCoopers (1999). Net to radically change health care industry. Available at http://www.nua.net.surveys/?f=VS&art_id=905355379&rel=true. Accessed: 10 October 2001.

Reuters (2000). Gender gap has almost disappeared in US. Nua Internet Surveys. Available at http://www.nua.net.surveys/?f=VS&art_id=905355546&rel=true. Accessed: 10 October 2001.

Rice, R. E. and Atkin, C. K. (eds) (2001). *Public Communication Campaigns*, 3rd edn. Thousand Oaks, Calif.: Sage.

Richards, B., Colman, A. and Hollingsworth, R. (1998). The current and future role of the Internet in patient education, *International Journal of Medical Informatics*, 50, 279–85.

Rippen, H. L. (1999). Criteria for assessing the quality of health information on the Internet (Policy paper), Health Summit Working Group, Mitretek. Available at http://hitiweb.mitretek.org/docs/policy.html. Accessed: 24 July 2000.

Robinson, T. N., Patrick, K., Eng, T. R. and Gustafson, D. (1998). An evidence-based approach to interactive health communication: a challenge to medicine in the information age, *Journal of the American Medical Association*, 280, 1264–9.

Roffman, D. M., Shannon, D. and Dwyer, C. (1997). Adolescents, sexual health, and the Internet: possibilities, prospects. and challenges for educators. *Journal of Sex Education and Therapy*, 22(l), 49–55.

Rudin, J. L. and Littleton, D. (1997). Searching for information on the World Wide Web – a guide for dental health professionals: part 1, *Compendium of Continuing Education in Dentistry*, 18, 930–2, 934, 936.

Sacchetti, R., Zvara, P. and Plante, M. K. (1999). The Internet and patient education-resources and reliability: focus on a selected urologic topic, *Urology*, 53, 1117–20.

Schnarch, D. (1997). Sex, intimacy. and the Internet, *Journal of Sex Education and Therapy*, 22, 15–20.

Shapiro, D. E. and Schulman, C. E. (1999). Ethical and legal issues in e-mail therapy, *Ethics and Behaviour*, 6, 107–24.

Sharf, B. F. (1997). Communicating breast cancer on-line: support and empowerment on the Internet, *Woman and Health*, 26(l), 65–84.

Silberg, W. M., Lundberg, G. D. and Musaccio, R. A. (1997). Assessing, controlling, and assuring the quality of medical informauon on the Internet: *caveat lector et vieivor* – let the reader and viewer beware, *Journal of the American Medical Association*, 277, 1244–5.

Simpson, R. L. (1996). Will the Internet supplant community health networks?, *Nursing Management*, 27(2), 20, 23.

Sonnenberg, F A. (1997). Health information on the Internet: opportunities and pitfalls, *Archives of Internal Medicine*, 157, 151–2.

Steiner, B. D., Reid, A. and Smucker, D. R. (1996). Developments on the Internet: a practical guide for primary care physicians, *Family Medicine*, 28. 128–33.

Stemmer-Frumento, K. (1998). InfoBeat ... consumer health information, *National Network*, 23(2), 14, 18.

Stevens, L. (1998). A primer on Internet-based patient education. *Medical Management News*, 6(7), 6–9.

Thomas, L. (1998). The arrival of the Internet, *Nursing Standard*, 12(21), 1.

Tomaiuolo, N. G. (1995). Accessing nursing resources on the Internet, *Computers in Nursing*, 13, 159–64.

Tomlin, A. C. (1998). Cheaper by the dozen: low cost consumer health resources, *National Network*, 23, 9–10.

Toomey, K. E. and Rothenberg, R. B. (2000). Sex and cyberspace – virtual networks leading to high-risk sex (Editorial), *Journal of the American Medical Association*, 284, 485–7.

Voge, S. (1998). NOAH–New York Online Access to Health: library collaboration for bilingual consumer health information on the Internet, *Bulletin of the Medical Library Association*, 86. 326–34.

W3C (1999). Web content accessibility guidelines 1.0. Available at http://www/w3/org/TR/1999/WAI-WEBCONTENT-19990505. Accessed: 10 July 2001.

Weiler, R. M. (1996). Creating a virtual materials and resources index for health education using the World Wide Web, *Journal of School Health*, 66, 205–9.

Weisbord, S. D., Soule, J. B. and Kimmel, P. L. (1997). Poison on line – acute renal failure caused by wormwood purchased through the Internet, *New England Journal of Medicine*, 337, 1483.

Wilkins, A. S. (1999). Expanding Internet access for health care consumers, *Health Care Management Review*, 24, 30–41.

Williams, B. (1999). Provider profiles on-line – making health care choices easier for consumers, *Tennessee Medicine*, 92. 253–4.

Wilmot, W. W. (1980). Metacommunication: a re-examination and extension. In Nimmo, D. (ed.), *Communication Yearbook 4*. New Brunswick, NJ: Transaction Books, 61–9.

Wootton, J. C. (1997). The quality of information on women's health on the Internet. *Journal of Women's Health*, 6, 575–81.

World Health Organization (1995). *Ad Hoc Committee on Health Research Relating to Future Intervention Options. Investing in Health Research and Development*, Geneva: WHO.

Wyatt, J. C. (1997). Commentary: measuring quality and impact of the World Wide Web, *British Journal of Medicine*, 314, 1879–81.

Young, K. S. (1999). Evaluation and treatment of Internet addiction. In Vandecreek, L. and Jackson, T. L. (eds), *Innovations in Clinical Practice: A Source Book*. Sarasota, Fla.: Professional Resource Press, 19–31.

34 Gendering health: men, women and wellbeing*

Lesley Doyal

Introduction

Differences between men and women are now beginning to receive greater recognition in the planning of health services. The appearance of these issues on the healthcare agenda owes a great deal to the tenacity of those women who have drawn attention both to the specificity of their reproductive health needs and to the discrimination they still experience in many of their medical encounters (Fee and Krieger, 1994; Kitts and Roberts, 1996; Stein, 1997; Doyal, 1998). More recently, some men have begun to express similar concerns, highlighting their difficulties in receiving effective and appropriate care (Caroll, 1994; Sabo and Gordon, 1995; Schofield *et al.*, 2000). Both women and (latterly) men have also highlighted the ways in which gendered social relations constrain their lives in unhealthy ways (Harrison *et al.*, 1992; Doyal, 1995; 2001; Sabo and Gordon, 1995; Huggins and Lamb, 1998; Working with Men, 2001).

However, there are still significant conceptual confusions about the meaning of the terms 'sex' and 'gender', and about the impact of maleness and femaleness on health and health care. The term 'gender' is increasingly used in National Health Service (NHS) planning, in the mistaken belief that it is simply a more modern or politically correct term for sex. In fact the term 'sex' refers to the biological differences between women and men, while 'gender' refers to the social differences (Oakley, 1972; Birke, 1986). Though they are sometimes difficult to separate in practice, the conceptual distinction between the two is important in debates about the development of more equitable policies.

Understanding sex differences in health and illness

Differences in their sexual and reproductive organs have dominated both common sense and biomedical thinking on men, women and health. These differences clearly generate particular health promotion needs for both sexes, though they are more important for women than for men. Unless they are able to control their fertility and give birth

---

* Commissioned for this volume. This chapter draws on material published by the author elsewhere (see Doyal, 2001).

safely, women can determine little else about their lives, and this is reflected in their greater use of related health services.

However, these obvious differences in reproductive physiology are not the only ones that are important in understanding male and female health needs. There is now growing evidence of the impact of a much broader range of biological variations on differences in patterns of health and illness between women and men (Wizemann and Pardue, 2001). It is clear, for example, that men are more susceptible to early heart disease than men while women are more susceptible to a range of auto-immune diseases including arthritis (Wizemann and Pardue, 2001). Thus the confinement of 'female problems' to the reproductive speciality of obstetrics and gynaecology leaves many important sex differences in biological functioning unacknowledged and unexplored. Many of these will be relevant to health promotion activities, and our understanding of them will need to be extended if services are to both sex- and gender-sensitive.

Social construction of gender differences in well-being: the case of women

But even if we learn more about these biological variations, this will give us only a partial picture of the impact of maleness and femaleness on human health and illness. Gender or social differences are also important. The daily lives of men and women often vary dramatically, and this can affect their health in fundamental ways. Yet these socially constructed variations often receive little attention from those trained within the bio-medical tradition. This in turn can lead to significant limitations on the appropriateness and effectiveness of the services they can offer.

To put things simply, all societies are divided along the 'fault line' of gender (Papanek, 1990). This means that men and women are characterized as different types of beings with different responsibilities and different entitlements. The most obvious example of this is the split between the public and the private – the symbolic relationship between women and domesticity that allocates to those who are female the major responsibility for domestic labour (Charles, 1993). It is also significant that in most societies these gender differences are reflected in inequalities between women and men in access to a wide variety of social resources (UNDP, 1995). Not surprisingly, these inequalities have a major impact on the health of both men and women, but so far it is only their impact on women that has been investigated in detail.

Economic inequalities mean that many women will have difficulty in acquiring the basic necessities for a healthy life. The degree of deprivation they experience will vary depending on a variety of factors including their race, class, and geo-political status – whether they live in a rich country or a poor country. But underlying these differences, the common thread of gender inequalities in income and wealth can have a significant impact on health (Doyal, 1995).

Cultural devaluation is also important, though more difficult to map. Because they belong to a group that is seen as being less valuable, women in many societies may find it difficult to develop the sense of their own self-worth that is essential for positive mental health (Busfield, 1996; Kandiyoti, 1998). This process of devaluation often begins in girlhood and continues in later life when activities such as caring are unpaid and lack status, while women in the workforce are paid lower wages and shown less respect than men (UNDP, 1995)

Can gender divisions pose a threat to men's health?

We have seen that gender divisions constitute a significant constraint on the capacity of many women to optimize their well-being. Can we say the same about men? Do gender divisions enhance or inhibit men's ability to realise their potential for health? Because it is women and their advocates who have led the debate on gender and well-being, the main focus has been on the ways in which the social structuring of patriarchy leads so many men to behave in ways that damage women's health (Doyal, 1995). However, new questions are now being raised about the possible health hazards of being a man.

Some of these questions arise from a (more or less) radical critique of contemporary constructions of masculinity which are assumed to be potentially damaging to the health of women as well as men (Harrison *et al.*, 1992; Sabo and Gordon, 1995; Cameron and Bernardes, 1998; Lloyd, 1998; Kraemer, 2000). Others take a very different approach, focusing on what they see as destructive and unwarranted attacks on men and their lifestyles (Lyndon, 1992). These arguments may sometimes appear to overlap, but they are, in reality, separate strands running through contemporary debates on masculinity in general, and men's health in particular (Hearn, 1993).

One of the most obvious links between gender divisions and men's health is to be found in the area of waged work (Waldron, 1995). The emergence of nuclear families and the 'male breadwinner' during the Industrial Revolution gave many men little option but to continue working in what were often extremely dangerous conditions (Hart, 1988). As a result, male rates of industrial accidents and diseases have historically been higher than female rates, with deaths from occupational causes more common among men than among women. As women enter new areas of work, many are beginning to encounter these traditionally male hazards (Messing, 1998). However, waged work continues to pose significantly greater health risks for men than for women (Waldron, 1995).

With urbanization and industrialization, men have been more likely than women to adopt unhealthy lifestyles – smoking and drinking in particular, as well as dangerous driving and risky sports. These have contributed to their higher rates of premature mortality, keeping their life expectancy below that of women in the same social group (Hart, 1988; Waldron, 1995). A new literature is now emerging which links these activities with the ideologies and practices constituting contemporary masculinity (Moynihan, 1998; Schofield *et al.*, 2000). Researchers have looked at young men in particular and the pressures many feel to conform to certain models of maleness (Canaan, 1996; Pleck and Sonenstein, 1991).

Similar arguments have been used about the high rates of male-to-male violence, especially in those parts of the world where it is at its most severe. In the inner cities of the United States, for example, young black men have been referred to as an endangered species because their life expectancy is declining (Gibbs, 1988). The interaction of contemporary masculinity with aspects of poverty, class and race is frequently deployed as the basis for explaining this disturbing phenomenon (Staples, 1995).

In the area of mental health, too some men are now beginning to make a link between their individual problems and wider gender divisions in society. Women have long complained about what they see as the incapacity of many men to participate fully in intimate and mutually supportive relationships. Some men are now beginning to acknowledge this problem and to blame it on the gender stereotyping that narrows the acceptable range of emotional expressivity among those claiming male identity.

The underlying presumption behind many of these arguments is that unreconstructed masculinity can be dangerous to the health of both women and men. This analysis is based in part on ideas from the new field of 'men's studies', which shares much of its theoretical framework with critical feminism (Kimmel and Messner, 1993; Sabo and Gordon, 1995; Hearn, 1998). It needs to be distinguished from the very different argument that men's problems derive not from traditional ideas about masculinity but rather from the disintegration of these.

One version of this argument stresses the secular changes in society – the rise of male unemployment combined with the entry of more women into the labour market and the increase in single-parent families (Sianne and Wilkinson, 1995; Willott and Griffin, 1996). These are said to have challenged men's sense of identity, causing significant mental health problems. The rapid rise in the number of suicides in young males, for example, has been linked to these trends (Charlton *et al.*, 1993; Aggleton, 1995).

However, more confrontational critics have placed the major stress not on broader social and economic change but on feminism itself – on women's demands for more resources, which are seen to lead to the neglect of men. The perceived failure to deal effectively with prostate cancer, for example, has been blamed on women's demands for higher levels of expenditure on breast cancer research (Kadar, 1994). More generally, men are said to have been displaced in the family and at work by women's vociferous campaigns for advancement, leaving them vulnerable and damaged (Lyndon, 1992). The solution is seen to lie in a return to traditional values, which, it is claimed, potentially could benefit both sexes.

It is clear that these are important and highly charged issues which cannot be resolved through the health service alone. Broader social change will be required, and we return to explore the potential for this in the final section. However, more work will also be needed in the field of health services in general, and health promotion in particular, if policies are to be designed which take gender issues seriously.

Sex and gender bias in medical practice

We have seen that both social (or gender) and biological (or sex) differences may affect the health needs of women and men. It is also clear that gender insensitivity in the health services themselves may affect differentially the ability of men and women to satisfy these needs. We can explore the implications of this in more detail by looking first at the creation of medical knowledge – at some of the basic assumptions built into the research process – and then at related aspects of the organisation of health care.

Sex and gender bias in funding priorities and in the methods of medical research received a great deal of attention during the 1990s, especially in the United States (US National Institutes of Health, 1992). There have been high visibility campaigns for more money to be spent on topics of specific relevance to women, with breast cancer being a particular focus for concern (Batt, 1994). At the same time, women's health advocates have stressed the need for mainstream medical research to pay more attention to both sex and gender differences (Auerbach and Figert, 1995).

The basis for these campaigns has been the fact that epidemiological studies and clinical trials have too often been based on the unstated assumption that men and women are similar physiologically in all important respects apart from their reproductive systems (LaRosa and Pinn, 1993; Mastroianni et al., 1994). Men are treated as being the norm and women as the 'other', with the result that many major studies have been carried out on all-male samples. Even when women are included as subjects, the variables of sex and gender are often not treated seriously in the analysis.

This bias can limit the effectiveness both of treatment and of preventive services, as recent debates about coronary heart disease has shown. Many of the most important studies in both the United Kingdom and the United States were based on predominantly male samples, reflecting the perception of heart disease itself as a men's problem. As a result, we know very little about the sex or gender appropriateness of many of the most common diagnostic, treatment and prevention strategies in this field (Sharp, 1998). Similar concerns have been voiced in relation to the diagnosis and treatment of HIV/AIDS, where so much of the early research was (understandably) based on the experience of gay men (Bell, 1992; Kurth, 1993).

Issues of sex and gender insensitivity have also been raised in the context of medical treatment itself, and again much of this criticism has come from women. In many countries there are still major inequalities in access to services (Timyan et al., 1993; Doyal, 1995). In the UK, the existence of the NHS has largely removed these financial constraints on access. However responsibilities such as caring for others can still limit women's capacity to use services on their own behalf. There is also evidence that the quality of care women receive may be limited by gender bias, both in clinical treatment and in the more subjective aspects of the medical relationship itself.

Clinical bias has again been especially evident in the context of heart disease. Studies in the USA have shown that the diagnostic process itself is not as accurate in women as in men (Foster and Mallik, 1998; Redberg, 1998; Travin and Johnson, 1997). This, in turn, may contribute to the tendency among clinicians to order fewer invasive diagnostic tests such as angiography for their female patients (Foster and Mallik, 1998; Tobin et al., 1987). Similar problems have been identified in the UK, where men in one region were found to be 60 per cent more likely than women with the same condition to be given an angiogram (Petticrew et al., 1993). Once they receive a diagnosis, women may also receive less intensive treatment than men when they have symptoms of the same severity (Weintraub et al., 1996). They have a higher mortality rate than men from CABG and a number of other operative procedures (Redberg, 1998; Sharp, 1998).

Turning to the more experiential aspects of care, women have been documenting their concerns about sexism in medical encounters over a long period (O'Sullivan, 1987; White, 1990; Doyal, 1995; Fisher, 1996). Women in the UK have reported particular difficulties in getting enough information from doctors and being able to act on it. They appear to be seen as less knowledgeable than men, less competent and less capable of complex decision making (Graham and Oakley, 1981; Roberts, 1985). As a result, female patients risk becoming the passive victims of doctor's ministrations, and for some this will be a distressing and demeaning experience (O'Sullivan, 1987).

This should not, however, be taken to mean that men always have unproblematic encounters with their doctors. Working-class men and black men in particular may also have difficult experiences, as may those whose sexual identities do not conform with what has been called 'hegemonic masculinity' (Connell, 1987). An unwillingness to admit weakness may prevent many men from taking health promotion messages seriously and from consulting a doctor when problems arise. Indeed, illness itself may especially be feared because of its capacity to reduce men to what one recent study has called 'marginalised masculinity' (Cameron and Bernardes, 1998).

The way forward: health for all?

We have seen that both biological differences between the sexes and socially constructed gender differences should be of concern to health planners. Issues of gender sensitivity therefore need to be built into all services to make sure that they meet the needs of both women and men. This will mean paying careful attention both to the clinical aspects of services as well as to the quality of human relations that form a central element in the process of health care. Women and men do need to be treated differently – where it is appropriate – but any differential must always be justifiable with reference to its appropriateness in meeting human needs in a better way.

If the gender bias in medical research is to be eliminated, study designs will need to include sex and gender wherever appropriate, and results will need to be analysed and disseminated in ways that recognize differences in their implications for women and men. To improve access to services, women (and some men) may need to have better transport and appropriate arrangements for the care of dependents. For both men and women there may also be a need to provide more services in the workplace and the community. Across the range of health care settings it is essential that women should not be humiliated by sexist behaviour, while men should not be expected to live up to stereotypical conceptions of heterosexuality and masculinity.

Health promotion policies in particular need to be gender sensitive if their messages are to be heard. Too many campaigns are addressed towards women in their roles as carers of others while ignoring their own well-being. Men too often feel that health is women's business, and that health promotion messages are not addressed to them. HIV/AIDS campaigns have exhorted both women and men to 'use a condom' without recognizing the very real differences in power and status that structure most medical encounters and limit many women's freedom of choice. There is therefore considerable scope for making health promotion messages more gender sensitive. But this will go only part of the way.

Effective health promotion will only be possible if policies are designed to reshape some of the more fundamental aspects of social organization. It is evident that if women are to optimize their wellbeing, many men will have to change the ways in which they behave – sharing resources and labour more equally, taking greater responsibility for domestic labour and emotional support, and protecting women from the major health risk of physical and sexual abuse (Berer, 1996; Doyal, 2000).

The development of more effective equal pay and sex discrimination policies, for example, could clearly be of value in tackling the economic and social inequalities that continue to damage some women's health. And some of these policies could benefit men as well as women. The provision of paid paternity leave, for example, as well as more flexible working conditions, would make it easier for men to develop the 'female' side of themselves through bridging the gap between home and work.

These changes in public policy could play a part in promoting gender equity in health (Doyal, 2000). However, they would still leave some of the most fundamental problems untouched. So long as masculinity continues to be defined in ways that are hazardous to health, too many men will continue to experience preventable diseases and even death. At the same time, too many women will continue to be damaged by the actions of male partners who continue to follow the scripts of masculinity (Doyal, 2001). These narratives will be difficult to reshape, since many men (and some women) are likely to resist changes in the most intimate areas of their daily lives (Faludi, 1992). But unless this can be achieved, gender inequalities will continue to be one of the major factors limiting the capacity of both women and men to realize their potential for health.

References

Aggleton, P. (1995). *Young Men Speaking Out*. London: Health Education Authority.

Auerbach, J. and Figert, A. (1995). Women's health research: public policy and sociology, *Journal of Health and Social Behaviour* (extra issue), 115–31.

Batt, S. (1994). *Patient No More: The politics of breast cancer*. London: Scarlet Press.

Bell, N. (1992). 'Women and AIDS: too little too late? In Bequaert Holmes, H. and Purdy, L. (eds), *Feminist Perspectives in Medical Ethics*. Bloomington, Ind.: Indiana University Press.

Berer, M. (1996). 'Men, *Reproductive Health Matters*, 7, 7–11.

Bird, C. (1994). Women's representation as subjects in clinical studies: a pilot study of research published in Journal of the American Medical Association in 1992. In Mastroianni, A., Faden, R. and Federman, D., Women and Health Research: *Ethical and legal issues of including women in clinical studies*, 2. Washington, DC: National Academy Press.

Birke, L. (1986). *Feminism and Biology*. Brighton: Wheatsheaf.

Busfield, J. (1996). *Men, women and madness: Understanding gender and mental disorder*. London: Macmillan.

Cameron, C. and Bernardes, D. (1998). Gender and disadvantage in health: men's health for a change, *Sociology of Health and Illness*, 18(3), 673–93.

Canaan, J. (1996). 'One thing leads to another': drinking, fighting and working class masculinities. In Mac an Ghaill, M. (ed.), *Understanding Masculinities*. Buckingham: Open University Press.

Carroll, S. (1994). *The Which? Guide to Men's Health*. London: Consumers' Association.

Charles, N. (1993). *Gender Divisions and Social Change*. Hemel Hempstead: Harvester Wheatsheaf.

Charlton, J. Kelly, S., Dunnell, K., Evans, B., Jenkins, R. (1993). Suicide deaths in England and Wales: trends in factors associated with suicide deaths, *Population Trends*, 71 (Spring).

Connell, R. (1987). *Gender and Power: Society, the person and sexual politics*. Stanford, Calif.: Stanford University Press.

Doyal, L. (1995). *What Makes Women Sick: Gender and the political economy of health*. London: Tavistock.

Doyal, L. (ed.) (1998). *Women and Health Services: An agenda for change* Buckingham: Open University Press.

Doyal, L. (2000). 'Gender equity in health: debates and dilemmas' *Social Science and Medicine* 51 :931-939

Doyal , L. (2001). Sex, gender and health: the need for a new approach *British Medical Journal*, 323, 1061–3 (3 November).

Faludi, S. (1992). *Backlash: The undeclared war against women*. London: Chatto & Windus.

Fee, E. and Krieger, N. (1994). *Women's Health, Politics and Power: Essays on sex/gender, medicine and public health*. Amityville, NY: Baywood.

Fisher, S. (1996). *In the Patient's Best Interest: Women and the policies of medical decision making*. New Brunswick, NJ: Rutgers University Press.

Foster, S. and Mallik, M. (1998). A comparative study of differences in the referral behaviour patterns of men and women who have experienced cardiac-related chest pain, *Intensive and Critical Care Nursing*, 14(4), 192–202.

Gibbs, J. (1988). *Young, Black and Male in America: An endangered species*. Dover, Mass.: Auburn House.

Graham, H. and Oakley, A. (1981). Competing ideologies of reproduction: medical and maternal perspectives on pregnancy. In Roberts, H. (ed.), *Women, Health and Reproduction*. London: Routledge & Kegan Paul.

Harrison, J., Chin, J. and Ficarrotto, T. (1992). Warning: Masculinity may be dangerous to your health. In Kimmel, M. and Messner, M. (eds), *Men's Lives*. New York: Macmillan.

Hart, N. (1988). Sex, gender and survival: inequalities of life chances between European men and women. In Fox, A. (ed.), *Inequality in Health within Europe*. Aldershot: Gower.

Hearn, J. (1993). The politics of essentialism and the analysis of the 'Men's Movements', *Feminism and Psychology*, 2, 405–10.

Hearn, J. (1998). The welfare of men? In Popay, J., Hearn, J. and Edwards, J. *Men, Gender Divisions and Welfare*. London: Routledge.

Huggins, A. and Lamb, B. (1998). *Social Perspectives on Men's Health in Australia*. Melbourne: Maclennan and Petty.

Kadar, A. (1994). The sex-bias myth in medicine, *The Atlantic Monthly*, 274, 66–70.

Kandiyoti, D. (1998). 'Bargaining with patriarchy', *Gender and Society*, 2(3), 274–90.

Kimmel, M. and Messner, M. (eds) (1993). *Men's Lives*, New York: Macmillan.

Kitts, J. and Roberts, J. (1996), *The Health Gap: Beyond pregnancy and reproduction*. Ottawa: IDRC.

Kraemer, S. (2000). The fragile male, *British Medical Journal*, 321, 1609–12.

Kurth, A. (ed.) (1993). *Until the Cure: Caring for women with AIDS*. London and New Haven, Conn.: Yale University Press.

LaRosa, J. and Pinn, V. (1993). Gender bias in biomedical research, *Journal of the American Medical Women's Association*, 48(5), 145–51.

Lloyd, T. (1998). *Men's Health. A Public Health Review*. London: Men's Health Forum.

Lyndon, N. (1992). *No More Sex Wars: The failures of feminism*. London: Sinclair Stevenson.

Mastroianni, A., Faden, R. and Federman, D. (eds) (1994). *Women and Health Research: Ethical and legal issues of including women in clinical studies*, Vols 1 and 2. Washington, DC: National Academy Press.

Messing, K. (1998). *One-Eyed Science: Occupational health and women workers* Philadelphia, Pa.: Temple University Press.

Moynihan, C. (1998). Theories of masculinity *British Medical Journal* 317, 1072–5.

Oakley, A. (1972). *Sex, Gender and Society*. London: Temple Smith.

O'Sullivan, S. (1987). *Women's Health: A Spare Rib reader*. London: Pandora Press.

Papenek, H. (1990). To each less than she needs, from each more than she can do: allocations, entitlements and values. In Tinker, I. (ed.), *Persistent Inequalities: Women and world development*. Oxford University Press.

Petticrew, M., McKee, M. and Jones, J. (1993) Coronary artery surgery: are women discriminated against?, *British Medical Journal*, 306, 1164–6.

Pleck, J. and Sonenstein, F. (eds) (1991). *Adolescent Problem Behaviours*. Hillsdale, NJ: Lawrence Erlbaum.

Redberg R. F. (1998). Coronary artery disease in women: understanding the diagnostic and management pitfalls, *Medscape Women's Health*, 3(5), 1.

Roberts, H. (1985). *The Patient Patients: Women and their doctors*. London: Pandora Press.

Sabo, D. and Gordon, D. (1995). *Men's Health and Illness: Gender, power and the body*. London: Sage.

Schofield, T. Connell, R., Walter, L., Wood, J., and Butland, D. (2000) Understanding men's health and illness: a gender relations approach to policy, research and practice, *Journal of American College Health*, 48, 247–57.

Sharp, I. (1998). Gender issues in the prevention and treatment of coronary heart disease. In Doyal, L. (ed.), *Women and Health Services: An agenda for change*. Buckingham: Open University Press.

Sianne, G. and Wilkinson, H. (1995). *Gender, Feminism and the Future*. London: Demos.

Staples, R. (1995). Health among Afro-American males. In Sabo, D. and Gordon, D., *Men's Health and Illness: Gender, power and the body*. London: Sage.

Stein, J. (1997). *Empowerment and Women's Health*. London: Zed Books.

Timyan, J., Griffey Brechin, S., Measham, D. and Ogunleye, B. (1993). Access to care: more than a problem of distance. In Koblinsky, M., Timyan, J. and Gay, J. (eds), *The Health of Women: A global perspecitve*. Boulder, Col.: Westview Press.

Tobin, J., Wassertheil-Smoller, S., Wexler, J., Steingart, R., Budner, N., Lense, L., Wachsprecs, J. (1987). Sex bias in considering coronary bypass surgery, *Annals of Internal Medicine*, 107, 19–25.

Todd, A. (1989). *Intimate Adversaries: Cultural conflict between doctors and women patients*. Philadelphia, Pa.: University of Pennsylvania Press.

Travin, M. and Johnson, L. (1997). Assessment of coronary artery disease in women. *Curr. Opin. Cardiol.*, 12, 587–94.

United Nations Development Programme (UNDP) (1995). *Human Development Report 1995*. New York: UNDP.

US National Institutes of Health (1992). *Opportunities for Research on Women's Health* (NIH Publication No. 92-3457). Washington, DC: US Department of Health and Human Services.

Waldron, I. (1995). Contribution of changing gender differentials in behaviour to changing gender differences in mortality. In Sabo, D. and Gordon, D. (eds), *Men's Health and Illness: Gender, power and the body*. London: Sage.

Weintraub, T. A., Paine, L. L. and Weintraub, D. H. (1996) Primary care for women, comprehensive assessment and management of common mental health problems. *Journal of Nurse–Midwifery*, 41(2), 125–38.

White, E. (1990). *Black Women's Health Book: Speaking for ourselves*. Seattle, Washington: Seal Press.

Willott, G. and Griffin, C. (1996). Men, masculinity and the challenge of long term unemployment. In Mac an Ghaill, M. (ed.), *Understanding Masculinities*. Buckingham: Open University Press.

Wizemann, S. and Pardue, M.-L. (2001). *Exploring the Biological Contribution to Human Health: Does sex matter?* Washington DC: National Academy Press.

Working with Men (2001). *Boys' and Young Men's Health: Literature and practice review* London: Health Development Agency.

35 The future of the health-promoting school*

Susan Denman, Alysoun Moon, Carl Parsons and David Stears

So, what does the future hold for health promoting schools? This article summarizes a number of key issues relating to the successful development of healthy schools. These include: ensuring that schools provide stability and structure for young people in a rapidly-changing world, and that they are viable settings for promoting the health of young people; the development of skills in citizenship and democracy that form part of a healthy school's curriculum and prepare young people to participate in their own health promotion-, the need for genuine partnerships in promoting health; the importance of a whole-school approach to health; links between healthy and effective schools; and, finally, building capacity and thereby sustainability.

There have been many changes in society in the UK over recent decades that are mirrored in other European countries. Moral, cultural and community frameworks have fragmented with successive generations in a postindustrial society. Some countries have been torn apart by war, and others have witnessed comprehensive changes in the ideologies that underpin them. The disintegration of the traditional family, whatever its cause, has resulted in children being put under stress, and often lacking the support of a caring, extended family. These changes have presented major challenges for those who are concerned to promote the health and well-being of children and young people, and will continue to do so in the future. They include the challenge of meeting the changing health-related needs of present and future youth populations in ways that are acceptable, appropriate and relevant. Within this challenge lies the crucial factor of government recognition of the need for financial investment in the health of young people in the future (Ziglio, 1998). Experience has shown already that, where health promoting schools receive adequate monies and resources, sustainability is supported and health promotion in school settings develops and grows. This applies to locally, nationally and internationally-based schemes, including the English National Healthy School Standard (NHSS) and the European Network of Health Promoting Schools (ENHPS).

* From Denman, S., Moon, A., Parson, C. and Stears, D., *The Health Promoting School: policy, research and practice* (2002), pp. 153–60, London, Routledge Falmer.

There is general recognition that schools themselves can offer stable environments within changing societies and provide young people with a security that is often absent in their home and external environment. The daily routines, responsibilities and opportunities to develop strong and supportive relationships with a range of adults can help to give structure and consistency to children's lives. School organization and management styles can support all aspects of a child's development – spiritual, moral, social and cultural – in a positive, safe and welcoming milieu. This in turn can provide support for the taught curriculum in PSHE (Personal, Social and Health Education) and Citizenship and, by implication, health promotion. The potential for partnerships with groups within the local community further strengthens this stability and helps to make schools viable settings for promoting health.

A stable, happy and health promoting environment in school, however, will depend on the health and well-being of the staff. It is important to consider the effects that sustained pressure for change on schools can have. In the UK, much of this centres on improving quality and educational achievement – legitimate goals for the health-pro-moting school because of their health-protecting effect. But too much pressure causes stress for adults, and this is likely to affect positive social interactions with pupils and the wider community. It is worth remembering that the health-promoting school is a utopian concept that is difficult to achieve, producing its own short-term pressures even though it may reap benefits in all aspects of school life in the future. Governments will need to recognize that if school staff are over pressurized and continuously stressed, there is little likelihood of their being able to establish and maintain the kind of environment that underpins the healthy-schools concept. Political support needs to be consistent. It is essential to signal the importance of the health-promoting school to schools and their communities, and to review urgently the degree to which schools have been able to integrate the healthy schools concept into the fabric of the school organization. It is easy to pay lip-service to the NHSS in England, for example, without investigating whether it has achieved full integration into schools, or whether more drastic measures are needed.

Effective partnerships are fundamental to public health practice and, in particular, to the future development of healthy schools. The principles of good partnership have been identified by Hardy and Hudson (1999) as:

- recognising and accepting the need for partnership;
- developing clarity and realism of purpose;
- ensuring commitment and ownership;
- developing and maintaining trust; and
- clear and robust partnership arrangements.

These principles provide a useful framework within which to develop partnerships, and will work well where all partners have consulted, worked out and agreed practical details and collaborate on their implementation. It is especially important for outside agencies working with schools to understand the constraints on progress and for both to set realistic aims and targets. All partnerships are process driven, and will require time for development. There are enormous challenges facing schools, communities and outside agencies in developing good partnerships. In areas targeted with resources, i.e. areas of deprivation, there is a need for much greater clarity of purpose, and better co-ordination and co-operation in order to make good use of resources and to achieve a greater sense of coherence in what is planned and implemented. Community development shows the most promise for a way forward, but schools will need to be more open and to be a resource for their communities, seriously seen in the community school movement of the 1970s – and in some parts of the UK more recently. Once again, consistent government support will be essential.

The English NHSS guidance document (DfEE, 1999a) identifies partnerships as the first of its three main sections – partnerships, programme management and working with schools. Partnerships are required that involve local health and education services, school staff, governors and pupils, and statutory and non-statutory community groups and agencies, Partnerships with parents too are important when dealing with matters relating to their children's health, particularly when sensitive issues are involved – for example sex and relationships education. Although the school setting is unique within the community, a school cannot work in a vacuum, and future attainment in the development of healthy schools will depend, at least in part, on the success of these partnerships.

The nature of partnerships at international and national level is an issue in terms of control and empowerment. The technical secretariat of the European Network of Health Promoting Schools, based at the (WHO) World Health Organization European Office in Geneva, has played an enabling role with national co-ordinators, organized pump priming to support national efforts and sought to bring national education and health ministries together to support a national scheme. At national level, there is the need for facilitating funding, a supportive framework and a legitimated status for health promotion in schools. A top-down model of the health-promoting school is inappropriate and would appear to be at odds with the notion of empowerment extolled by the Ottawa Charter, prompting questions about the degree of centralization and the balance between control and empowerment of local agents. It is important to be aware that countries are often selective in the parts of the health-promoting school project they seek to implement, depending on their own cultural and philosophical mores. A major challenge for the future will be for the healthy-schools movement to address the tension that exists currently at all levels – local, national and international – between rhetoric about empowerment and the importance of involving pupils as partners, and the sometimes prescriptive nature of the protocols that are sent into schools.

It is clear that schools need to be truly democratic institutions and to reflect the work being done in the curriculum. This means that children will be involved in decision making within school, and more widely within their communities. For example, there is some promising work being done by primary care groups in England. In discharging their duties regarding health improvement, they are holding community consultation events and asking residents to identify their concerns. Many have included children and young people in that process. Following needs assessment, the key question is how to tackle these concerns. What could be the contribution of the school among the many contributions needed from individuals, groups, families and organizations? Arguably this kind of approach will give children a better sense of their wider community, and the school's, and their place within it.

Skills development within PSHE, citizenship and democracy education provides a foundation for healthy schools which will also equip young people for life beyond the school gate and in the future. It is best achieved through a range of teaching styles and active learning processes appropriate to pupils' age, ability and level of maturity. The management styles and ethos of the school will also contribute to skills development by providing pupils with opportunities to practise and consolidate the application of their learning. Work undertaken by schools in Denmark in this area over recent years reported outcomes that have changed the location of real power and control within society (Jensen, 1999). The grasp of action competence is fundamental to the process of empowerment if young people are to make positive decisions about their health behaviour – a move from mere tokenism to actual control. In this sense, skills development will help to fulfil the requirements of the Ottawa Charter that health promotion should not only provide healthy choices but also empower those involved to make appropriate decisions about their health. The role of advocacy is key in school health promotion, whereby individuals and groups, both within schools and in the wider community, work together to achieve change for the good of each other. Once again, the success of these aspects of a health promoting school will depend upon the school being a democratic institution that communicates with and involves all its stakeholders in its planning and implementation.

A whole school approach to health education and promotion is discussed with confidence and extolled a great deal, bur achieved with difficulty (Moon, 1999). Yet it remains at the core of a healthy school and its proper definition and application need to be understood and put into practice if the healthy schools movement is to prosper in the future. It is based on the premise that health education and promotion will be much easier if their principles underpin all that happens within the school, and if they involve actively all those connected with the school. Healthy eating messages, for example, will be conveyed and reinforced through what is taught in the classroom, what is provided in school canteens and tuck-shops, school policy relating to the use of external caterers, and the active contribution of pupils, parents and people at home. A whole school approach will involve the whole school community (pupils, staff, parents, governors and community partners) in policy development and in physical, social and cultural activities.

In practice, however, it has been very difficult to involve the whole school community when time constraints are tight and there are many other demands on busy teachers, governors and parents. The perception still held by many that health education and promotion in schools is of low status means that there is still a danger that one enthusiast who is on the staff will be left with the responsibility of introducing and implementing a healthy schools programme. The time has come, however, to recognize that this is not enough, and a broader-based and comprehensive approach to health promotion in schools is needed if healthy schools are to be sustained.

It is clear that, while a whole-school approach to health promotion is central to the healthy-schools movement, it cannot be achieved overnight. Leadership and commitment by senior management in schools are essential and it will take a great deal of planning, time and hard work. It may be helpful for each school to explore the concept of a whole-school approach for itself, define it realistically within what is possible and achievable, and identify ways in which it can be realized. The roles of parents and the community in achieving a whole-school approach must not be underestimated.

There are indications that there may be an association between the health of young people and their level of educational achievement (Hopkins, 1995; Young, 1998) and that there may be links between a health-promoting school and an effective school (Novello *et al.*, 1992; Boddington and Hull, 1996). Samdal *et al.* (1998) have highlighted the potential contribution of programmes such as the ENHPS to creating a school environment that students perceive to be safe and justly organized and, in turn, to improving students' educational experience and enhancing their well-being and health. There are similarities between the aims of a healthy school – for example, effective partnerships, skills development – and the factors identified by Rutter *et al.* (1979) as characteristics of effective schools. More research is needed, but the suggestions that 'healthy schools create healthy students' and that, in turn, healthy students will be better able to learn, are axiomatic.

Achieving effective schools where learning is enhanced and academic improvements accomplished is of prime educational importance In all societies. The links between healthy and effective schools provide a sound basis for the future support and development of health promoting schools and need to be exploited.

The factors involved when considering the sustainability of a health promoting school initiative are closely linked with capacity building and include the following:

- Funding flexible enough to support schools from all levels of society at different levels of achieving health promoting status and with differing and wide-ranging needs;
- Education and training of teachers who are the main contacts at the interface between school and communities and will represent the health promoting school to outsiders;
- Flexibility to adapt to changing circumstances and constraints and to step outside right schedules and boundaries to offer realistic and appropriate support;
- The curriculum having a symbiotic relationship with the school environment and what takes place in school; and
- Evidence-based practice to underpin future developments; that is, an outcome of internal monitoring and evaluation carried out and owned by the stakeholders.

The need for *funding* and resources has been highlighted already. It is not enough that the healthy-schools development has become a strong political issue, in the UK and elsewhere. Denman *et al.* (2002) highlighted the roller-coaster pattern of political commitment and strategic policy development of health education and promotion since the 1950s. Verbal support and encouragement, whether given at government or local level, will not provide schools with the subject status, time, skills and resources needed to implement the requirements of a national or European scheme. The lack of funding is linked undoubtedly to the low status accorded to health education and promotion, and this has become a fundamental obstacle to progress. A major step would be for funding bodies to recognize that a school in a deprived area will need much more support than one in a 'middle class' district, where parents and the community are already actively involved. Schools should be given the freedom to use their funds creatively to achieve their own unique alms and objectives. While acknowledging the need for firm political commitment at all levels, the future sustainability of health-promoting schools is dependent on concrete resources and adequate funding to match the rhetoric.

Education and training of all school staff, especially teachers, in health education and promotion, and in the development of, for example, a whole school approach, is crucial to the future success of healthy schools. For teachers, training is needed at initial teacher education level and through in-service training when appropriate. A lack of training leads to a lack of understanding of the concept and its potential significance in the lives of those in school. It is worth recording the need for politicians and those in positions of power in any government or community to receive education about the health-promoting school, what it involves for schools in their communities and their roles in helping schools to achieve health-promoting status.

Flexibility is essential, because the health-promoting schools initiative will not succeed if the requirements and guidelines for its implementation are too rigid and circumscribed. Each country will have a mixture of similar and different local and individual school needs, and the scheme must be sufficiently flexible and adaptable to meet those needs. In the same way, some countries may have more resources and assets available for distribution to schools than others, and this will affect the work undertaken and the outcomes.

The curriculum, particularly those parts relating to PSHE and relationships education, forms the cornerstone of the health-promoting school and is also linked with the need for flexibility. The health-related aspects that support the development of a healthy school will need to be dynamic and progressive, skills-based and specific to different localities so that it will meet the differing needs of pupils in rapidly changing environments and equip them to make healthy choices and decisions for themselves.

Evidence-based practice highlights the need for the assessment and evaluation of healthy schools, particularly at individual school level, in order to provide evidence of effectiveness and success. There is no longer a need for expensive large scale national and regional evaluation initiatives, and the future focus must be on school-based evaluation. There is, none the less, a need for the urgent development of rigorous, sensitive, appropriate, tried and tested evaluation tools. Unless the health-promoting schools initiative can be shown to have a positive impact on the health and well-being of those in schools, and thereby on the wider community, then its sustainability in the future is in doubt. However, RCTs (Randomised controlled trials) are difficult to apply to the health promoting school in the search for causality. Depending on the objectives of an intervention, evaluation may consider all or some of the following at all levels of the school: policy, organizational development, partnerships, process and outcome – at the level of the school. At project level, the success of recruitment strategies, programme reach (diffusion), organizational change, partnership development, audit and other areas as necessary will need to be investigated. Schools are at different stages in developing as health promoting environments. Setting the health-promoting school within a development planning cycle will require schools to monitor their progress. Evaluation needs to fit the objectives and reflect the complexity and scope of the health-promoting school. The most appropriate model is action research, in which the teacher, who knows the school and how it functions, is a reflective practitioner. An evaluation carried out internally will be ongoing, sustainable and much more empowering than one imposed from outside the school.

There was a rapid growth of healthy schools or health-promoting school initiatives in the 1990s, and it seems likely that this will continue while governments or international bodies continue to support their development. The concept of the health-promoting school, however, is complex and hard to implement in ways that involve all stakeholders, despite its apparent simplicity and potential for practical application. Identifying the components of a whole school approach and putting them into practice can be fraught with difficulties, albeit surmountable, and is dependent on a variety of factors, both internal and external to the school. Nevertheless, there is sufficient evidence now to show that a carefully structured and supported framework for intervention can have positive health-related effects and outcomes on school ethos, management structures and practice, the curriculum, and, to a greater or lesser extent, on some pupil behaviour.

The future of health promoting schools looks promising. There is still much work to be done and real, sustained commitment to funding needed from governments, but, with the support and impetus of local, national and international initiatives, it seems likely that the day will come when 'Every child and young person in Europe ... will have the opportunity of being educated in a health promoting school' (WHO, 1998).

References

Boddington, N. and Hull, T. (1996). *The Health Promoting School: Focusing on health and school improvement*. London: Forbes Publications.

Denman, S., Moon, A., Parsons, C. and Stears, D. (2002). *The Health Promoting School: Policy, Research and Politics*, London: Routledge Falmer.

DfEE (1999a). *National Healthy School Standard – Guidance*, London: Department for Education and Employment.

Hardy, B. and Hudson, B. (1999). *What Makes a Good Patnership? A partnership assessment tool*. Leeds: The Nuffield Institute for Health.

Hopkins, D. (1995). Healthy schools, healthy students, development strategies for school effectiveness. In Pierrs D. (ed.), *Towards an Evaluation of the European Network of Health Promoting Schools (The Eva Project)*. Brussels: Université Libre de Bruxelles.

Jensen, B. B. (1999). Evaluation of Danish schools, *First ENHPS Evaluation Conference Report, Thun, Switzerland*. Copenhagen: ENHPS.

Moon, A. (1999). Does a healthy schools award scheme make a difference? The evaluation of the Wessex Healthy Schools Award. Unpublished Ph.D. thesis, Department of Public Health Medicine, University of Southampton.

Novello, A. C., Degraw, C. and Kleinman, D. V. (1992). Healthy children ready to learn: an essential collaboration between health and education, *Public Health Report*, 107, 1.

Rutter, M., Maughan, B. and Ouston, J. (1979). *Fifteen Thousand Hours*. London: Open Books.

Samdal, O., Nutbeam, D., Wold, B. and Kanna, L. (1998). Achieving health and educational goals through schools – a study in the importance of school climate and the students' satisfaction with school, *Health Education Research*, 13(3), 383–97.

WHO (1998). *The Health Promoting School – An investment in education health and Democracy, report of the first conference of the European Network of Health Promoting Schools*, Thassaloniki-Haldiki, Greece 1–5 May 1997. Copenhagen: World Health Organization.

Young, I. (1998). *Can schools make a difference?*, Unpublished discussion paper for the Health Education Board for Scotland.

Ziglio, E. (1998). *Repositioning Health Promotion: Research Implications*, Paper presented at the First UK Health Promotion Research Conference, April 1998, Heriot-Watt University, Edinburgh.

36 Think globally, act locally*

Peter Townsend

. . . [M]uch of the problem of increasing poverty and instability in the United Kingdom derives from failure to collaborate not just in Europe but more generally in the world to (i) regulate the power of multinational corporations and financial institutions; (ii) democratize international agencies like the World Bank and the International Monetary Fund; and (iii) buttress the living standards (and hence productivity and health) of the poor throughout the world by establishing a new 'International Welfare State' which would include universal services like education and health as well as forms of universal social security. This would offset or balance some of the excesses of the new international market . . .

The trend towards greater social polarization has first to be slowed and then reversed. Policies for the United Kingdom have to take better account of global causes of local problems, devise new forms of international collaboration to reduce poverty in rich and poor countries alike, and establish equitable conditions of employment and growth . . .

Structural trends

In too many countries in the world, both rich and poor, inequalities grew fast during the 1980s and early 1990s. The latest reports from UNDP and the International Fund for Agricultural Development show that a majority of the poorest countries in the world are experiencing an increase in poverty which is not explained by population changes or flagging growth of their economies. Countries such as Bangladesh, the Philippines, Kenya and Mexico experienced both an absolute and a proportionate increase in the extent of poverty, as measured by international agencies between 1965 and the end of the 1980s. Their problems are an amalgam of debt, inadequate and misconceived aid policies advocated by the IMF and the World Bank, and stunted opportunities within the international market . . .

In the United Kingdom, the richest 20 per cent had disposable income after housing costs in 1979 amounting to 35 per cent of the national total (CSO, 1994). By 1989 this had grown to 41 per cent and in the next two years, 1990–1, reached 43 per cent . . .

* From *European Labour Forum* (Summer 1994), 2–8.

By contrast, the poorest 20 per cent had a disposable income in 1979 amounting to 10 per cent of the national total. This diminished to 7 per cent by 1988–9 and to 6 per cent in 1990–1. This fall represented a loss to the poorest 11 million people of £17 billion a year. For the average household in this group of the population this represents a loss of £3,000 each year . . .

Europe

Trends in other European countries have not been so marked. In some there is not much evidence of structural changes, but in others, like the Netherlands, Belgium, Spain and even Sweden, similar trends are beginning to make themselves felt. The point which needs to be seized is that the causes are international as well as national. There is, for example, the growing power of the IMF and the World Bank. Their policies have become increasingly monetarist, and their loans increasingly conditional on national implementation of those policies. The two are embodied in 'structural adjustment' policies which are a prime cause of polarization and of poverty. There is a close connection between these agencies' policies for the Third World and their policies for the First World. The quasi-monetarist policies of deflation, deregulation, privatization, cuts in public expenditure, cuts in personal income taxation and withdrawal from the welfare state are being applied in rich and poor countries alike. Governments everywhere have been, and are being, forced to acquiesce. Clear examples in the 1990s were afforded by many Latin American and African countries, but also by the Commonwealth of Independent States and other Eastern European countries.

The rapidly growing power of multi-national corporations, the largest of which now have an annual financial turnover bigger than middle-sized nation states, such as Saudi Arabia, is a related factor. The effects of both these international forces can be seen at local and regional level. For example, the problems of drug addiction in inner cities is directly attributable to the operations of multinational drug empires which the international community shows little capacity to control. Again, hundreds and thousands of redundancies in specific areas are attributable to the closure of modern industrial plants in some of the rich countries, so that they may be reopened in countries where labour costs are smaller. Government intervention to moderate the damage is inhibited by free market ideology . . .

The loss of pension rights provides another example. The growing number of company mergers and take-overs by multinational companies has revealed gaps in national laws which do not provide full protection of occupational pension rights and have had a devastating effect on the pension expectations of thousands . . .

National government policies have reinforced, and in some instances anticipated, deflationary divisive international policies. They have been causing destructive forms of social polarization. Evidence of the harmful social effects of this polarization are reported every day: increases in thefts, burglaries and crimes of violence; high rates of homelessness; increased numbers of bankruptcies and repossessions; unnecessarily high rates of premature mortality and disability; deteriorating public services and deteriorating standards of council housing.

The key strategy

What can be done to halt the international and national slide? A start might be made with a collaborative programme of *social development* . . . Government must act internationally in the first instance to protect economic and social health. This will mean working with European allies to argue for the introduction of forms of regulations for multinational corporations: closing loopholes in cross-national taxation; protecting home-based companies and individual employees by means of more democratic company laws nationally and internationally; promoting international trade union links; facilitating the internationalization of democratic pressure groups; facilitating cross-national links between city authorities; and, in particular, taking new initiatives to foster First World–Third World relationships. To such a strategy must be added measures to monitor the development of multinational companies; and to democratize the IMF and the World Bank in ways which are deliberately intended to raise the representation of Third World populations, but also the social interests of poorer groups in all the rich countries. The international problem is not one just of the exclusion of Third World countries It is now also the problem of the exclusion of the poorest fifth or two fifths of the populations of rich countries. The asylum of refugees and the considerate treatment of temporary workers in Europe are prime examples . . .

International social insurance

What can be done in Europe to buttress development and minimize poverty and unemployment? What is needed is a renewed commitment to underpin the security of the waged and non-waged populations. A number of European countries have a deeper commitment to social insurance schemes than does the United Kingdom . . . Levels of benefits are often much higher than in the United Kingdom and were not cut back to the same extent in the 1980s. The change from the earnings-related to the price-related formula of the retirement pension, and abolition of earnings related sickness and unemployment benefit, together with the reduction in scope of both sickness and unemployment, are the major examples. While social insurance systems throughout Europe vary widely, it is inconceivable that European economic development will not be predicated upon some harmonization of existing schemes.

The likelihood is that for both political and economic reasons contributory insurance will be stabilized, with income support or social assistance being reformulated to cope with much larger number of migratory workers and retirees. For reasons of social stability as well as to provide a basis for high productivity, the United Kingdom's strategy should be to emphasize the former.

Universal benefits in the United Kingdom are at a cross-roads. The problem is not that they should be made more selective but that their role should be greatly improved to suit modern conditions. This means better provision for interruptions in employment, part-time employment, migratory labour and populations, and coverage for the hard work of those involved in the care of children, and disabled and elderly persons. The problem is not to defend an old institution for the sake of tradition and familiarity but to use an efficient, economical and socially integrative mechanism to new advantage . . .

A modernized version of social insurance has to be seen as an integral part of a wider policy of economic and social development. This is partially, but not fully, recognized in the EU's (European Union's) Social Chapter. The Social Chapter provides for workers to have a right to social security benefits of a sufficient level; and for those excluded from the labour market to have a right to a guaranteed level of resources. Inevitably there will be sharp arguments about the definition of these entitlements, but confirmation of the link between contribution and benefits will help to lift some of the downward pressures of fiscal competition. The strengthening of social insurance is a long term and not a short term element of social policy, which will provide a partial defence against temporary pressures to undercut wages and employment. Incidentally, social insurance also provides an example of the better usage of the principle of subsidiarity – by allowing connections to be made between national, regional and local schemes affecting relations between governments and subsidiary organizations of workers and employers.

Secure state pensions for the elderly

Income support does not reach more than a million elderly people who are entitled to that support. The basic state pension has already fallen from 20 per cent to 15 per cent of average male earnings. It is predicted to fall to 8 per cent in the twenty-first century unless government policies are changed. European and UK evidence demonstrates public willingness to incur higher taxes to improve the standard of living of the elderly. Some of the evidence from the 9th Report on *British Social Attitudes* deserves to be quoted:

> not only do the British reject *cuts* in public spending in health and education: a majority claims to support *tax increases* to finance more spending on welfare services . . . Indeed, 1991 saw the largest year-on-year rise in the survey series' history in the proportion of respondents claiming to be willing to see higher taxes to pay for more social spending . . . (Since 1983 those supporting the idea of increasing taxes and spending more has increased from 32 per cent to 65 per cent.)
>
> The favourite priority for more spending has always been retirement pensions . . . The most striking change in recent years has been an increase in support for more spending on child benefit . . .

A key component of policy must be to raise the basic state pension relative to earnings, and then to restore the annual earnings related formula. The increase should be higher for the over 75s and should be related to an increase in the disability living allowance for those who are moderately or severely disabled. At ages 65–74 a higher rate of tax should be applied to those with a disposable income of more than three times the basic state pension. The privatization of the state earnings-related pension scheme should also be opposed, but a phased introduction of a regionalized and locally accountable successor for younger age groups should be investigated as a priority.

The additional costs of a modernized and revitalized scheme for social insurance could be met partly by extending the national insurance contribution to the top of the earnings scale, and partly by selective cuts in tax expenditure . . .

Basic income for child and disability support

If modernized social insurance can play a new part in providing security and protection for those in the labour market in a form which is both proven and popular, and yet also serves the social and economic objectives of European union, the needs of the larger number who are outside the labour market have to be recognized. There are elderly and disabled people, especially women whose benefit is very small and whose income needs to increased. But there are also many younger people providing many hours of support to families and to disabled relatives and others whose work, and financial needs, are not recognized in the market economy. An organized and industrious society must be based on principles which go much wider than the vagaries of the market. Levels of reward for work performed in the interests of society and of economic growth deserve public scrutiny, discussion and approval. This feature of democracy has hitherto attracted too little attention. The extent of inequalities in the wage system, and trends in those inequalities, of course deserve regular examination. But other inequalities cannot be ignored. The provision of social insurance for those in the wage system has to be balanced by adequate child care and disability care payments to those engaged in equally demanding, if not more demanding work, despite the fact that they do not receive a conventional wage . . .

Minimum wage

The features of social polarization which have been documented in this chapter show how different are the conditions of the, 1990s compared, say, with the 1950s and 1960s. In the aftermath of action on the Beveridge Report, social insurance (together with social assistance in a subsidiary role) was believed to meet the problem of poverty. Today the depression of low wages, together with the casualization of employment and the much larger numbers holding part-time employment, highlights the importance of minimum wage, or minimum earnings guarantee, legislation. A decent minimum wage is a necessary condition of productive and good quality work, but also of employment incentives and social stability. In the conditions of the so-called secondary labour market it is a particular necessity.

But, like proposals targeted on the poorest outside work, proposals for the poorest inside work are not enough. Schemes for a minimum wage have to be related to the evolution of the national (and international) wages system. Action on one cannot be effective without action on the whole. All wages and salaries are part of a hierarchy of earnings. Action at any level will only be effective if action is taken (by corporations no less than by governments) to modify the entire structure. This applies especially to topmost earnings – which set the pace, or the example, for the evolution of the entire structure. The justification for absurdly high salaries and substantial perks is too rarely debated. The problem of the undeserving rich is treated lightly, when in fact it is far more of a threat to social order and responsibility than the problem of the so-called 'undeserving poor'.

In the 1970s criticisms of narrowly conceived incomes policies were just. In today's conditions, when multinational companies are creating greater wage inequalities among their workforces, and when the bargaining rights of unions have been greatly reduced, the formulation of any statutory (and maybe international) incomes policy has to be very different . . . Proposals for a minimum wage are meaningless unless set within a reconstituted and modern income policy. This has to include guidelines in principle for the structure of wages and their development in a democracy.

In conclusion

National strategy to enhance economic and social development should therefore take full account of the problems being created by international market and financial forces, including the role of the international agencies.

A national and European social contract

This would be a UK version of the European Social Chapter which would extend as well as illustrate, in nationally specific form, the agreements involved in that chapter. It would specify proposals for the integration of international company law, the monitoring of information about multinational companies, revision of the democratic constitutions, and principles of accountability, of international agencies, and the rights and responsibilities of citizens and employee and employer organizations, as well as develop a national model of collaborative action within Europe to promote social development.

Democratization of international agencies as well as of rich and poor nation states

The representation of the nations who are not members of the G7 nations – which account for only 12 per cent of world population – on the executive and other committees of the agencies should be increased. The G7 nations currently account for more than 50 per cent of the voting powers of the executive boards of the World Bank and the IMF. There is also the well-documented problem of the 'democratic deficit' of the European Parliament, and the weak powers as well as representativeness of many national Parliaments. Renewed efforts to strengthen democratization at local level are also necessary to social development. In the United Kingdom, local government has been seriously weakened since 1979, and quangos have been created without adequate elected representation on governing bodies. The rights of citizens must be reinforced in both respects. Democratization is part and parcel of social development

Modernized social insurance

This would build on the basic state pension, the state earnings related pension, the disability living allowance, and child benefit. Costs would be met by raising the national insurance earnings ceiling, targeting of mortgage tax relief and of the married couple's allowance (and the restriction of subsidy for personal pensions), and the restructuring of tax expenditures generally to leave the tax system itself more progressive and more logical. Savings in income support would be made from an expansion of social insurance.

Basic income for child and disability support

In modern conditions of greater equity between men and women the skills of women can only be recognized by ensuring a basic participation income outside as well as inside paid employment, as conventionally defined. In the interests of economic and (not only social) development a basic income for both child care and disability care has to be paid. That income has to be complemented with a more adequate level of child benefit and disability income.

[The last two] recommendations would of course need to be implemented in conformity with the earlier recommendations. The contributory element of social insurance would be widened to cover more comprehensively those with intermittent, part-time and occasional earnings, those seeking asylum, and visitors and migrant workers. There would be non-contributory rights to benefit on the part of those working in occupations of national importance but not attracting a conventional wage, or only attracting a wholly inadequate wage. Once childcare, disability care and other care payments are introduced or improved, non-contributory rights for those attracting those payments would be reduced.

Minimum and maximum earnings

In the interests of maximizing revenue as well as conditions and quality of work, guidelines for the evolution of the wage system need to be laid down. This could take the form of a minimum earnings guarantee and conditions for increases in high earnings.

A new charter of collective and individual worker rights

More account would have to be taken of the collective as well as individual interests of workers. These would have to be framed in relation to general worker-rights within the European Union – as they were implemented during the 1990s and into of the twenty-first century. The individualization of pay in rich countries through schemes for performance-related and skills-related pay, have tended to depreciate employee rights, as well as lower already low levels of pay. The restoration of definitions of collective worker rights will be a necessity in the middle and late 1990s . . .

The agenda for the achievement of social justice is indeed dauntingly large. An international perspective is inescapable.

37 From healthy cities to locality based initiatives: margin to mainstream*

Michael P. Kelly and Amanda Killoran

Introduction

This chapter considers recent developments in the public health of urban and city settings in Britain. The story begins in the early 1980s with the Healthy Cities project (Davies and Kelly, 1993a). This project aimed to develop partnerships at the level of the municipality, and to promote healthier urban environments via community development principles. It was adopted by a number of British cities. *The Health of the Nation* (Secretary of State for Health, 1991) launched by the Conservative Government in 1992, represented England's first national health strategy. Although it expected and anticipated the development of local health partnerships and strategies at local level, evaluation showed that it had limited impact because of its narrow disease-based approach, lack of resourcing and process flaws (Department of Health, 1998). The World Health Organization (WHO) Healthy Cities initiative had there-fore already been in place for some time as an organizing principle in a number of English towns and cities when this strategy was introduced. The Healthy Cities project had an international momentum, and in many areas continued to provide a focus for interagency strategies that recognized the wider determinants of health, even after the introduction of *The Health of the Nation*. However, some local successes notwith-standing (Davies and Kelly, 1993a), the locality approach tended to remain marginal to the mainstream business of the delivery of public health and to healthcare provision more generally.

In 1997, the incoming Labour government brought with it a radical shift in national health policy. A socio-economic model of health was fully embraced, and tackling health inequalities became a central com-mitment. The White Paper *Saving Lives: Our Healthier Nation* (OHN) (Department of Health, 1999) set a framework for the pursuit of a broad public health strategy that aimed to improve health, particularly of those worst off in society. The new policy context changed fundamen-tally the nature and position of locality-based health initiatives. The

---

* Commissioned for this volume.

landscape of locality-based health responses was transformed, and many of the principles underpinning Healthy Cities are now part of official policy and the new diversity of approaches. The Healthy Cities project has been superseded by neighbourhood renewal, local strategic partnerships, Health Action Zones, *Surestart*, and the methodology of health impact assessment (Department of Health, 1999, 2000, 2001). The underlying philosophy of the new arrangements is empirical, has a concern with the reduction of inequalities at its heart, and tries to base itself on evidence.

In large part, the transformation in the landscape is a result of changes in government policy and these will be described below. However, there were a number of inherent problems with the philosophy and practice of the Healthy Cities approach, which contributed to its marginalization. This chapter begins by considering some of these, drawing on earlier work about Healthy Cities and its philosophy (Davies and Kelly, 1993b; Kelly *et al.*, 1993; Kelly *et al.*, 1997).

Healthy cities and the postmodern turn

The Healthy Cities movement began with commitments to breaking conventional discipline-bound research methods and paradigms and to inter-sectoral and participative methods of working. This was based on the underlying guiding principles of Health for All, the new public health and health promotion (WHO, 1986, 1988). The new public health and health promotion deliberately represented themselves as multi-sectoral, multi-disciplinary, socio-ecological, low resource, participative and empowering (Ashton and Seymour, 1988; Bunton and Burrows, 1995). The new public health stressed that positive health is a quality of individuals and social groups that is self-defined rather than imposed by others. The degree to which it might be measured, quantified and scrutinized with reference to conventional canons of evidence was not only called into question, but also to a large degree denied. The emphasis on positive health was highly distinctive.

Historically speaking, the idea of positive health had gained popularity through the critiques of rationalist medicine. Writers such as Szaz (1972), Illich (1975), McKeown (1976) and Friedson (1970) had questioned, in different ways, the underlying rationalist principles of medicine and of medical advance. This seemed to fit well with the WHO's definition of health as not merely the absence of disease but rather a state of complete physical, mental and social well being (WHO, 1946). Consequently, within heath promotion, health came to be defined less as a physical condition and more as an ability to achieve potential and to respond positively to the challenges of the environment (Nutbeam, 1986). In these terms, health was seen as a resource for everyday life, not merely the object of living. It was a positive concept because it empha-sized social and personal as well as physical capabilities. This vision of health was based on aesthetic and moral values. Health and disease were not conceptualized as two ends of a continuous spectrum. They were identified as belonging to two quite different universes of discourse, one modern and scientific, and the other postmodern and subjective (Kelly *et al.*, 1993).

Adherents to the Healthy Cities approach sought to turn the scientific enterprise upside down. They wanted to bring together communities, service providers, researchers and planners (Davies and Kelly, 1993b). They wanted communities to define the research problems and to deter-mine delivery priorities. What the Healthy Cities philosophy tried to articulate was the abolition of the discipline boundaries between the social and biological sciences, making the subject matter contingent based on a view of knowledge as tentative, modifiable, probabilistic and reversible (Kellner, 1988). There were always interesting tensions in this approach (see, e.g., Davis and Kelly, 1993a). Once communities were brought into the research and delivery process in meaningful ways, and scientists and other stakeholders no longer defined conventional research or management problems, the nature of what the question should be and whose version of the truth should be applied to evaluate the answer immediately became matters of dispute.

It may be argued that Healthy Cities, Health for All, the new public health and health promotion were a product of the postmodern turn (Kelly *et al.*, 1993, 1997; Kelly and Charlton, 1995). The term 'post-modern' and its derivatives 'postmodernism' and 'postmodernity' have been debated at length by social theorists (Giddens, 1991, 1992; Callinicos, 1999; Delanty, 1999). In essence, the terms refer to a variety of major social and cultural disjunctions that happened in different fields of human cultural and scientific activities during the twentieth century. Postmodernism was a critique of three ideas or assumptions characteristic of modern advanced industrial societies. These three bedrock ideas were as follows. First, by virtue of a shared rationality, knowledge and science are linked inextricably to the political and bureaucratic levers of power. Second, through the advance of science and technology, social progress will also occur. Third, through science, underlying truths about the nature of material and human life will be revealed (Lyotard, 1984; Seidman and Wagner 1992). These beliefs in science and progress were the cornerstones of modernism and the modern world (Whitehead, 1926). The critique came to be termed post-modernism.

According to postmodern thinking, reality is not rational but is chaotic, uncertain and open-ended (Featherstone, 1988). In postmoder-nity, rationality and irrationality merge together with truth and false-hood. The difference between lay beliefs and expert knowledge is

rendered meaningless, and the privileged position of scientific knowledge and expertise is called into question (Kelly and Charlton, 1995).
These and related ideas exerted a profound influence in the latter part of
the twentieth century, directly and indirectly, in a variety of fields. They
also seemed to be concordant with a range of other political and social
movements such as environmentalism and consumerism, as well as
certain types of liberation politics. This was especially so in health promotion. Postmodern ideas chimed with the notion that bio-medically-
based health care (i.e. that was professionally led, based on expertise and
relied on high technology) was quintessentially modernist, and more
importantly, fundamentally oppressive.

Healthy Cities and Health for All were political activities. The principles of the *Ottawa Charter for Health Promotion* (WHO, 1986) were political principles, demands for the prerequisites of health were political not
scientific, and the doctrine of positive health is an aesthetic and moral
principle. In such political processes, meta-narratives (Lyotard, 1984)
must give way to micro-narratives. More precisely, the postmodern
approach of Health for All and Healthy Cities had to describe the lives of
men and women as they lived and experienced them (Kelly, 1990). It
needed to grasp the complexities of their thoughts and actions as they
moved through stressor-rich environments and attempted to come to
some kind of accommodation with them. That accommodation with
them would have been microbiological and internal. It would have been
psychological and inter-personal. For the purposes of understanding
these adaptation processes, it was useless to abstract. Abstraction is a
modernist principle. The postmodern solution should have been to integrate the holistic involvement in all these spheres of human existence.

The writings of Antonovsky (1996) were not infrequently invoked as a
justification for the postmodern approach in health. Antonovsky's work
(1985, 1987) challenges the dominance of what he called the pathogenic
approach. This encourages us to *not* to try to find the origins or causes of
pathology (be they bio-medical or social). He advocated instead an
approach, that would seek to find the origins of health. He wanted to
know how and under what circumstances health could flourish and be
created. Antonovsky termed this approach salutogenesis, meaning the
identification of the origins of health. It was proposed as a viable paradigm for health promotion research, and practice for the Healthy Cities
movement (City of Copenhagen, 1994). Modern contemporary cities,
which were the product of deliberate human planning, so the argument
went, nevertheless produced human misery, in urban sprawl, amid pollution, social problems, crime, homelessness and inequalities.
Contemporary cities and all their problems seemed to give the lie to the
rationalist hope of social engineering on a grand scale to produce human
happiness. The salutogenic approach was, or appeared to be, critical for
the Healthy Cities movement, because it suggested that the goal or

purpose was to understand the origins of health with its success bench-marked by an enhanced quality of life.

From the margins

By the time the new Labour Administration was elected in May 1997, the intellectual as well as the political climate had shifted from post-modern contemplation and doubt to something more empirical, evidence based and realistic. 'Did it work?' became a guiding principle for the new administration, coupled with a concern about delivery. As far as public health was concerned, inequalities in health were placed firmly at the centre of debate within and beyond the Department of Health. Significantly, Sir Donald Acheson was commissioned to produce a report on inequalities in health (Acheson, 1998) and the pieces were soon in place for a strategy to tackle inequalities. Several publications form the basis of the strategy (Department of Health, 1999, 2000, 2001). The *Our Healthier Nation* White Paper (OHN) (Department of Health, 1999) artic-ulated explicitly the need 'to improve the health of everyone, particu-larly the worst off, taking into account the social, economic and environmental factors affecting health'. To do this, a rationalist approach, quite at odds with the postmodern thinking of the earlier period, required the construction of an up-to date map of the evidence base for public health and health improvement; the commissioning of research and evaluation to support and strengthen the evidence base; the setting of standards based on the evidence for public health and health promotion practice; and the targeting of health promotion and those worst off in order to narrow the health gap.

In *The NHS Plan* (Department of Health, 2000) there is a concentration on health services and their delivery structures. There is less of a concern with the socio-ecological determinants of health, which were high-lighted in OHN. *The NHS Plan* is explicitly part of the government's modernization programme. The emphasis in the plan on building the service for the patient/consumer brings modernization and service delivery together. The emphasis on partnerships between health and social care in the plan is the point at which it gives practical substance to the broader socio-economic determinants of health.

Chapter 13 of the plan is about improving health and reducing inequalities. Several key areas are highlighted. These are infant and childhood mortality; child poverty; *Surestart;* cancer; and coronary heart disease (CHD), with an emphasis on cancer prevention via screening especially for breast, cervical and colorectal neoplasms. There is a focus on teenage pregnancy, antenatal and neonatal screening, and HIV. The importance of reductions in smoking, improving diet and nutrition (with a special emphasis on fruit and vegetable consumption) are noted.

Reducing obesity and increasing physical activity are signalled as being very important. Drug and alcohol misuse and associated crime are mentioned. Potential ways of dealing with these problems are linked to partnerships with local authorities in respect of neighbourhood renewal, the Healthy Communities Collaborative and a leadership programme for health visitors. Mental health is highlighted. In respect of CHD, smoking is targeted as a critical area, with a strong emphasis on speeding up treatment and getting more people into surgery. Finally, special provision for the elderly population is pinpointed with an emphasis on dignity, privacy, good supportive palliative care and extending access to services. This is the language of rationalism, realism and delivery, and is underpinned by an empirical approach.

The empirical approach is typified by the Department of Health's *A Research and Development Strategy for Public Health* document (Department of Health, 2001). The principles enshrined in this are: a systematic approach to using scientific evidence for public health; and the provision of high quality research evidence that will be used to improve the health and well-being of the population as a whole, and to reduce inequalities in health. New organizations such as the Health Development Agency and the National Electronic Library for Public Health were constructed to deliver the evidence base.

Against this background there has been a proliferation of 'area-based' initiatives that have health-related objectives designed to target those worst off and test innovative practice. Area-based initiatives are a combination of national programmes that target particular client groups, with resources spatially concentrated into especially needy places (for example, Health Action Zones, Healthy Living Centres, Employment Action Zones, Education Action Zones and *Surestart*); and initiatives that are intended to change the nature of an areas and to engage with all the communities who live there (for example, New Deal for Communities and most Single Regeneration Budget (SRB) schemes) (Stewart *et al.* 2001). Any particular area has a complex mix of initiatives which pursue health-related outcomes as prime or subsidiary objectives. Examples of initiatives with prominent health objectives are highlighted below.

Health Action Zones (HAZs) are distinctive in their breath of objectives and geographical scale, and were intended to be trailblazers; pioneering innovative approaches to reducing health inequalities and modernizing health services. They cover about a third of the English population living in the most deprived areas of the country. The first-wave HAZs were established in April 1998, followed by fifteen second wave sites in April 1999. HAZ funding amounted to about a 1 per cent to 1.5 per cent addition to the revenue allocation of health authorities in zones. The zones vary widely in nature, size and complexity. Merseyside, the largest HAZ, with a population of 1.4 million, is almost eight times larger than Luton, the smallest of the HAZs. An initial mapping exercise undertaken as part of the national evaluation identified over 200 programmes and 2,000 projects, with the majority of activity focused on addressing the root causes of ill health, including employment, housing and education issues.

The Healthy Living Centre Initiative was launched in January 1999 with the aim of promoting good health, targeting disadvantaged areas and groups, and reducing inequalities in health. The initiative is managed by the New Opportunities Fund and has a budget of £300 million of Lottery money. HLCs are planned to be accessible to 20 per cent of the most disadvantaged sectors of the population by 2002. There is no blueprint for projects, but they are expected to involve communities and users in design and delivery.

Surestart is contributing to the cross-government programme to tackle child poverty and social exclusion. The principal aim is to work with families and children in some of the most deprived areas of England, and in particular to promote the development of pre-school children to give them the best possible start before they go to school. *Surestart* aims to promote the physical, intellectual and social development of babies and young children – particularly those who are disadvantaged. It focuses on children aged between 0 and 4, and parents and parents-to-be. Interim targets, to be attained by 2004, are in the areas of re-registration on child protection registers, smoking reduction among pregnant mothers, speech and language problems, and workless households Typical *Surestart* catchment areas are small, and programmes offer enhanced child care, play and early learning opportunities and better access to health services, as well as training for parents. By 2001 there were 437 programmes in operation, approaching the target of 500 by 2004. An action research study, commissioned by the Department of Transport, local government and regions, focused on six locations, where a range of area-based initiatives (AIBs) had been established, to identify learning for collaboration and co-ordination.

The Government's Spending Review 2000, which set targets to improve outcomes in public services in deprived neighbourhoods, gave further impetus to the development of local strategies, concerned with improving the health and well-being of communities. For the first time, government departments, local authorities and health agencies are being judged on their performance in the areas where they are doing worst rather than on the national average. Furthermore, the national *Strategy for Neighbourhood Renewal* expects improvements of mainstream services to produce better outcomes in the most deprived areas in terms of more jobs, reduced crime, better educational attainment, improved health and better housing. Local strategic partnerships have been established to bring together key stakeholders from the public, private, voluntary and community sectors to develop an overarching framework for an area, in the form of community strategies. They are expected to rationalize the number of partnerships in areas and achieve more effective integration of AIBs.

A Neighbourhood Renewal Fund is being allocated to tackle deprivation in the most deprived neighbourhoods, and kickstart the neighbourhood renewal process in eighty-eight local authorities in the most deprived areas of England. *The NHS Plan* commits the health sector to contributing to Local Strategic Partnerships and neighbourhood renewal through Health Improvement and Modernization Programmes. Another initiative is New Deal for Communities. New Deal for Communities (NDC) partnerships have to tackle five key issues: poor job prospects; high levels of crime; educational under-achievement; poor health; and problems with housing and the physical environment.

In 2002–3 several other activities will get under way, including local health equity audits and the development of the heath poverty gauge, and all this will take place within a reorganized Primary Health Care structure in which the delivery of specific inequalities targets relating to life expectancy and to infant mortality will be an integral part of will be expected to be delivered at local level.

Conclusion

The shift of the locality approach to the mainstream flows from political changes and developments. However, while there are very important continuities in the policies now in place, the discontinuities between the older philosophy and the new, rationalist, evidence-based approach could hardly be more marked. Contemporary initiatives are based on the *a priori* assumption that evidence can be gathered and can be put to use to make a difference. The nihilism that denied the importance of evidence has been overtaken by a more reasoned approach. There is an orientation to the delivery of services, albeit in partnership, but the possibility of doing it better is not denied.

The academic arguments have changed too. One of the most eloquent exponents of the new realism in the field of public health is John Bunker. He advocates an end to the dichotomy between the social and medical models, and especially the end to the untested and largely untestable proposition that clinical medicine plays no part in the improvement in the health of the public. In 1994, with colleagues, he published in the *Millbank Quarterly* a paper entitled 'Improving Health: Measuring the Effects of Medical Care'. The argument was a direct challenge to those who argued (as was common in the Healthy Cities movement) that improvements in the health of populations were the result of improvements in the social and economic infrastructure – housing, nutrition, sanitation and so on – rather than improvements in medicine. While not denying that these things are important, Bunker assembles the case that *together* medical advances *and* general social and economic conditions significantly affect the improvements in life expectancy and quality of life (Bunker *et al.*, 1994). In a further elaboration on the theme, Bunker (2001) suggested that the frequent argument that clinical medicine has been insignificant in the improvement of the health of the public is unfounded. He notes that the theses of Dubos (1962, 1980), Illich (1975) and McKeown (1976), need serious re-evaluation. While their critiques were compelling, they were able to advance their argument in the absence of any serious data that could have been used to counter their points. He concedes that their arguments may have had some force in the first half of the twentieth century, but that it has become increasingly difficult to sustain, in the face of evidence now available. He identifies benefits caused by surgery, certain types of screening, immunization, and a variety of drugs, on increased life expectancy. He also argues that while the wider determinants play a very important role, their causal pathways are very complex and the proper scientific evaluation of their effectiveness is tricky. That is, of course, not a reason for not doing it, and retreating into a postmodern relativism. It is the reason for a systematic and rational approach to the evidence. Locally based initiatives have a vital role to play. The challenge is not to mount a critique of the possibility of change, but rather to derive culturally sensitive and methodologically rigorous ways of developing the evidence base to facilitate the understanding of the most appropriate and suitable ways of achieving health improvements at local level.

References

Acheson, D. (1998). *Independent Inquiry into Inequalities in Health Report*. London: The Stationery Office.

Antonovsky, A. (1985). *Health, Stress and Coping*. San Francisco: Jossey Bass.

Antonovsky, A. (1987). *Unravelling the Mystery of Health: How people manage stress and stay well*. San Francisco: Jossey Bass.

Antonovsky, A. (1996). The salutogenic model as a theory to guide health promotion, *Health Promotion International*, 11(1), 11–18.

Ashton, J. and Seymour, H. (1988). *The New Public Health: The Liverpool Experience*. Milton Keynes: Open University Press.

Bunker, J. (2001). *Medicine Matters After All: Measuring the benefits of medical care, a healthy lifestyle, and a just social environment*. London: The Stationery Office/The Nuffield Trust.

Bunker, J. P., Frazier, H. S. and Mosteller, F. (1994). Improving health: measuring effects of medical care, *The Millbank Quarterly*, 72, 225–58.

Bunton, R. and Burrows, R. (1995). Consumption and health in the 'epidemiological' clinic of late modern medicine. In Bunton, R., Nettleton S. and Burrows, R. (eds), *The Sociology of Health Promotion: Critical analyses of consumption, lifestyle and risk*. London: Routledge.

Callinicos, A. (1999). *Social Theory: A historical introduction*, Cambridge: Polity Press.

City of Copenhagen (1994). *Healthy City Plan of the City of Copenhagen, 1994–1997*. Copenhagen: Copenhagen Health Services.

Davies, J. K. and Kelly, M. P. (eds) (1993a). *Healthy Cities: Research and practice.* London: Routledge.

Davies, J. K., and Kelly, M. P. (1993b). Healthy cities: research and practice. In Davies, J. K. and Kelly, M. P. (eds) *Healthy cities: research and practice.* London: Routledge, 1–13.

Delanty, G. (1999). Social *Theory in a Changing World: Conceptions of Modernity.* Oxford: Polity Press.

Department of Health (1998). The Health of the Nation – A policy assessed. Two reports commissioned for the Department of Health from the Universities of Leeds and Glamorgan, and the London School of Hygiene and Tropical Medicine. London: The Stationery Office.

Department of Health (1999). *Saving Lives: Our Healthier Nation.* London: The Stationery Office.

Department of Health (2000). *The NHS Plan: A plan for investment, a plan for reform.* London: The Stationery Office.

Department of Health (2001). *A Research and Development Strategy for Public Health.* London, The Stationery Office.

Dubos, R. (1962). *Torch of Life.* New York: Simon and Schuster.

Dubos, R. (1980). *Man Adapting,* New Haven, Conn.: Yale University Press.

Featherstone, M. (1988). In pursuit of the post-modern: an introduction, *Theory, Culture and Society,* 5, 195–221.

Friedson, E. (1970). *Professional Dominance: The social structure of medical care,* Chicago, Ill.: Aldine.

Giddens, A. (1991). *Modernity and Self-identity: Self and society in the late modern age.* Cambridge, Polity Press.

Giddens, A. (1992). Uprooted signposts at the century's end, *The Times Higher Education Supplement* (17 January), 21–2.

Illich, I. (1975). *Medical Nemesis.* London: Calder and Boyars.

Kellner, D. (1988). Post-modernism as social theory: some challenges and problems, *Theory, Culture and Society,* 5, 239–69.

Kelly, M. P. (1990). The role of research in the new public health, *Critical Public Health,* 3, 4–9.

Kelly, M. P., Davies, J. K., and Charlton, B. G. (1993). Healthy Cities: a modern problem or a postmodern solution? In Davies, J. K. and Kelly, M. P. (eds), *Healthy Cities: Research and practice.* London: Routledge, 159–67.

Kelly, M. P., Davies, J. K., Charlton, B. (1997). Healthy Cities: a modern problem or a post-modern solution? In Sidell, M., Jones, L. Katz, J. and Perbedy, A. (eds), *Debates and Dilemmas in Promoting Health: A reader.* London: Open University/Macmillan, 353–62.

Kelly, M. P. and Charlton, B. G. (1995). The modern and post-modern in health promotion. In Bunton, R., Nettleton, S. and Burrows, R. (eds), *The Sociology of Health Promotion.* London: Routledge.

Lyotard, J. F. (1984). *The Post-modern Condition: A report on knowledge* (trans. G. Bennington and B. Massumi). Manchester: Manchester University Press.

McKeown, T. (1976). *The Role of Medicine: Dream, mirage, nemesis?* London: Nuffield Provincial Hospitals Trust.

Nutbeam, D. (1986). Health promotion glossary, *Health Promotion,* 1, 113–27.

Secretary of State for Health (1991). *The Health of the Nation: A consultative document for health in England* (Cmnd 1523). London: HMSO.

Seidman, S. and Wagner, D. G. (eds) (1992). *Post Modernism and Social Theory.* Oxford: Blackwell.

Shustermann, R. (1988). Post-modernist aestheticism: a new moral philosophy, *Theory, Culture and Society,* 5, 337–55.

Stewart, M. *et al.* Collaboration and Coordination of Area-Based Initiatives. (2001). University of the West of England, Office of Public Management, University of Newcastle.

Szaz, T. (1972). *The Myth of Mental Illness: Foundations of a theory of personal conduct,* London: Paladin.

Whitehead, A. N. (1926). *Science and the Modern World.* Cambridge University Press.

WHO (1946). *Constitution.* New York: World Health Organization.

WHO (1986). *The Ottawa Charter for Health Promotion.* Ottawa: WHO, Canadian Public Health.

WHO (1988). *Research Policies for Health for All.* Copenhagen: WHO.

38 Health promotion as an investment strategy: a perspective for the twenty-first century*[1]

Lowell S. Levin and Erio Ziglio[2]

Introduction

Health promotion should be positioned at the heart of social and economic development, and be perceived increasingly as a health investment strategy. This is the approach chosen by the European Office of the World Health Organisation (WHO/EURO) to position health promotion for the twenty-first century (World Health Organization, 1995; Ziglio and Krech, 1996; Ziglio *et al.*, 2000).

The Ottawa Charter's action domains

Since the 1980s the Ottawa Charter for Health Promotion (WHO, 1986) has had a remarkably wide acceptance as a strategic 'checklist' for health promotion, if not as a formal strategy. The Charter incorporates elements of traditional concern (personal health skills) with the more recent attention given to community action and environmental and public policy issues. Further, the Charter focuses on the key functions of enabling, advocacy and mediation. The five action domains are: building healthy public policy; creating supportive environments; strengthening community action; developing personal skills; and reorientating health services.

Beyond the principles set out in WHO documents such as the *Health for All* strategy and in the *Ottawa Charter for Health Promotion* lies the real challenge to apply them in practice in increasingly complex societies (WHO/EURO, 1996, 1998). These societies invariably have immediate priorities, such as economic competitiveness and fiscal soundness, and their social institutions are directed towards achieving those priorities. Specifically, the challenge is therefore to find ways of deploying investment for health to reinforce such priorities and, conversely, to enhance people's health – equitably and sustainably – through the medium of social and economic development.

---

* Commissioned for this volume.

For twenty-first-century health promotion, our energy can therefore be applied most productively to working out how health promotion can be integrated effectively into mainstream social and economic development and have its influence visible in relevant programmes, regulations and wide-ranging public policies. The success of this strategy will quite clearly depend heavily on health promotion expertise which is based on the most valid theoretical constructs of the social and behavioural sciences, organizational behaviour and social development sciences. What would be useful, indeed critical, for twenty-first-century health promotion, is to organize an international record of intervention efforts, including their contextual circumstances, strategies applied, logistical and technical aspects, and observations of their impact, e.g. cost benefit, cost effectiveness, diffusion, etc. Without such a knowledge base, health promotion will lack the traction necessary to move towards a strategic theme that could guide its general advance and at the same time encourage national, regional and local variations.

Such a knowledge base would be a requisite for research, which would have known denominators (populations) and numerators (resources) and known independent variables (interventions, programmes or policies) and dependent variables (health and socio-economic change). Since health promotion can be framed conceptually in broad terms of social development well beyond the limits for a bio-clinical model, it is necessary to document its impact on a wide range of decisions in diverse policy areas. Here, it is not only a matter of documentation, but also a justification for sustainable inter-sectoral involvement.

The goal is to demonstrate the synergistic contribution of its component parts to a holistic, equitable improvement in the health and well-being of the population. The focus should not be on evaluating the impact of isolated interventions as end points, but rather on the relationship of a given intervention to the other components of the health promotion strategy. Such an analysis might indeed provide a fresh assessment of the validity of theories underlying its several components.

Health as a human, social and economic investment

Population health is, by and large, determined by social, demographic and economic factors and public policies well beyond the traditional remit of medicine, or even public health (Wilkinson, 1996; Bartley et al., 1997; Blane et al., 1997; Cornia, 1997). Throughout history, the greatest improvements in people's health have arisen mainly from social and economic improvements which also promote health (McKeown, 1971, 1976; Marmot, 1998). Conversely, a healthier population can make a more productive contribution to overall development, and requires less social support in the form of health care and welfare benefits. Therefore, investment aimed at securing positive health and well-being also brings social and economic benefits for the whole community.

The Investment for Health (IFH) approach is a practical approach based on these interlocking facts. It is based on the rationale that resources are best applied in a way that both attacks the main causes of ill-health in a credible, effective and ethical manner, and furthers the achievement of goals for social and economic development.

Priority social and economic policy areas – such as education, income maintenance, workplace regulation, housing, transport, agriculture and communications – as well as private initiatives, have a profound influence on health. Governments have great potential to improve or worsen people's health through their policy decisions in these areas. This applies increasingly to the private sector. Great harm can be done to health by misguided public policies and private initiatives alike. The IFH approach offers practical measures to prevent this – by building social and economic strength alongside health improvement for the population in an equitable, empowering and sustainable way.

The IFH approach therefore calls for a new form of partnership. In today's complex world, action for the promotion of health cannot come from the healthcare sector alone. It needs to be built on strong cross-sector alliances between health and health care, social development, and equitable and sustainable economic development.

In summary, IFH is a deliberate attempt to address the main 'causes' of health in a credible, effective and ethical manner that engages other sectors of society as well as the healthcare sector (Ziglio et al., 2000). The approach develops policies and programmes that are based on, and address, key determinants of health. Such determinants are linked mainly to economic and social factors (World Health Organization, 1997; Ziglio, 1998). Stimulating and securing the self-interest of other relevant sectors of society is critical. Positive changes for health should be facilitated at both individual and community level. Therefore, unhealthy life conditions (e.g. poverty, inequalities and social exclusion) should be modified, and not only bio-medical risk factors!

Finally, it should be emphasized that IFH does not take a narrow view of solely utilitarian aspects of investment and economic trade-offs. It places the protection and promotion of the health of the population firmly within a human rights perspective, as well as an indictor of human and social development. Thus IFH is not confined to mere issues of costs–benefit analysis of selected prevention and health promotion programmes. Indeed, Investment for Health focuses on maximization of assets for health. Similarly, IFH is sensitive to the removal of social, economic and environmental barriers to the promotion of health. These adverse conditions can be associated with a wide range of factors, including lack of democracy and infringement of human rights, the burden of the external debt of many developing countries, or the unequal distribution of resources and opportunities for social and personal development.

Reframing communication

Health promotion at this moment of rapid change in the world's political and economic order must define its potential in a way strong enough to withstand the vagaries of shifting political boundaries and populations, international and civil conflicts and the fearful, sometimes cynical, withdrawal of people from sharing their resources or committing themselves to co-operative social action. In both developed and developing countries, there is an atmosphere of uncertainty and anomie that dampens enthusiasm for long term investments to secure health and well-being.

The challenge now is to adapt the Ottawa Charter *principles* to twenty-first-century realities. This is the case when the opinions and perspectives of new partners in health promotion must command attention; particularly those of the lay community, legislators and policy makers (see Levin *et al.* 1994, pp. 1–4). These new partners may possess little or no sophistication or primary interest in health *per se*. Nevertheless, it is *their* construction of reality that must frame health promotion action. The exchange of ideas, experiences, and information among these partners in health promotion is often far from ideal, however. Indeed, there is often substantial miscommunication between parties of unequal social status or political power, or between groups with different demographic characteristics such as age, gender, ethnicity and race. Differences in conceptual language are often daunting. Consider the conceptual vocabularies of educators, environmentalists, policy analysts and community organizers. Where is the common denominator of meaning they may assign to such notions as empowerment, equity, participation, or even health? What aspects of communication theory or social marketing theory pertain here?

Clearly, health promotion will have to be inventive, will of necessity have to test a variety of new techniques and fora for dialogue and consensus building. What is presented here is an exceptional opportunity to create what may be called collaborative or adaptive communication; namely, communication that leads to a common understanding and harmonious, mutually beneficial interaction between action domains of the Ottawa Charter and their link with public policy sectors.

Many experts in health promotion feel uneasy about working in policy and programme sectors where concepts and technologies are unfamiliar and/or where they perceive a potential ethical conflict of values (e.g. saving money versus saving lives). Misunderstandings on both sides of the equation have limited tests of health promotion's potential in key areas of public policy. Can health promotion respond opportunistically without jeopardizing its integrity? What aspect of social change theory pertains here? What strategic advice is available to increase the possibility of success? What are the implications for preparing the health promotion workforce to have an effective influence on public policies outside the health sector?

New thinking for multi-sectoral action

The 'Investment for Health' programme and related demonstration projects of WHO/EURO are designed to explore collaborative communication, option appraisals and other issues mentioned earlier. These demonstration projects began in 1994. They have as their primary goal the strengthening of the capacity of national, regional and local authorities to identify public policy areas relevant to the solution of priority health concerns and to modify those policies, singly or in concert, to achieve and sustain health gains (WHO/EURO, 1994, 1995a, 1996; Ziglio et al., 2000).

In brief outline, the health investment strategy involves the following processes. Community groups and health authorities contribute perspectives on health concerns and opportunities, prioritize them, and then break down the agreed list of priorities into their more detailed aspects. Each aspect is then 'located' on a 'health gain map' which relates them to the most relevant policy areas (e.g. education, transportation, housing, communications, income maintenance, medical care, agriculture, tourism, environment). Finally, possible policy intervention choices are assessed against criteria that include matters of equity, empowerment, sustainability, accountability, acceptability and fiscal feasibility, among others (WHO/EURO, 1995a, 1996; Ziglio et al., 2000). The aim is to identify mutual concerns and policy options, to seek grounds for conflict resolution.

A variant of the above health investment strategy was first developed by WHO/EURO (Health Promotion and Investment Programme) in Slovenia in 1996 (WHO/EURO, 1996, 2002). The objective was to undertake a system-wide assessment of health promotion resources (current and potential) at country level: human resources, management infrastructure, financial resources and political support. The assessment, undertaken as a demonstration, was commissioned by the Slovenian Parliament and was thus free of any bias or obligation to any ministry or special group. The proposals for health investment that resulted, while reflecting the options of a vast array of agencies and voluntary interest groups, were arrived at independently and were assiduously politically neutral.

It is clear that we need more investment-for-health approaches which can respond to a wide range of circumstances: political, cultural and at the level of socio-economic development. The task is to make the investment process empowering of those involved, and a process which will have long-lasting development benefits beyond immediate health investment decisions.

The WHO/EURO Investment for Health Projects are helping to clarify, and in some important respects redefine, the role of the health sector in promoting health. It is essentially an oversight role, where the prime concern is to ensure that a holistic approach to health promotion takes into account the social *and economic* determinants of health, be they at the individual, community, or policy level. These determinants are referenced in operational terms by the Ottawa Charter (World Health Organization, 1986; see also WHO/EURO, 1984). Indeed, there are few precedents for a managerial role in social, much less health, development, where multiple public policy and agency inputs are orchestrated. Even the World Bank's 'structural adjustment' strategy provides only limited oversight confined to economic and fiscal policies and their related programmes (World Bank, 1993, 1995).

The circumstances of promoting health in an open system, with multiple players, agendas and citizen participation, simply make the application of most of the existing management theories inappropriate (see Grossman and Scala, 1993; see also Bennis *et al.*, 1994; Senge, 1990). Experience with the Investment for Health demonstration projects offers a unique opportunity to build a theory of management within the open system approach to health promotion (see Ashton, 1992; Ziglio *et al.*, 1995). Some insights into such a managerial role have been organized for the above-mentioned projects, but these remained largely anecdotal.

The task now is to standardize observations relevant to the management role in comprehensive health promotion efforts. Thus we can begin to generate testable hypotheses as a basis for forming a theoretical perspective as a practical tool for advancing this role. We are seeking defining management strategies that empower populations; reduce health inequities; estimate available resources; respond to consumer preferences; set programme and policy priorities; assign intersectoral action; design interventions; organize collaborative efforts; build professional capacity; and assess cost–benefit and cost effectiveness as well as peripheral impact. This is a formidable paradigm shift from current management in public and private sectors!

Twenty-first-century challenges

Now is a propitious time for health promotion to position itself for the challenges ahead. In doing so, there is a need to play a stronger and more effective role in examining the options for health promoting investments, and recommending the appropriate legislative and other relevant initiatives to achieve a truly comprehensive and sustainable health promoting policy. Is health promotion prepared to accept this challenge in Europe and elsewhere? The vision is there. Now we need to produce an inventory of the analytic and political skills available; upgrade professional education programmes; and undertake the research and demonstrations required to bring the health promotion resource up to an appropriate standard.

In the light of the above, there are a number of tough questions which people committed to twenty-first-century health promotion should address. Some of the most relevant are:

- Where are those health investments in public policies with the greatest promise of benefits?
- Who will identify them?
- What kind of data and policy-relevant information will be required?
- What new analytical skills will be needed to evaluate the cost and benefit implications for health investments?
- How will investment options be presented in order to ensure political acceptability?
- How will public policies be monitored and publicized to achieve public review and critique of their health implications?

Conclusions

As the investment for health perspective becomes a major orientation for health promotion, additional research and training needs will become obvious. Fewer distinctions will be made between the concepts of health and general well-being and thus we can expect a more productive and harmonious integration of effort among all relevant public policies. Health, and particularly the speciality of health promotion, can serve as the nexus for this new convergence of policy resources in health investment. Health promotion has to respond to and influence a rapidly changing world. The catalogue of disciplines upon which it has to base its practice must expand to meet new challenges and new opportunities.

For IFH principles to be applied effectively, traditional policy making approaches must change. New commitment and skills to work both within and, most importantly, outside the health sector, and new skills of policy analysis and assessment will all be needed. Lessons learnt in WHO demonstration projects, as well as the national IFH appraisals outlined in this chapter, have shown that the challenges of moving from an understanding of IFH to implementing it should not be underestimated. It is a huge step from believing that the connections between health, economic and social development are real, to getting others, including ourselves, to change the way we work. Change is difficult, and the forces of inertia are strong, but the potential benefits of IFH are enormous. So how can the ground be prepared for cultivating IFH in practice? There are some essential developments that need to happen (Ziglio *et al.*, 2000):

1 There needs to be political priority given to health. Health can no longer be seen just as a matter for doctors, nurses, their patients and the Ministry of Health. This needs to be more than a commitment in principle and words. – politicians need to develop a better understanding of the factors that determine health and illness and what can be done to address them. For Ministries of Health this presents an unrivalled opportunity to take a leadership and advocacy role within government, encouraging colleagues with other portfolios to see the relevance of the health agenda to their own sphere of activity and interests, and supporting them to develop the right, and political skills, to make decisions that improve health.

2 Beyond political priority there also needs to be clear accountability for health improvement across policy sectors and departments. 'Health for all is the business of all' has become a cliché. As in business, so in politics: there must be accountability for results. If ministers, policy makers and managers are to be held to account for their successes and failures in health improvement, there will need to be more effective ways of measuring health. Unless we can measure improvements there can be no accountability. Most countries collect data on mortality and morbidity, but few focus on positive health indicators. So, with accountability comes the development of systems, processes and analytical tools to assess health and health impacts of policy options.

3 There needs to be a public understanding of health and how the health of the population can be promoted and sustained. Public opinion is too easily captured by hospitals and illness. Public understanding and commitment to investments that promote health will be essential if politicians are to be able to make the necessary but difficult decisions.

4 There are always competing options when decisions are made on an investment. This is equally true for IFH. Some options may be obvious; others less so. The more IFH is explored, the greater the range of options that will be uncovered. There needs to be recognition of the trade-offs between health, economic and social development outcomes. Not all stakeholders who have an influence on health have health improvement as their main priority. Associated with this is an urgent need for decision-making processes that allow those in different sectors to understand and make those trade-offs in their decisions.

5   At all levels of society, skills need to be developed in working across sectors. Each sector of society has its own interests, goals, resources and ways of working. Common action to improve health requires common ground – shared ideas, resources, a place to meet. These do not just happen – there must be stimulation and processes to bring people, and other resources, together.

6   New incentives need to be developed. Sectors will not co-operate because someone says that it is a good idea. They must see benefits for their own remit, and see incentives sufficient to justify policy adjustments that may promote health. Political drive, tax breaks or special reward schemes might be needed – imagination and negotiation certainly will.

7   A clear picture of what an IFH strategy can deliver needs to address not only what is possible at state or civil level, but also what individuals and communities can do. Bottom-up approaches that mobilize community resources can be sustainable, but they need to have a context within which to work.

8   New infrastructures may be required to support Investment for Health. But these cannot run in parallel with outmoded systems. Far more important is the adaptation of the current infrastructure to sustain IFH.

9   A new data set of Investment for Health indicators should be developed. There is still a paucity of health/salutogenic indicators (as distinct from disease/pathogenic indicators) used at the global, national and local level. Such indicators ought to include measures relating to the determinants of, and assets for, health. National, regional and local governments should publish regular reviews of progress on health improvement and social and economic development against clear indicators of success.

10 Crucial to all the above is a willingness to learn about how to make IFH work. Here, WHO has a unique and fascinating role in facilitating cross-fertilization of ideas, practical experiences and research findings across countries and governments.

Note

1   This chapter is based on an earlier article written by the authors, (1996) 'Health promotion as an investment strategy: considerations on theory and practice', *Health Promotion International*, 11(1), (1996), 33–9, Oxford University Press; and on Ziglio, E., Hagard, S., McMahon, L., Harvey, S. and Levin, S. L. Investment for Health – Technical Report, 5th International Conference on Health Promotion, Mexico City, 5–9 June, (2000). Washington, DC: Pan American Health Organization.

2   The views expressed in this chapter are those of the authors and not necessarily those of the organizations for which they work.

References

Ashton, J. (1992). *Healthy Cities*. Buckingham: Open University Press.

Bartley, M., Blane, D. and Montgomery, S. (1997). Socioeconomic determinants of health: health and the life course: why safety nets matter. *British Medical Journal*, 314(4), 1194–6.

Bennis, W., Parikh, J. and Lessem, R. (1994). *Beyond Leadership: Balancing economies, ethics and ecology*. Cambridge Mass.: Blackwell.

Blane, D., Brenner, E. and Wilkinson, R. G. (1996). *Health and Social Organization – Towards a Health Policy for the 21st Century*. London: Routledge.

Cornia, G. A. (1997). Labour market shocks, psychosocial stress and the transition's mortality crisis. Research in progress, October 1997. Helsinki: United Nations University, WIDER.

Grossman, R. and Scala, K. (1993). *Health Promotion and Organisational Development*, European Health Promotion Series, 2. Copenhagen: World Health Organization, Regional Office for Europe.

Levin, S. L., McMahon, L. and Ziglio, E. (eds) (1994). *Economic Change, Social Welfare and Health in Europe*. Copenhagen: World Health Organization, Regional Office for Europe.

Marmot, M. (1998). Improving the social environment to improve health, *The Lancet*, 351(1), 57–60.

McKeown, T. (1971). A historic appraisal of the medical task. In McLachlan, C. and McKeown, T. (eds), *Medical history and medical care: A symposium of perspectives*. London: Oxford University Press.

McKeown, T. (1976). *The Role of Medicine: Dream, mirage or nemesis?* London: Nuffield Provincial Hospital Trust.

Senge, P. M. (1990). *The Fifth Discipline – The art and practice of the learning organisation*. New York: Doubleday.

Wilkinson, R. G. (1996). *Unhealthy Societies*. London: Routledge.

World Bank (1993). *Investment in Health. The world bank in action*. Washington DC: The World Bank.

World Bank (1995). *Investing in People: the world bank in action*. Washington DC: The World Bank.

World Health Organization (WHO) (1986). *Ottawa Charter for Health Promotion*. World Health Organization, Health and Welfare Canada, Canadian Public Health Association. Ottawa Charter for Health Promotion, Ottawa, Ontario, Canada (November 21). Copenhagen: World Health Organization, Regional Office for Europe.

World Health Organization (1995) *Health in Social Development*. WHO Position Paper, World Summit for Social Development, Copenhagen, March. Geneva: WHO.

World Health Organization (1997). *The Jakarta Declaration on Leading Health Promotion into the twenty-first Century*. Copenhagen: World Health Organization.

WHO/EURO (1984). *Health Promotion: A discussion document on the concept and principles*. Copenhagen: World Health Organisation, Regional Office for Europe.

WHO/EURO (1994). *Investment in Health in the Valencia Region: Mid-term report*. Copenhagen: World Health Organizations, Regional Office for Europe, Health Promotion and Investment Unit.

WHO/EURO (1995a). *Securing Investment in Health: Report of a demonstration project in the provinces of Bolzano and Trento*. Copenhagen: World Health Organisation, Regional Office for Europe, Health Promotion and Investment Unit.

WHO/EURO (1995b). *First Meeting of the European Committee for Health Promotion Development – Dublin, Ireland, 14–16 March 1995. Summary report*. Copenhagen: World Health Organization, Regional Office for Europe, Health Promotion and Investment Unit.

WHO/EURO (1996). *Investment for Health in Slovenia.* Copenhagen: World Health Organization, Intersectoral Health Development Unit, Health Promotion and Investment Programme.

WHO/EURO (1998). *Health 21 – Health for all in the 21st Century,* European Health for All Series No. 5. Copenhagen: World Health Organization.

WHO/EURO (2002). *Review of Finland Health Promotion Policy.* Venice: WHO European Office for Investment for Health & Development (forthcoming October 2002).

Ziglio, E. (1998). Key issues for the new millennium. *Promoting Health: The Journal of Health Promotion for Northern Ireland,* 2, 34–7.

Ziglio, E. and Krech, R. (1996). Bruchenschlag zwischen Politik und Forschung in der Gesudheitsforderung. In Rutten, A. and Rausch, L. (eds), *Gesunde Regionen in Internationaler Partnerschaft: Konzepte und Perspekitven.* Webach-Gambur, Germany: G. Conrad, Verlag für Gesundheitsforderung.

Ziglio, E., Rivett, E. and Rasmussen, V. (1995). *The European Network of Health Promoting Schools: Managing innovation and change. Report prepared by the Technical Secretariat of the European Network of Health Promoting School.* Copenhagen: World Health Organization, Regional Office for Europe, Health Promotion and Investment Unit.

Ziglio, E., Hagard, S., McMahon, L., Harvey, S. and Levin, S. L. (2000). *Investment for Health – Technical Report,* 5th International Conference on Health Promotion, Mexico City, 5–9 June. Washington, DC: Pan American Health Organization.

Index